Antibiosis and Host Immunity

Antibiosis and Host Immunity

Edited by
Andor Szentivanyi and
Herman Friedman
University of South Florida College of Medicine
Tampa, Florida
and
Günther Gillissen
Rhein.-Westfälische Technische Hochschule
Aachen, Federal Republic of Germany

PLENUM PRESS • NEW YORK AND LONDON

Library of Congress Cataloging in Publication Data

International Symposium on Antimicrobial Agents and Immunity (1985: Siena, Italy)
Antibiosis and host immunity.

"Based on the proceedings of the International Symposium on Antimicrobial Agents and Immunity, held May 2–4, 1985, in Siena, Italy"—T.p. verso.
Satellite symposium of the Third International Conference on Immunopharmacology, held in Florence, Italy, May 6–10, 1985.
Includes bibliographies and index.
1. Antibiosis—Congresses. 2. Antibiotics—Immunology—Congresses. 3. Immunity—Congresses. I. Szentivanyi, Andor. II. Friedman, Herman, 1931- . III. Gillissen, G. IV. International Conference on Immunopharmacology (3rd: 1985: Florence, Italy). V. Title. [DNLM: 1. Antibiotics—immunology—congresses. 2. Host-Parasite Relations—congresses. 3. Immunity—drug effects—congresses. QV 350 I6035a 1985]
QR99.I58 1985 616.07'9 87-18514
ISBN-13: 978-1-4612-9058-2 e-ISBN-13: 978-1-4613-1901-6
DOI: 10.1007/978-1-4613-1901-6

Based on the proceedings of the International Symposium on Antimicrobial Agents and Immunity, held May 2–4, 1985, in Siena, Italy

Softcover reprint of the hardcover 1st edition 1987
A Division of Plenum Publishing Corporation
233 Spring Street, New York, N.Y. 10013

PREFACE

This book contains 32 chapters based on the corresponding papers delivered at the International Symposium on Antimicrobial Agents and Immunity, held in Siena, Italy on May 2-4, 1985 as a Satellite Symposium of the Third International Conference on Immunopharmacology, held in Florence, Italy on May 6-10, 1985.

As editors we express our profound appreciation and gratitude to the authors who have contributed so richly to this volume, and we think that it may not be too much to hope that a new cadre of investigators and students will share this gratitude for these records of experience and insight into antibiotic and host-parasite interactions. We owe a very special gratitude to Mrs. Christine Abarca for her outstanding editorial assistance in the preparation of this book.

Andor Szentivanyi, M.D.
University Distinguished Professor
Departments of Pharmacology
and Internal Medicine
University of South Florida
College of Medicine
Tampa, Florida

Herman Friedman, Ph.D.
Professor and Chairman
Department of Medical Microbiology
and Immunology
University of South Florida
College of Medicine
Tampa, Florida

Günther Gillissen, M.D., Ph.D.
Professor and Chairman
Department of Medical Microbiology
Faculty of Medicine
RWTH, Aachen, F.R.G.

CONTENTS

SECTION I
HISTORICAL BACKGROUND AND INTRODUCTORY OVERVIEW

SECTION II
INFLUENCE OF ANTIBIOTICS ON BACTERIA AS RELATED TO HOST IMMUNITY

SECTION III
INFLUENCE OF ANTIBIOTICS ON HOST DEFENSES IN VIVO

SECTION IV
ANTIMICROBIAL EFFECTS ON PHAGOCYTIC FUNCTION OF POLYMORPHONUCLEAR LEUKOCYTES, MONOCYTES, AND MACROPHAGES

SECTION V
ANTIMICROBIAL EFFECTS ON HUMORAL AND CELLULAR LYMPHOCYTE RESPONSES

SECTION VI
RELATIONSHIP BETWEEN IMMUNE STIMULATORS AND ANTIBIOTICS

SECTION I
HISTORICAL BACKGROUND AND INTRODUCTORY OVERVIEW

IMMUNOMODULATORY EFFECTS OF SOME ANTIBIOTIC-INDUCED CHANGES IN BACTERIAL AND HOST DETERMINANTS

Andor Szentivanyi[1], Herman Friedman[2], Günther Gillissen[3] and Judith Szentivanyi[4]

[1]Departments of Pharmacology and Therapeutics and Internal Medicine, [2]Medical Microbiology and Immunology, and [4]Comprehensive Medicine, University of South Florida College of Medicine, Tampa, Florida and [3]Department of Medical Microbiology, Faculty of Medicine, RWTH Aachen, F.R.G.

More than 3,000 years ago, ancient peoples stumbled on the discovery that some molds could cure some diseases. The Egyptians, the Chinese, and Indians of Central America used molds to treat rashes and infected wounds. But it was not until the summer of 1928 that Sir Alexander Fleming grasped the meaning and possible significance of a small mishap in his laboratory. Fleming noted that bacteria growing in culture in the vicinity of a contaminating mold were lysed. Originally classified as _Penicillium rubrum_, the mold was later shown by Thom, an outstanding American mycologist, to be _Penicillium notatum_. A decade later, a group at Oxford led by Florey and Chain isolated a crude preparation of the bactericidal agent from cultures of _Penicillium notatum_, and subsequently demonstrated the dramatic effect of this component on a variety of bacterial infections.

In this historical example, one microorganism, a mold, was capable of killing other microorganisms, that is certain bacterial cells. This recognition led to the concept of "antibiosis" and to the naming of the substances that are responsible for the phenomenon "antibiotics" in 1942. The name, antibiotic, is derived from two Greek words meaning "against life."

The discovery of penicillin initiated an era of unusually rapid advances in studies on antibiotics, and their total number by now is in excess of 3,000 that represent about 1,300 antibiotic groups. At the same time, there has been little change in the central concept of antibiotic action that is that of "selective toxicity" which is based on the antibiotic's capacity to exploit differences between the biochemistry of the bacterium and that of the host. In this way, the growth of the bacterial cell is selectively inhibited, or the microorganism is killed, supposedly without damage to the host cells. In the case of penicillins, their selective action is due to their inhibition of bacterial cell wall synthesis, an effect that cannot occur in mammalian cells since they lack a cell wall. This explains the selective action of the penicillins, but not their relative lack of toxicity, since there are other antibiotic inhibitors of bacterial cell wall synthesis that are quite toxic for the cells of the host.

Thus, by conclusion *a posteriori*, the idea of selective toxicity as the historically developed concept of antibiotic action views the ideal antibiotic as one that has no adverse effects on the host, but is destructive to the bacterium. There is no ideal antibiotic, but penicillin G in the nonallergic patient represents the closest approximation of the ideal. Historically, therefore, penicillin became the model antibiotic, and the acknowledgement of an antimicrobial agent as an "antibiotic" became patterned after penicillin resulting in research on antibiotic action essentially directed toward the bacterial cell.

Borrowing an example from another biological field, we wish to briefly mention the developmental background of the concept of chemical versus electrical transmission of the nerve impulse through the synaptic cleft or neuromuscular junction from one to another neuron. The seminal contribution to this problem was the finding of Otto Loewi in 1921 who demonstrated the phenomenon of chemical transmission by transferring the ventricular fluid of a stimulated frog heart onto a nonstimulated frog heart, thereby showing that the effects of the nerve stimulus on the first heart were reproduced by the chemical activity of the solution flowing onto the second heart. This experiment led to the chemical identification of acetylcholine which became the first accepted neurotransmitter. Patterned after this model transmitter, certain interdependent criteria have been developed to identify junctional transmitters, but also to prevent some overly enthusiastic investigators to use this term to cover new candidates as transmitter molecules before sufficient data are available to assure their transmitter status. While such caution in any scientific inquiry is an elementary consideration, the set of criteria, requiring fulfillment for assignment of transmitter status, would provide a perfect fit only for acetylcholine. Analogous circumstances apply to the original concept of antibiotic action. These circumstances became considerable handicaps in the evolution of our understanding of neurotransmission and/or antibiosis, and in the latter case explain why the bacterium remained the almost singular focus in the exploration of the effects of these agents in the mammalian host. In the last few years, however, a considerable body of experimental evidence has emerged in the literature clearly showing that antibiotics not only react with the microorganism to which they are directed but also affect the host in a variety of ways including critically important parameters of the immune response. Thus, there is a growing recognition that a triangle of three equally important factors appears to be responsible for the effectiveness of chemotherapy, i.e., the infecting agent, the chemotherapeutic drug used and the host. The material of this volume is another attempt to demonstrate the essential validity of this view.

Although the objective of research on antibiotics in general is to determine how such drugs can be used in the therapy of infectious diseases to eradicate bacteria from the site of infection, most investigations on these drugs and their effects on bacteria have been carried out at antibiotic concentrations equal to or greater than the minimum inhibitory concentrations (MIC's), or the minimum bactericidal concentrations (MBC's). At concentrations lower than the MIC, antibiotics produce effects which are not milder than those seen at the MIC, but which are qualitatively different. At these levels of concentrations, the antibiotic actions are not considered to be on the multiplication mechanisms, but rather on the modification of bacterial morphology and ultrastructure and their ultimate influences upon the host's anti-infectious mechanisms. In recent years, in vitro observations on the effects of subinhibitory concentrations of antibiotics have gathered momentum and showed modifications of bacterial membrane morphology, physico-chemical and serological properties associated with changes in their susceptibility to phagocytosis and killing of polymorphonuclear phagocytes as well as alterations of immunogenic determinants. For these reasons, Section II is designed to focus primarily on the bacteria in relation to the influence of antibiotics on host immunity.

Thus, the lead chapter of Section II discusses the physico-chemical alterations produced by subinhibitory concentrations of beta-lactam antibiotics on the outer membrane of E. coli. It is shown by Opferkuch and associates that the antibiotics did not induce changes in the expression of outer membrane proteins, in the polymerization of LPS O-side chains, or in the phospholipid (PL) profile. In contrast, analysis of the outer membrane by sucrose density ultracentrifugation revealed significant differences between drug-treated and untreated bacteria. They were due to quantitative differences in their protein, LPS, or PL content representing different areas on the bacterial surface. In addition, immunization with outer membrane vesicles from bacteria elicited an antibiotic dependent high anti-protein or LPS response as well as an increased bacterial adherence to macrophages combined with an enhancement of the chemiluminescence reaction. Studies described in the subsequent chapter by Stubner were designed with the assumption that differences in phagocytosis are due to different compositions of the bacterial cell wall. To verify these assumptions, lectins and lectin-receptors of beta-lactam resistant and susceptible Pseudomonas aeruginosa strains were determined and their relation to the attachment of human polymorphonuclear granulocytes were studied. It was found that bacterial attachment to PMN depended only on the lectins and not on other carbohydrates on their surface. Furthermore, significant differences in carbohydrate and lectin distribution on the various strains were found with an indication that the resistant strain possesses less surface lectins and, therefore, its phagocytosis is less effective. Another dimension of the nature of bacterial attachment and its modification by antibiotics is discussed with respect to the role of glycocalyx by Lambe and his associates. The glycocalyx is a structure of bacteria consisting of a capsule and exopolysaccharides, or slime, which may be attached to the bacterial cell, or detached into the surrounding milieu. Glycocalyx-enclosed bacterial microcolonies are formed on smooth and irregular surfaces; the microcolonies may develop into solid biofilms. The possibility has been raised that glycocalyx serves as a protective mechanism for the bacterial cell since it may interfere with phagocytosis by masking peptidoglycan, enveloping teichoic acid which enhances opsonization, and consuming complement. Using a rabbit model of osteomyelitis, in which the normal bone surface is significantly altered by copious glycocalyx adhering to the bone, subinhibitory concentrations of clindamycin were shown to inhibit this adherence, and prevent the development or cure of an already existing acute osteomyelitis.

In another chapter of this section, LaGrange and associates are presenting evidence that pretreatment of Pseudomonas aeruginosa with subinhibitory concentrations of antibiotics changed the morphologic and ultrastructure of the bacteria. Their significant cellular alterations were accompanied by changes of surface characteristics, the antibiotic-treated bacteria being more able to absorb specific antibodies. This increased expression of antigenicity was also accompanied with higher immunogenicity, and the cell wall alterations induced by subinhibitory concentrations of beta-lactam antibiotics seemed to be associated with an increased expression of specific epitopes on the bacterial surface. Complementary to these observations are the findings of Siegmund-Schultze and associates described in the next chapter. Over the past several years, this group has been investigating the quantitative and qualitative characteristics of the immune responses to surface components of antibiotic-treated bacteria. More specifically, they studied immune responses to antigens from the outer membrane of gram-negative bacteria, and how these responses to antigens can be modulated by complexing the antigens, i.e., LPS, with other components of the outer membrane. They have used a model system consisting of defined complexes produced from isolated, purified components of the bacterial form of Proteus mirabilis strain VI, and various forms of this strain with progressive cell wall defects (filament form, unstable spheroplast L-form, and stable protoplast L-form) induced by beta-lactam antibiotics. The cell walls or protoplast membranes isolated and complexed from these forms were then administered to mice and the secondary IgM and IgG subclass responses to LPS measured showing characteristically different patterns of antibody class and subclass production depending on the combination of components used. In the closing chapter of Section II, Friedman and Warren report that pretreatment of E. coli with subinhibitory concentrations of semisynthetic penicillins, but not Penicillin G, markedly increases its susceptibility to antibody mediated complement dependent bacterial lysis as well as to phagocytosis by macrophages. The latter which had ingested these organisms also showed higher levels of immunogenic cell surface components of the bacteria as compared to phagocytes which had ingested untreated bacteria.

Section III that deals with the influence of antibiotics on host defenses in vivo covers a broader range of interacting mechanisms than the preceding section. The topic of the first chapter by Paul G. Quie revolves around the issue of host defenses in patients with identifiable defects in their immune systems. It is pointed out that knowledge of components of the immune system most seriously compromised in individual patients does not allow informed empiricism for making therapeutic decisions. Consequently, microbial identification and antibiotic sensitivity testing are critically important when caring for such immunocompromised patients. Precise bacterial identification is required since relatively toxic antibiotics may be necessary and recurrence of infection is a frequent clinical problem. Also prolonged hospitalization in such cases favors colonization with multiple resistant strains of microbes and continued development of new antimicrobials effective against unusual or resistant organisms is necessary. Bistoni and associates discuss in their chapter an effort to evaluate the hypothesis that the immunoactive effects of amphotericin-B may contribute significantly to its overall antifungal activity in vivo. For this purpose, they have investigated the impact of amphotericin-B treatment on mouse resistance to systemic Candida albicans infection; moreover, experiments were also performed in vitro to ascertain whether exposure of candidacidal effectors to amphotericin B may influence their cytotoxic potential. It was found that a single administration of amphotericin-B was followed by a dramatic increase in the in vivo resistance of the animals to candida infections, an effect which was mirrored by a remarkable modification in in vitro functions of cells with anti-candida reactivity. Wiemer and associates describe their experiences with the effect of antibiotics on the serum resistance of Enterobacteriaceae. As is known, resistance to the bactericidal activity of serum is an important virulence factor of gram-negative bacteria inasmuch as it is responsible for the ineffectiveness of a main host defense mechanism that is the attack and killing by the complement system. The studies presented in the chapter indicate that some of the newly developed beta-lactam antibiotics, especially imipenem, do in fact decrease the serum resistance as far as the serum resistance of certain strains of gram-negative organisms are concerned. This phenomenon of induced serum-sensitivity of bacteria is dose-dependent and completely reversible. Furthermore, the usual biochemical target that is the penicillin-binding protein of these antibiotics does not appear to be responsible for the phenomenon of induced serum sensitivity. Although it was also determined that the bactericidal activity works via the antibody-dependent classical pathway, the serum protein responsible for the effect could not as yet be identified.

A theoretical analysis of measuring the uptake and antibacterial effects of antibiotics within cells is presented by Charles S. F. Easmon. It is concluded that no one method by itself is satisfactory for these kinds of measurements. Properly controlled functional assays of intracellular killing must form the base work but it should be combined with more quantitative assays that do not rely on intracellular targets. In this regard, use of radio-labelled agents alone does not provide information whether intracellular antibiotics are biologically active. On the other hand, the precise intracellular localization of antibiotics can be determined by cellular disruption with differential centrifugation using marker enzymes to identify intracellular organelles.

Brandely and associates, following a concise historical review of the capacity of Suramin (Germanin R, Bayer) to inhibit the reverse transcriptase of animal retroviruses and its potential effectiveness against human non-oncogenic retroviruses associated with AIDS, examine the effects of this agent on the mouse immune system. Their findings suggest that this agent will not substantially benefit patients with late stage AIDS, but there may be a rationale for using this drug early in the disease associated with pro-host immunotherapy in order to restore both the retrovirus-induced immune effects and the immune alterations connected with the Suramin treatment itself. As discussed by Mario R. Escobar, recent accumulated knowledge of the molecular biology of viruses has opened the way to more rational approaches to the development of more potent and more selective antiviral agents. Some of these which effectively inhibit viral replication may also possess, however, significant immunosuppressive activity. Only in a few instances have antiviral agents been investigated for their interaction with the immune system. Studies in his laboratory have been undertaken to explore the immunoreactive dimension of such antiviral agents. In these investigations, a correlation between the minimal antiviral concentration of the agent required to inhibit replication in cell culture and its minimal immunosuppressive concentration measured by lymphocyte responsiveness to mitogens or certain viral antigens has revealed different levels of efficacy (i.e., highest antiviral effect and lowest immunosuppressive activity): highest level as in the case of acyclovir (ACV) and bromovinyldeoxiuridine (BVDU) for HSV-1; moderate level as in the case of ribavirin, idoxuridine (IDU) and vidarabine (Ara-A), and, lowest as in the case of trifluridine (TFT). Since the herpes viruses HSV,VZV, CMV, and EBV are of great importance as the etiologic agents of severe viral infections in immunocompromised patients, Erik DeClercq presents extensive additional information on the new antiviral drugs and therapeutic modalities that have recently been developed to treat these diseases. Of these, only ACV and Ara-A are at present licensed for the treatment of HSV and VZV infections of immunosuppressed patients. Intravenous or oral ACV can also be used for prevention of HSV infections in cases of severe immunosuppression such as occurs in bone marrow transplant recipients. However, oral ACV has not been shown to be effective against VZV infections. Conversely, BVDU is a more potent inhibitor of HSV and VZV replication than ACV or Ara-A, and nontoxic for bone marrow progenitor cells and lymphocytes at doses far in excess of those required to inhibit HSV or VZV replication. Open clinical studies indicate its usefulness in infections caused by these viruses. For the treatment of CMV and EBV infections no particular drug can at present be recommended. Finally, in the closing chapter of this section, Ghione and associates discuss studies on type I interferon production in experimental animals or cells of pediatric patients treated with commonly used antibiotics.

Organization of the material included in Section IV is guided by the consideration that there are mainly two functional, morphologically different phagocytic cell populations in blood responsible for defense against infection, the polymorphonuclear leukocytes (also called neutrophils, granulocytes, PMN's) and monocytes, both deriving from precursor cells in the bone marrow. Thus, Section IV deals with the various antimicrobial effects on the phagocytic activities of these two cell types starting out with a discussion of the influence of tetracyclines on granulocyte functions by Gnarpe and associates. This chapter indicates that there are pronounced differences between the effects of the different tetracyclines: the highly lipid soluble preparations causing a marked depression of both the PMN undirected and directed migration as well as on the rate of internalization of opsonized yeast cells. These effects are most likely due to chelated binding of divalent cations, primarily Ca^{2+}, but also Mg^{2+} being essential for membrane transportation and deformability. Grassi and Fietta from their in vitro studies on PMN locomotion conclude that no apparent correlation exists between the mechanism or the type of action of various antibiotics and the effect on PMN function. Moreover, the interference of these agents with chemotaxis does not relate exclusively to the capacity of the antibiotic to penetrate phagocytic cells. In addition, unexplained differences in displaying this effect seem to exist among derivatives belonging to the same family of antibiotics. With respect to in vivo significance of in vitro findings, it is apparent that some phenomena observed in vitro may have little significance at the clinical level, possibly because of the presence of some currently unknown protective factors. Another aspect of their studies concerns the mechanism by which antibiotics affect PMN chemotaxis in those situations when they do. In their laboratories, a new technique has been established that is based on the consideration that following exposure of PMN's to chemoattractants one of the first steps in the cellular activation sequence is membrane potential changes. Utilizing the fluorescent probe $DiOC_5$ that is sensitive to such changes they found that several antibiotics that inhibited in vitro chemotaxis at therapeutic concentrations, had no effect on chemoattractant-induced membrane potential changes in PMN's. In contrast, amphotericin-B irreversibly inhibited PMN-membrane potential changes even at concentrations lower than the therapeutic levels and most importantly this effect was not achieved through interference with the binding of chemoattractants to their PMN-membrane receptors. Since opsonization of a bacterium is necessary for phagocytosis, in those cases where an enhanced uptake after exposure to subinhibitory concentrations of antibiotics can be shown to occur, the phenomenon may be due to changes in the structure of antibody binding or complement activating sites. In the studies of Veringa and Verhoef, therefore, S. aureus was opsonized in heated antiserum to inactivate the complement system and test the influence of antibodies alone, and conversely the bacteria were opsonized in serum of a patient with an antibody deficiency syndrome, to test the effect of complement alone. Using the heated antiserum as an opsonic source, the clindamycin-treated bacteria were taken up by PMN's more readily than the controls, indicating that clindamycin in subinhibitory concentrations enhances antibody-dependent phagocytosis, and when agammaglobulinemic serum was used as the opsonic source clindamycin also enhanced complement-dependent phagocytosis by PMN's. The clindamycin-treated bacteria were also better killed by the PMN's once they were ingested, and evidence was obtained indicating that the enhancing effect of clindamycin on phagocytosis was dependent on the presence of a certain amount of protein A on the bacterial cell surface. Enhancement of phagocytosis by clindamycin, furthermore, was shown to take place in bacterial strains that are protein A-rich, and appeared to be the outcome of an inhibition of protein A synthesis by the antibiotic. Reduction of the amount of protein A on the bacterial cell surface, therefore, appears to improve the possibilities for opsonization by complement and antibodies. In a subsequent chapter, Curtis G. Gemmell gives an extensive account of the pathogenecity of different bacteria and the possible consequences of the interaction between these antibiotic-damaged organisms and cells of the reticuloendothelial system in vitro and in vivo.

A recently completed clinical trial done under the auspices of the National Cancer Institute of Canada provided clinical efficacy data for ticarcillin/tobramycin (tic/tob) versus ticarcillin/moxalactam (tic/mox) in the treatment of febrile neutropenic patients. Having these clinical data, and using sera from leukemic patients containing chemotactic inhibitors, the effects of these drug combinations on PMN chemotaxis were tested by Lionel A. Mandell using an in vitro system that more closely approximates the in vivo situation. This model employs drug combinations originally used in their clinical trial (tic/tob, tic/mox) added to PMN's from normal donors in a chemotactic inhibitor-free in vitro system. Under these conditions, significant inhibition of chemotaxis is seen. When a chemotactic inhibitor (C5a, BF) was present, however, testing of the foregoing drug combinations produced results that correlated with the clinical outcome in infected patients treated with the same antibiotic combinations. From studies on the effect of beta-lactam antibiotics on the bactericidal activity of PMN's against E. coli discussed by Axel Dalhoff in the next chapter, the conclusion emerges that the degree of filamentation due to the exposure of E. coli and some other bacteria to various beta-lactams is directly correlated to the increased intraleukocyte killing of these microorganisms. It is also demonstrated that the bactericidal effect is antagonized by alpha-methylmannoside, thus indicating that the probable site of action of the antibiotic lies in its interference with the mannose-sensitive adhesions of E. coli. In investigations forming the material of the preceding chapters, phagocytosis by PMN's was studied in monocultures of bacteria, whereas in a clinical setting infections caused by mixed cultures of bacteria may occur. It is of interest therefore, that the chapter of Shah and associates provides some information on the phagocytic activities of human PMN's against mixed cultures containing gram-negative and gram-positive organisms such as E. coli, K. pneumoniae, and S. aureus. It appears that in the presence of S. aureus, the rate of phagocytosis and killing of both E. coli and K. pneumoniae was markedly reduced. The preferred phagocytosis of S. aureus was also observed in phase contrast microscopy and has been documented on video (copies are available on request to the author). The reason for this phenomenon is at present not understood.

Antibacterial activity of monocytes and macrophages against S. aureus and Klebsiella pneumoniae with or without latamoxef is discussed by Just and associates. In their studies, blood-born monocytes, incubated on Teflon membranes, underwent transformation into macrophages in a period of four to eight days, which was confirmed by parallel macrophage surface marker determinations, cytochemistry, and antitumor activity. Monocytes killed a significantly smaller proportion of each of the two bacterial strains investigated than did monocyte-originated macrophages obtained from the same individuals indicating that the ability to kill bacteria seems to increase with the macrophage maturation process. Comparing the killing rate of bacteria that had been incubated with normal human pooled serum, heat-inactivated serum, or HBSS-gel without serum, most rapid antibacterial killing was observed by mature macrophages when normal serum was used as opsonin suggesting that heat-labile factors may have a role in increasing the rate of bacterial phagocytosis by macrophages. While in these experiments the phagocytic activity of human macrophages grown from blood monocytes was examined, Schroten and associates in the subsequent chapter provide evidence that alveolar macrophages, obtained by lung lavage from guinea pigs, could ingest and kill virulent, encapsulated K. pneumoniae without opsonization. Macrophage killing of this bacterium was increased by subinhibitory concentrations of gentamycin, and phagocytosis by these macrophages was considerably augmented in the presence of specific antibodies to surface components of the bacteria. In addition, evidence is also provided for enhanced uptake of the bacteria after co-cultivation of the macrophages with autologous lymphocytes prior to phagocytosis. This logically leads us to a more detailed discussion of antimicrobial effects on humoral and cellular lymphocyte responses presented in the next section of this volume.

In the first chapter of Section V, Hahn and associates describe the effects of two recently developed quinolones, Doxycyclin (a tetracycline derivative), and a new beta-lactam antibiotic (HR221) on two immune parameters: 1) specific interaction of T-cells with antigen presented by macrophages in vitro, and 2) delayed type hypersensitivity to sheep red blood cells in mice. Taken together, their findings show that beta-lactams and quinolones at therapeutic concentrations do not inhibit T-cell mediated functions, T-cell proliferation and DTH. Doxycyclin showed suppressive effects, both in vitro (at concentrations slightly higher than therapeutic ones), and at supratherapeutic doses in vivo as well. Wittke and associates investigated the impact of different concentrations of antibiotics (tetracycline, cefmenoxime, ceftazidime, and clavulanic acid) on the blast formation of maximally and moderately mitogen-stimulated as well as of non-stimulated splenic murine lymphocytes by measuring ^{3}H-thymidine incorporation. Based on their experiences, it might be expected that the stimulative effects seen with tetracycline, cefmenoxime, and clavulanic acid, achieved by therapeutic concentrations, actually play a role at least during long-term treatment with these agents. Except for ceftaxidime, the dosage required for a depression of lymphocyte transformation is beyond the therapeutic level (tetracycline, cefmenoxime) or only reachable for a short period of time following bolus injection (clavulanic acid) and may thus be of lesser importance for antibiotic treatment.

Clot and Pelous examined the activity of three cephalosporins (cefadroxil, cefalexine, and cefaclor), a tetracycline (doxycycline), and a macrolide (josamycine) on T-cell subsets and functions in relation to a mitogen. It was found that cephalosporin and cefadroxil, in particular, were able to stimulate prostaglandin-producing T-suppressor cells which may explain the parallel decrease of mitogen responsiveness seen in these studies. Such data may account for the relative paucity of allergic reactions associated with the use of cefadroxil. This cephalosporin could limit or decrease IgE production by stimulating suppressor cells. The chapter by Pocidalo and associates evaluates the effects of two antibiotic families, macrolides and new quinoline carboxylic acid derivatives on mitogen-stimulated human peripheral blood mononuclear leukocyte responses. Having demonstrated that erythromycin, spiramycin, ciprofloxacin, pefloxacin, and oflaxacin suppressed significantly lymphocyte transformation to mitogens, it was also found that thiol compounds as antioxidant agents, essentially 2-Mercaptoethanol provided partial protection of the depressed immune responses induced by high antibiotic concentration. The authors advanced the hypothesis that this type of antibiotic immune injury could be partly mediated by an oxidant injury. The mechanism of this injury could be related to an oxidant metabolite which is derived from the antibiotic demethyl metabolites. The drugs that are able to protect the critical cells participating in the organization of an immune response from an oxidant stress could then represent a new family of immunomodulator agents.

Section VI deals with the relationship between immune stimulators and antibiotics in general, starting out with a discussion of amphotericin-B (AmB) as a model murine immunostimulant by Little and associates. Several studies in their laboratories have shown that in many mouse strains, AmB or its derivative, amphotericin-B methyl ester (AME), can stimulate cell-mediated as well as humoral immunity with a potency comparable to complete Freund's adjuvant. In their studies reported here, they provide new evidence that optimal stimulation of lymphocytes by AME in vitro requires the participation of accessory cells. In addition, they show that the immunostimulation of lymphoid cells by AmB or AME can be related to the formation of reactive oxygen metabolites, especially H_2O_2. They also conclude that the immunostimulant effects of AmB may play a significant role in the therapeutic efficacy of AmB in the treatment of systemic fungal infections. The objective of the studies described in the chapter by Gunther Gillissen was to further explore immunological side effects of antibiotics through their possible influence on the synthesis of immunomodulatory pharmacological mediators by the cells of the immune network. Specifically, the effect of cefotaxime, cefoxitin, and cefaclor have been examined in vitro as well as in vivo on the synthesis of PGE2 and IL1 production by macrophages and on PGE2 sensitivity of thymocytes. In vitro as well as in vivo, cefotaxime enhanced PGE2 production, and PGE2 resistance of thymocytes has also been increased by cefotaxime compared with cefoxitin both in vitro as well as in vivo. Furthermore, cefaclor in vivo induced a similar change of PGE2 resistance of thymocytes as did cefoxitin. IL1 production of macrophages has particularly been increased by cefotaxime in vitro and, to a smaller degree, by cefoxitin. In vivo experiments showed that cefotaxime and cefaclor augmented IL1 production considerably whereas cefoxitin had no effect. DeSimone and Hadden present a comprehensive review of the immunomodulatory effects of isoprinosine and NPT 15392. It is pointed out that at present two classes of compounds are considered thymomimetic: inducers of thymic hormones or thymic hormone-like substances (e.g., levamisole) and simulators of the action of the thymic hormones (i.e., isoprinosine and NPT 15392). Their review focuses on this second category. Isoprinosine is licensed for clinical use in 70 countries. Although relatively high doses are required, isoprinosine is not generally toxic and is consistent in its immunopharmacologic actions. NPT 15392 is an experimental drug under development and on a weight basis this drug is more potent by a factor of 10-1000 than methisoprinol and has more prolonged actions in vivo. In addition to inducing T-cell differentiation and modulating mature T-cell function, these substances induce B-cell differentiation, potentiate gamma-IFN, IL1 and IL2 production, increase natural killer cell activity and phagocytic cell function. These effects might be interpreted by postulating that both drugs act through a receptor shared by T-cells, B-cells, NK cells, granulocytes, and macrophages, inducing modification of as yet unknown enzymatic pathways. The two agents could be allosteric modifiers of inosine or hypoxanthine-utilizing enzymes giving rise to active analogs of xanthine and uric acid which regulate in turn the activity of ADA, PNP, 5'-nucleotidase inosine dehydrogenase or HGPRT. The closing chapter of Section VI. by Parant and Chedid discusses the effects of muramyl dipeptides on host immunity and other defense mechanisms. Following their extensive review the authors conclude that the synergistic combination of various MDP's and antibiotics represents an important contribution leading to a decrease in ED_{50} values of antibiotics and to an increase in the efficacy of muramyl peptides to stimulate nonspecific mechanisms of resistance. Such an application may be considered against various types of infections to lower the dose of the antibiotics that may possess significant inherent toxicity or immunosuppressive effect. A case in point is the example of a _Leishmania donovani_ infection, in which a combined therapy with an antimonial drug and lipophilic muramyl peptide was found to be more effective than either of the two treatments applied individually. Moreover, the synergistic action of macrophage-activating factor (MAF) and MDP's in therapeutic studies against cancer metastases may open a new horizon of research by taking advantage of the opportunity offered by modern biotechnology to produce cytokines.

In closing this overview, it seems that the critical effects of antibiotics on immunity presented in this volume could be compared to discontinuous points lying in one plane. This reflects the fact that there has been no systematic investigation of this field, and in no case do the fragmentary facts available permit a complete and comprehensive description of the immunoregulatory activities of antibiotics. The contributors and the editors of this volume believe that extensive additional investigations in this very young field of scientific inquiry will soon provide a more cohesive account of the entire spectrum of antibiotic and host interactions.

SECTION II
INFLUENCE OF ANTIBIOTICS ON BACTERIA AS RELATED TO HOST IMMUNITY

THE INFLUENCE OF SUBINHIBITORY CONCENTRATIONS OF ANTIBIOTICS ON THE BACTERIAL SURFACE WITH RESPECT TO HOST DEFENSE MECHANISMS

W. Opferkuch, K. H. Büscher, H. Leying, M. Pawelzik, and S. Suerbaum

Ruhr-Universität Bochum
Medizinische Mikrobiologie und Immunologie
Bochum, F.R.G.

INTRODUCTION

It is well known that a successful treatment of bacterial infections depends on an effective host defense system. This observation presupposes either that the antibiotic treatment reduces the number of bacteria in a given infection and that the remaining bacteria are subsequently eliminated by the host-defense system, or that antibiotics render bacteria more susceptible to host defense mechanisms. In addition, it is well established that β-lactam antibiotics interfere with peptidoglycan synthesis and that this is combined with changes in the shape of bacteria. Several authors (2,3,12) have pointed out that there is a mutual influence between peptidoglycan and membrane synthesis, but the arrangement and composition of the outer membrane under the influence of β-lactam antibiotics have so far not been investigated adequately.

However, some reports indicate that changes may occur in cell envelope macromolecules (4,12,16). The question whether β-lactam antibiotics alter structures of the bacterial cell envelope is relevant, if the second of the hypotheses mentioned is to be confirmed. The aim of this study was therefore to investigate whether treatment of *E. coli* with subinhibitory concentrations of β-lactam antibiotics induces measurable physico-chemical alterations of the outer membrane and whether these changes are accompanied with changes in the interaction of bacteria and host-defense mechanisms.

The main difficulty in this project is the comparison of the reaction of antibiotic treated and untreated bacteria (see also Lorian et al., this volume). Taking these results into account we tried to design experiments which allowed us to circumvent this problem and use, if possible, outer membrane vesicles. In our study we investigated four parameters:

1. Composition of the outer membrane
2. Adherence of unopsonized bacteria
3. Chemiluminescence
4. Immunogenicity

MATERIALS AND METHODS

Bacteria

E. coli WF 96, serogroup 07:K1:H6 was obtained from St. Mary's Hospital, London; D 509, serogroup 086 and D 539, serogroup not determinable, were obtained from Dundee, University of Scotland.

Reagents

The following antibiotics were used: Latamoxef (Lilly), Cephaloridine (Lilly), Mezlocillin (Bayer), Ciprofloxacin (Bayer), Piperacillin (Cyanamid), Imipenem (MSD), Aztreonam (Squibb), Mecillinam (Leo-Pharmacia), Ticarcillin (Beecham), Cefuroxime (Hoechtst).

Preparation of Bacterial Membranes

Membranes were prepared according to Kroll et al. (9) by sucrose density ultracentrifugation. Bacteria were grown to an optical density of about 0.5 at 578 nm, centrifugated and washed once with phosphate buffered saline. Subsequently, the bacteria were suspended in 5 ml 0.05 M HEPES (N-2-hydroxy-ethylpiperazine- N'-2-ethanesulfonic acid) (pH 7.2) containing 0.75 M sucrose and 50 µg of egg white lysozyme (Sigma Chemical Co., St. Louis, MO, U.S.A.) per ml. After 10 minutes of incubation the plasmolysed bacteria were lysed by transferring them into 120 ml of distilled water containing 1 mg DNase (Serva Feinbiochemica, Heidelberg, Germany). After this, membranes were separated from soluble material by ultracentrifugation (1 hr, 130,000 g, 4° C). Subsequently, outer and inner membrane vesicles were isolated by sucrose density ultracentrifugation (16 hrs, 120,000 g, 4°C). During the fractionation of the gradients, the absorbance at 278 nm was continuously monitored with a Uvicord (LKB). The density of the fractions was determined by refractometry.

Determination of Bacterial Adherence

Fresh Mueller-Hinton broth containing 10 µCi ^{14}C acetate/ml was incubated with 1/100 g of a labeled overnight culture (10 µCi ^{14}C acetate/ml). After 3 hrs growth with or without antibiotics, the bacteria were harvested by centrifugation (2000 x g, 10'), washed once with HEPES-buffer, and the control culture was adjusted to a concentration of 1.5×10^8, 2×10^8, or 2×10^9 bacteria/ml. Cpm of these suspensions were determined and the antibiotic treated cultures were adjusted to the same cpm value as the control. 0.5 ml of these suspensions were incubated with a macrophage monolayer, prepared according to the method of Vosbeck et al. (15). After 20 minutes of incubation at 37°C, the monolayers were washed four times with HEPES-buffer. In order to determine the attachment of the bacteria to the cells, the macrophages were lysed with 1 ml of distilled water containing 1% SDS. An aliquot (50 µl) of these suspensions was transferred into 2 ml scintillation liquid (KL 372, Zinsser) and measured in a liquid scintillation counter.

Chemiluminescence Assay

Measurement of the luminol-dependent chemiluminescence was done according to Muller et al. (11): 1×10^6 purified macrophages in 0.5 ml Dulbecco's PBS supplemented with 1% v/v amino acids (Biochrom, Berlin, F.R.G.), 1% non-essential amino acids (Biochrom), 0.5 mM 1-glutamine (Biochrom), 1 mg/ml bovine serum albumin (Sigma Chemicals, Munich, F.R.G.) and 2.5 mg/ml glucose were incubated for 10 minutes at 37°C in the presence of 5×10^{-5} M luminol before the addition of 60 µg outer membrane material. The resulting chemiluminescence response was registrated continuously by use of a six-channel luminometer (LB 9595, Berthold, Wildbad, F.R.G.).

Immunization of Mice

50 µg (dry weight) of outer membrane vesicles were suspended in 0.5 ml of sterile PBS. Directly after vigorous agitation solutions were injected intraperitoneally into male B6D2 mice of age 8-10 weeks.

Direct Plaque Assay

The IgM-producing cell responses to LPS were measured by the hemolytic plaque-test using a modification of the thin-layer assay described by Mishell and Shigii (10). Briefly, 50 µl of a 10% v/v suspension of SRBC sensitized with alkali-treated LPS (2 mg/ml SRBC) (14) from E. coli WF 96 and 50 µl of a 1:3 dilution of guinea pig serum in MEM-Hank's without carbonate (Biochrom, Berlin, F.R.G.) supplemented with 1.16 mM Na_2HPO_4 and 1.19 mM $MgCl_2$ (MHP) were added to 600 µl of 0.6% w/v agarose (Miles, Elkhart, U.S.A.) in MHP. Immediately after this, 0.1 ml of a dilution of spleen cells in MHP were added, the mixture was poured directly into a petri dish and spread on the surface.

Assay of Humoral Antibodies Against Outer Membrane Proteins (ELISA)

Outer membrane proteins were diluted in carbonate-bicarbonate-buffer (pH 9.6) and were coated for 2 hrs onto polyvinyl chloride microplates (Falcon). Afterwards, remaining binding sites were saturated with BSA.

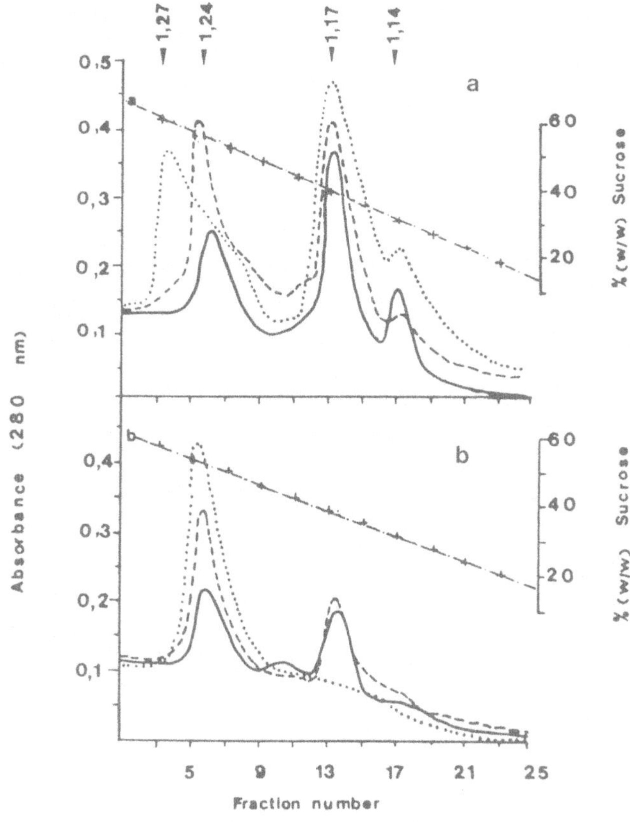

Figure 1. Distribution of membrane vesicles of E. coli WF 96 grown in the absence (a) or presence (b) of imipenem for 150 min (-), 210 min (--), 300 min (..) after sucrose density ultracentrifugation.

Serum dilutions were prepared in PBS containing 1 mg/ml BSA (Sigma Chemicals Co., St. Louis, U.S.A.) and 0.5% Tween 20 and were reacted for 2 hrs with the antigen on the microplates. Goat anti-mouse immunoglobulin (IgM + IgG) peroxidase conjugate (Medac, Hamburg, F.R.G.) was then reacted in the plates for 2 hrs. Plates were washed three times between each step with PBS-Tween-20-buffer. Thirty minutes after the addition of the substrate H_2O_2 and o-phenylendiamine (Sigma) the optical density was measured at 450 nm in a Dynatech ELISA reader.

RESULTS AND DISCUSSION

The Composition of the Outer Membrane

From Figure 1 it can be seen that in the late log phase 4 bands are generated within the sucrose gradient. The first two peaks represent outer membrane vesicles (buoyant densities 1.27 and 1.24 g/cm^3). The second two bands represent cytoplasmic membrane (CM) vesicles (buoyant densities 1.17 and 1.14 g/cm^3) as ascertained by measurement of the NADH oxidase activity, a marker enzyme of the cytoplasmic membrane.

In different growth phases the two first membrane fractions are formed in different amounts. After 150 minutes, that is in the early log phase, only the lighter outer membrane fraction could be isolated, while in the early stationary phase the dense OM peak was quantitatively more strongly developed. In the lower part of Figure 1 the distribution of membrane vesicles from E. coli WF 96 after incubation in culture medium containing

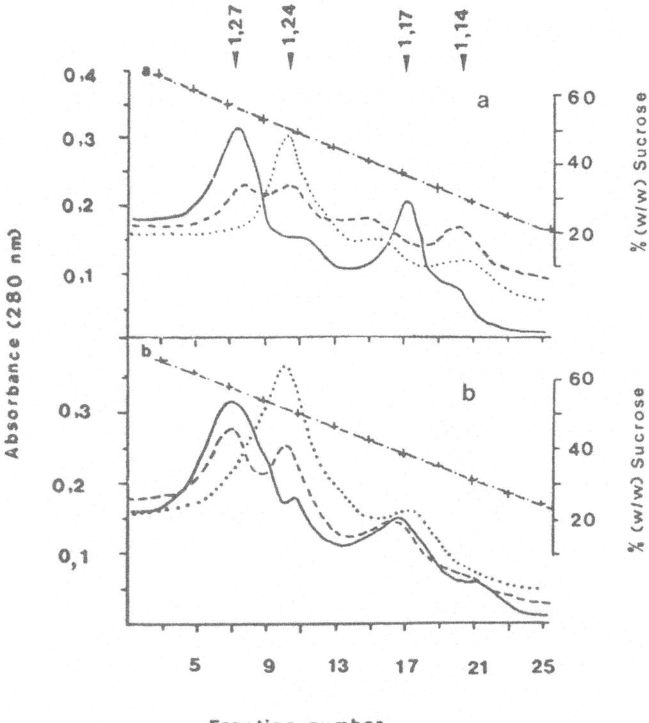

Figure 2. Distribution of membrane vesicles of E. coli WF 96 grown in the absence (-) or presence of 1/12 MIC (--), 1/6 MIC (..) imipenem (a) or aztreonam (b) after sucrose density ultracentrifugation.

1/4 MIC imipenem is shown, where in all growth phases only the OM peak with the lower buoyant density was formed.

The effect is also dependent on the concentration of the antibiotic (Figure 2). The β-lactam antibiotics caused a dose-dependent quantitative shift from the dense OM peak to the lighter one. While without antibiotics mainly the peak with a density of 1.27 g/cm^3 is found, with 1/12 MIC of the respective antibiotic the dense and the lighter peak is formed. In 1/6 MIC of the drugs only the OM fraction corresponding to the buoyant density of 1.24 g/cm^3 was formed within the sucrose gradients. Comparable results were obtained with other β-lactam antibiotics like mecillinam, lamoxactam, piperacillin and ticarcillin. An SDS-PAGE analysis of the proteins present in the four membrane peaks revealed that the CM peaks contained only traces of the major outer membrane protein bands. The two OM peaks were very similar with respect to their protein pattern (Figure 3).

The question whether the different membrane peaks isolated by sucrose density ultracentrifugation have different functional significance remains to be answered. But the assumption that the different membrane fractions reflect the heterogeneity of the OM as it occurs on living bacteria seems to be likely, because the distinct membrane fractions show different labeling kinetics in pulse-chase experiments with ^{3}H-glycerol as precursor of phospholipids and N-acetyl-D-^{14}C-glucosamine as precursor of lipopolysaccharides.

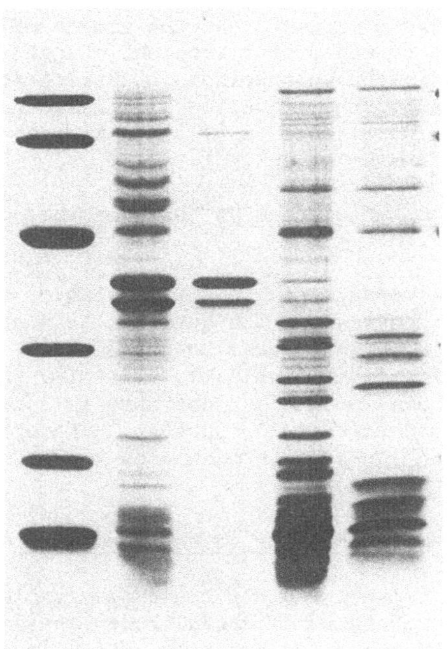

Figure 3. SDS-PAGE of the four peaks (I,II, III, IV) obtained after sucrose density ultracentrifugation of whole membranes of E. coli WF 96. The following proteins from Pharmacia (electrophoresis calibration kit) were used as molecular weight standards (Ref): phosphorylase b (94,000), bovine serum albumin (67,000), ovalbumin (43,000), carbonic anhydrase (30, 000), soy bean trypsin inhibitor (20,100), and alpha-lactalbumin (14,400). The gel was stained with coomassie brilliant blue R 250.

Table 1. Influence of 1/4 MIC of Antibiotics on the Adherence of *E. coli* Strains to Macrophages

Strain	Cefuroxime	Moxalactam	Aztreonam	Imipenem
WF 96 (MS^+/MR^+)	75	88	61	31
D 539 (MS^+/MR^+)	130	140	118	80
D 509 (MS^+/MR^-)	213	133	222	100
B 875 (MS^+/MR^-)	304	320	360	173

The values are expressed as % deviation in comparison to the control (control = 100%).

We could not detect any differences between drug treated and untreated cells as regards the quality of the OM proteins, lipopolysaccharide patterns, estimated by SDS-PAGE, or the migration properties of phospholipids in thin-layer chromatography. Although the exact quantitative contribution of proteins, lipopolysaccharides, and phospholipids to the OM composition remains to be determined, it seems likely that all β-lactam derivatives used caused alterations in the quantity and arrangement of the membrane constituents.

Preliminary experiments suggest that the amount of LPS and the phospholipid portion in respect to the protein content changes. This fact may be explained by the inhibition of phospholipid translocation as found in pulse-chase experiments. Finally, the amount on K1-polysaccharide is diminished in the presence of 1/4 MIC imipenem to 59% in comparison to the untreated control.

The Influence of β-lactam Antibiotics on the Adherence of E. coli to Macrophages

The adherence to macrophages is the first step of an "unspecific", non-opsonin-mediated phagocytosis. The question is whether this non-opsonin-mediated phagocytosis can be influenced by antibiotics. Two main results were obtained in this experiment (Table 1). Firstly, while strain WF 96 showed no significant change or a clear decrease in adherence, another strain (B 875) showed a more than three-fold increase. The other two strains were in between. Secondly, an increase in adherence was mainly seen with filament forming antibiotics.

The Influence of β-lactam Antibiotics on the Chemiluminescence Reaction

It was interesting to know whether these observations also have some biological meaning. Therefore we extended these experiments and tested the luminol-dependent chemiluminescence reaction (CL). In order to exclude any influence of the morphology of the bacteria (filaments, round cells) on the activation of phagocytes, outer membrane vesicles were used to stimulate the macrophages. Outer membrane vesicles from *E. coli* WF 96 were capable of inducing a significant chemiluminescence response of macrophages. This chemiluminescence was markedly increased if the bacteria had been pretreated with antibiotics (Table 2). In this case, the best stimulation was found if outer membrane vesicles from bacteria grown in the presence of imipenem were used. The amount of chemiluminescence was dependent on the amount of outer membrane vesicles used for stimulation. The differences between chemiluminescence induced by outer membrane vesicles from bacteria treated with antibiotics and that induced by non-treated bacteria could not be over-

Table 2. Luminol-Dependent Response of *P. acnes* Activated Macrophages to Different Outer Membrane Vesicles (OM)

Stimulus[1]	Counts/15 min. x 10^6
None	3.7
OM WF 96	26.8
OM WF 96-piperacillin[2]	53.7
OM WF 96-mezlocillin[2]	58.1
OM WF 96-lamoxactam[3]	115.0
OM WF 96-imipenem[3]	136.0
OM WF 96-aztreonam	93.0

[1] 80 µg OM/10^6 macrophages
[2] 1/6 MIC
[3] 1/4 MIC

come by increasing the amount of the stimulant, because different plateaus of chemiluminescence were reached with the respective stimuli.

As *E. coli* WF 96 expresses different types of fimbrial (6) and shows mannose-sensitive as well as mannose-resistant hemagglutination, it was interesting to know whether treatment of bacteria with different antibiotics has a selective influence on one type of adhesion. As can be seen from Figure 4, the increased stimulatory effect of outer membranes from antibiotic pretreated cells was mainly due to the participation of mannose-sensitive adhesins, whereas mannose-resistant adhesins were either not influenced or even slightly depressed as in the case of lamoxactam.

Inhibition experiments with superoxide dismutase and studies of the lucigenin-dependent chemiluminescence as well as measurement of superoxide anion by cytochrome C reduction showed that there was no liberation of superoxide anion by macrophages in response to outer membrane vesicles, indicating that there was no stimulation of the O_2 generating NAD(P)H-oxidase. Even pretreatment of bacteria with antibiotics could not lead to the activation of this enzyme.

Immunostimulation

It has been demonstrated by Karch & Nixdorff (7), Ruttkowski and Nixdorff (13) and Karch et al. (5) that the quantity as well as the subclass composition of the immune response against lipopolysaccharide from *Proteus mirabilis* can be influenced over a wide range by complexing with proteins, phospholipids, or both. In complexes of antigens, especially in liposomes associated with various antigens (1), mutual adjuvant effects, depending upon quality as well as quantitative contribution of the antigens, modulate the immune response against the single constituents of such complexes.

In the experiments presented here the primary immune response was measured against outer membrane proteins and lipopolysaccharide induced by an immunization with outer membrane vesicles from untreated bacteria and from bacteria of strain WF 96 grown in the presence of 1/4 MIC of lamoxactam, aztreonam, mezlocillin and imipenem, either by a direct plaque assay or an ELISA test for humoral antibodies. The immunization was done with 50 µg of outer membrane vesicles. The dose of 50 µg vesicles was chosen because it was sufficient to induce a maximal response against LPS. Immunization with

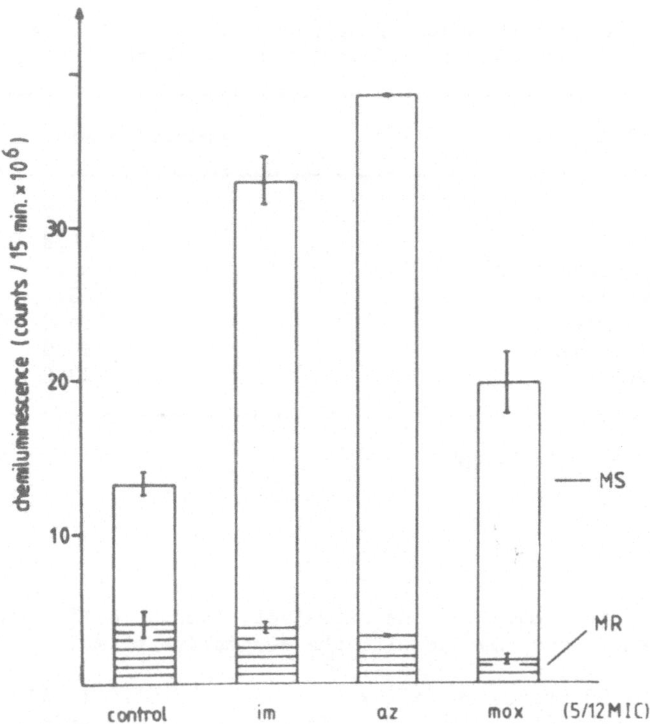

Figure 4. The influence of antibiotic treatment on the mannose sensitive and mannose resistant activation of marophages. Openbars: mannose sensitive CL; hatched bars: mannose resistant CL.

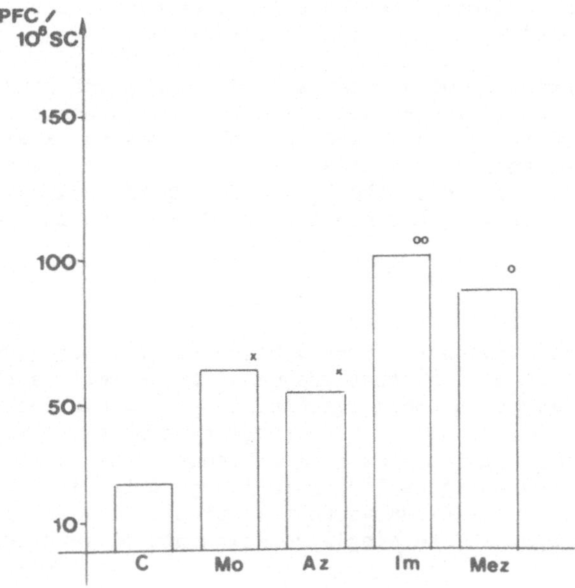

Figure 5. Antibody producing cell responses against LPS on day 5 after immunization with 50 μg of outer membrane vesicles from control bacteria (C) and moxalactam (Mo), aztreonam (Az), imipenem (Im), and mezlocillin (Mez)-treated bacteria. PFC values are the results from 3 separate experiments. x = no significant difference ($p>0.05$); o = significant increase ($p<0.02$); oo = significant increase ($p<0.001$).

vesicles from imipenem- and mezlocillin-treated bacteria induced an about four-fold increased antibody-producing cell response against LPS as compared with control vesicles ($p<0.001$ and $p<0.02$, respectively) (Figure 5). For aztreonàm and lamoxactam there were no significant effects. These results even gain in significance when one considers that the outer membrane vesicles prepared from antibiotic-treated bacteria all contain less lipopolysaccharide [estimated by KDO determination (8)] than control vesicles.

In addition, the sera of the animals were tested for antibodies against outer membrane proteins by an ELISA test (Figure 6). Whereas antibody concentrations did not show significant differences after immunization with vesicles from lamoxactam-, imipenem-, and mezlocillin-treated bacteria, immunization with vesicles from aztreonam-treated bacteria induced significantly higher ($p<0.02$) concentrations of antibodies against outer membrane proteins as compared with control vesicles. Outer membrane preparations showed only slight differences of protein content, so that this effect, too, is probably due to an increased immunogenicity of the outer membrane protein when incorporated in vesicles from aztreonam-treated bacteria.

Therefore, growth in subinhibitory concentrations of antibiotics can apparently change the immunogenic properties of bacterial surface components, probably by changing the quantitative contributions of the different compo-

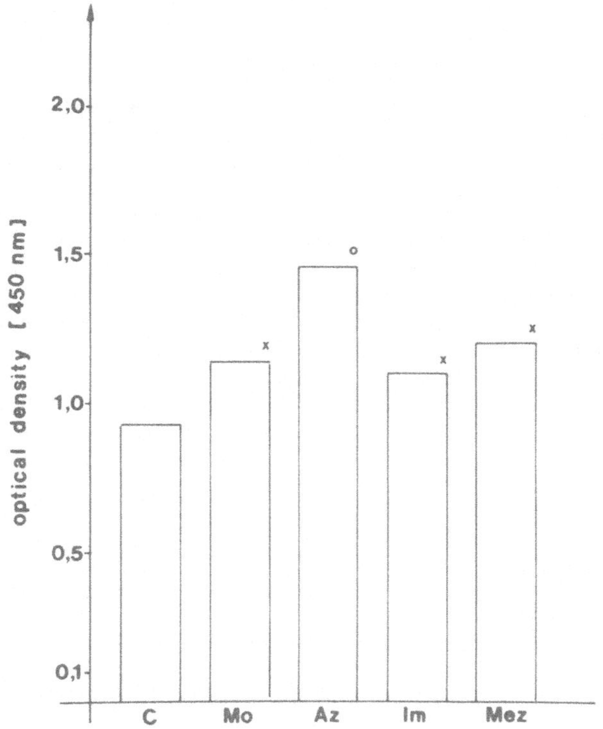

Figure 6. Comparison of concentrations of antibodies against outer membrane proteins (ELISA) after immunization with 50 µg of outer membrane vesicles from control bacteria (C) and moxalactam (Mo), aztreonam (Az), imipenem (Im) and mezlocillin (Mez)-treated bacteria. Values are given as mean optical densities of ten sera per group at one representative dilution (1:128). x = no significant difference ($p>0.05$); o= significant increase ($p<0.02$).

nents to the outer membrane, thus changing the epitope densities and the molecular surroundings of the different immunogens.

SUMMARY

It must be assumed that treatment of bacteria with subinhibitory concentrations of antibiotics leads to changes in the composition and structure of the outer membrane of bacteria and thereafter to changes in their interaction with host defense mechanisms. In order to test this hypothesis, E. coli (strain WF 96, D 509, D 539, B 875) were grown in 1/4 MIC of several β-lactam antibiotics; their outer membrane composition, the immunogenicity of outer membrane vesicles, the adherence to macrophages and the chemiluminescence reaction were studied. The following results were obtained: treatment of E. coli with subinhibitory concentrations of β-lactam antibiotics did not induce changes in the expression of outer membrane proteins nor in the polymerization of the LPS O-side chains. Furthermore, the phospholipid profile, as assessed by thin-layer chromatography, appeared identical thus indicating that there was no change of the qualitative composition of the outer membrane constituents of antibiotic-treated E. coli. In contrast to these observations the analysis of the outer membrane by sucrose density ultracentrifugation revealed remarkable differences between drug-treated bacteria and untreated controls. While the outer membranes of untreated bacteria showed a major fraction with a buoyant density of 1.27 g/cm^3 and a minor fraction with a buoyant density of 1.24 g/cm^3 at the late log phase, the outer membranes of antibiotic treated bacteria showed only one major fraction corresponding to the buoyant density of 1.24 g/cm^3.

As both fractions contained qualitatively the same outer membrane proteins it must be concluded that their differences in density were due to quantitative differences in their protein, LPS or PL content, and both fractions represent different areas on the bacterial surface. In addition to these physico-chemical changes of the outer membrane it could be shown that immunization with outer membrane vesicles prepared from antibiotic-treated bacteria elicited a higher anti-protein or LPS response depending on the antibiotics used. Another example for the influence of antibiotics on the host-parasite relationship includes adherence of non-opsonized bacteria to macrophages and the subsequent chemiluminescence reaction. With β-lactam antibiotics it could be shown that in general the adherence was increased. The extent of increase was dependent on strain and antibiotic used. This increase was combined with a marked enhancement of the chemiluminescence reaction.

REFERENCES

1. A. C. Allison and G. Gregoriades, Liposomes as immunological adjuvants, Nature 252:252 (1974).
2. J. Amaral, Effect of subminimal inhibitory concentrations of mecillinam on the synthesis of DNA, RNA and protein of Salmonella typhimurium: A proposed mechanism of action, Rev. Infect. Dis. 1:813 (1979).
3. J. L. Brissette, G. D. Shockman and R. A. Pieringer, Effects of penicillin on synthesis and excretion of lipid and lipoteichoic acid from Streptococcus mutant BHT, J. Bacteriol. 151:838 (1982).
4. R. James, Identification of an outer membrane protein of Escherichia coli, with a role in the coordination of desoxyribonucleic acid replication and cell elongation, J. Bacteriol. 124:918 (1975).
5. H. Karch, J. Gmeiner and K. Nixdorff, Alteration of the immunoglobulin G subclass responses in mice to lipopolysaccharide: effects of nonbacterial proteins and bacterial membrane phospholipids or outer

membrane proteins of Proteus mirabilis, Infect. Immun. 40:157 (1983).

6. H. Karch, H. Leying, K. H. Buscher, H. P. Kroll and W. Opferkuch, Isolation and separation of physicochemically distinct fimbrial types expressed on a single culture of Escherichia coli 07:K1:H6, Infect. Immun. 47:549 (1985).
7. H. Karch and K. Nixdorff, Antibody-producing cell responses to an isolated outer membrane protein and to complexes of this antigen with lipopolysaccharide or with vesicles of phospholipids from Proteus mirabilis, Infect. Immun. 31:862 (1981).
8. Y. D. Karkhanis, J. Y. Zeltner, J. J. Jackson and D. J. Carlo, A new and improved microassay to determine 2-keto-3-deoxy-octonate in lipopolysaccharide of gram-negative bacteria, Anal. Biochem. 85:595 (1978).
9. H. P. Kroll, S. Bhakdi and P. W. Taylor, Membrane changes induced by exposure of Escherichia coli to human serum, Infect. Immun. 42:1055 (1983).
10. B. B. Mishell and S. M. Shigii, eds., "Selected Methods in Cellular Immunology," Freeman, San Francisco (1980).
11. S. Muller, F. Falkenberg, R. A. Fromtling, A. M. Fromtling and V. Klimetzek, Signals of chemiluminescence emitted by spleen cells and bone marrow macrophages after stimulation with mitogens and particulate substances, in: "Bioluminescence and Chemiluminescence," M. A. de Luca and W. D. McElroy, eds., Academic Press, New York (1981).
12. H. J. Rogers and P. F. Thurman, Interrelationships between wall and membrane synthesis, in: "The Target of Penicillin," R. Hackenbeck, J. V. Holtje and H. Labischinski, eds., Walter de Gruyter, Berlin, New York (1983).
13. E. Ruttkowski and K. Nixdorff, Qualitative and quantitative changes in the antibody-producing cell responses to lipopolysaccharide induced after incorporation of the antigen into bacterial membrane phospholipid vesicles, J. Immunol. 124:2548 (1980).
14. S. Schlecht and O. Westphal, Uber die Herstellung von Antiseren gegen somatische (O-) Antigene von Salmonellen. II. Mitteilung: Untersuchungen uber Hamagglutinintiter, Zbl. Bakt. Hyg. Abt. I, Orig. 205:487 (1967).
15. K. Vosbeck, H. Handschin, E. B. Menge and O. Zak, Effects of subminimal inhibitory concentrations of antibiotics on adhesiveness of Escherichia coli in vitro, Rev. Infect. Dis. 1:845 (1979).
16. P. W. Taylor, H. Gaunt and F. M. Unger, Effect of subinhibitory concentrations of mecillinam on the serum susceptibility of E. coli strains, Antimicrob. Agents Chemother. 19:786 (1981).

LECTINS AND LECTIN RECEPTORS ON β-LACTAM RESISTANT AND SUSCEPTIBLE <u>PSEUDOMONAS</u> <u>AERUGINOSA</u> STRAINS: SIGNIFICANCE FOR ATTACHMENT AND INTRACELLULAR KILLING BY HUMAN PMN

G. Stübner

Institut für Bakteriologie und Hygiene
Krankenhaus Nordstadt
Hannover, F.R.G.

INTRODUCTION

Polymorphonuclear granulocytes (PMN) constantly come in contact with particles in a large number, but they attack and ingest only a few, because their plasma membrane bears structures that recognize specific molecules on the surface of the particles, and therefore, they are able to discriminate between ordered well known and disordered foreign structures (8). In recent years, evidence has been accumulated suggesting that sugar binding proteins, the lectins, being present on bacterial surfaces may serve as attachment moieties of certain pathogens to sugar residues on a variety of animal cells (3,6,10,13,14,17,18).

Today lectins are defined as carbohydrate binding proteins of non-immune origin with no detectable enzymatic activity which agglutinate cells or precipitate glycoconjugates, which recognize and interact with specific mono- or oligosaccharides (9). Bacteria possess many surface components which may serve as receptors for lecithins; e.g., lipopolysaccharides, capsules and group specific antigens and hydrophobic sites of proteins (17). The purpose of this study is to prove the presence of specific sugars and lectins on outer membrane structures of bacteria and on the plasma membrane of human PMN, and to evaluate their significance for attachment and intracellular killing.

EXPERIMENTAL DESIGN

The experimental design is based on three assumptions:

1. Sugar residues on bacteria and PMN are detectable with specific lectins.
2. PMN localized carbohydrates react with bacterial lectins.
3. For phagocytic uptake only those sugars and lectins are important which âre specifically corresponding to the lectins and carbohydrates on the PMN plasmamembrane.

MATERIAL AND METHODS

Bacteria

Two Pseudomonas aeruginosa strains from clinically proven infection (uti) were isolated before (strain 319014 S) and after antibiotic treatment (strain 319014 R). The strains are biochemically and serologically identical (serotype 3, pyocin type 5 y). Existence of a plasmide was excluded by Prof. Laufs/Hamburg. The sensitive and the resistant strain as well produces identical β-lactamases with differences in the amount of production. Therefore, it could be concluded that resistance was acquired by chromosomally determined change in regulation of β-lactamase activity (16).

Isolation of PMN

PMNs were prepared by density gradient sedimentation according to a modified procedure of Bøyum's (2) method (15). Briefly: 7 ml blood was withdrawn from a healthy volunteer into EDTA precoated tubes. 1 ml EDTA blood was piled on 3 ml Amipaque (Schering AG, Berlin)- Lymphoprep (Nyegaard & Co., Oslo)-solution and allowed to sediment for 90 min at 4°C. Due to careful subsequent addition of 1 ml 20% Humanalbumin (Behringwerke AG, Marburg) the plasma separated into three phases. The upper phase containing thrombocytes and lymphocytes and the phase below containing Humanalbumin were discarded and the granulocytes which concentrated in the interface were carefully collected with a pipette. Thereafter PMNs were washed twice and the pellet was resuspended in RPMI 1640 (Seromed-Biochrom, Berlin) and adjusted to a concentration of 2×10^6 cells/ml. A 94-97% viability was proved by trypanblue exclusion.

Table 1. Lectins of the Taxonolectin™-system, Their Carbohydrate Specificities and Binding Sites

Lectin		Sugar specificity	Binding sites
ConA	Concanavalin A	αDMan>αDGluc	4
TKA	Trichosanthes kinlowii	DGal	2
PNA	Arachis hypogaea	βDGal> DGalNac Gal in term, position	4
DBA	Dolichos biflorus	αDGalNac	2
STA	Solanum tuberosum	oligomers containing (1-4)βDGlucNac	2
LFA	Limax flavus	?	2
UEA I	Ulex europaeus	αLFuc	?
LCH	Lens culinaris	αDMan>αDGluc> DGlucNac	2
GS I	Griffonia simplicifolia	DGal, DGalNac	4
SBAS	Glycine max.	αDGalNac>αDGal	4
GS II	Griffonia simplicifolia	βDGluc Nac in term, position	4
WGA	Tritium vulgaris	βDGlucNac, (DGlucNac)$_2$	2
PHA-L	Phaseolus vulgaris	DGal(1-3,4),GlucNac, βDGal Nac	4
Lotus	Lotus tetragonolobus	αLFuc>αDGal>αGalNac	4

Adapted from Lis and Sharon (12); Goldstein and Hayes (7).

Lectin Receptors

Lectin-receptors on PMN and bacteria were proved semiquantitatively by use of the Taxonolectin[TM]-system (E. Y. Lab, San Mateo, U.S.A.) which enabled us to classify sugars on cell surfaces based on 14 lectins from different origin and different carbohydrate specificity. The lectins and their sugar specificities are outlined in Table 1. The system is based on the principle that a lectin, specifically corresponding to a sugar, is added to the cell suspension; the sugar residues are linked by the lectin and an agglutination reaction occurs (Figure 1).

Quantitative Determination of Lectins

Quantitative determination of lectins bound to the cells was carried out with a method first described by Connelly et al. (4) based on the fact that lectins can be inhibited by specific sugars. Chromatographically pure preparations of rhodamine conjugated lectins (E. -Y. -Lab., San Mateo, U.S.A.) were dissolved in p-buffer pH 7.4 and calibration curves covering concentrations from 25 µg to 250 µg/ml were recorded with a Perkin Elmer Fluorescence Spectrophotometer at excitation wavelength 555nm. Bacteria and PMN respectively were incubated with lectins in the absence and presence of the specific sugars. The difference between the lectin concentrations in the supernatant is the amount of lectin bound specifically. The lectin concentration of 100 µg/ml was chosen because this concentration is high enough to saturate all binding sites as our own preliminary examinations showed.

The amount of lectin molecules bound specifically to one bacterium or to one PMN was calculated by the following equation [adapted from (12)]:

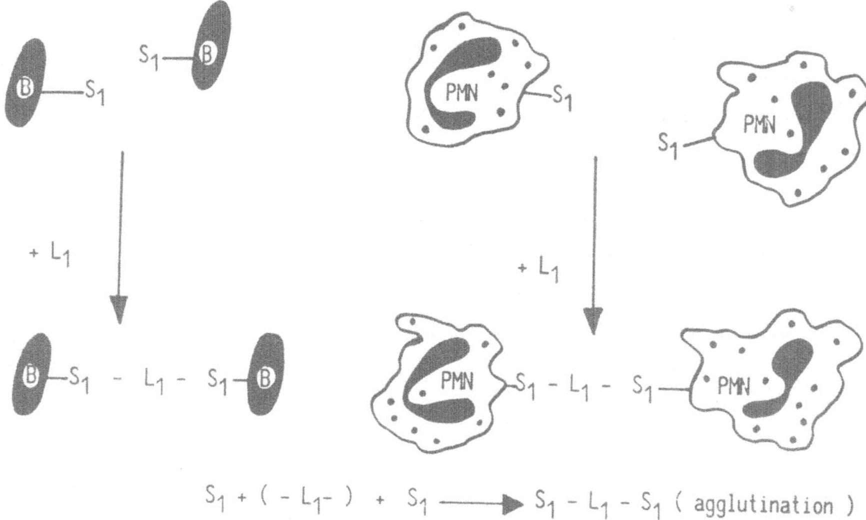

Figure 1. Identification of carbohydrates on cell surfaces with the Taxonolectin[TM] system. If lectin specific to a sugar on bacterial or PMN surface is added, an agglutination reaction occurs. S_1 = sugar residue 1; L_1 = lectin corresponding to S_1. 100 µl bacterial suspension containing 10^9 cfu/ml from logarithmic phase - respectively 100 µl PMN suspension (10^7 cells/ml) is filled into the wells precoated with 100 µg lectin. After 20 min. incubation time at 37°C the panels were rotated slightly by hand and the agglutination reaction is noted on a score card.

$$L_B = \frac{(r_1 - r_2) \times 6.02 \times 10^{23} - 10^{-3}}{nc \times mw}$$

Thereby, mw = molecular weight of the lectin; n_c = number of cells; (r_1 - r_2) = difference of lectin concentration in the presence and the absence of specific sugar, respectively;

$\frac{1}{mw} \times 10^{-3} = 1$ µg/ml.

Phagocytic Assay

Equal volumes (each 1.25 ml) of untreated or specific sugar pretreated bacteria (100 µg/ml, 10 min., 37°C) are added to equal volumes of PMN (ratio bacteria: PMN = 10:1; = 2×10^7 cfu/ml bacteria: 2×10^6 cells/ml PMN). Immediately following and after 15 min incubation at 37°C a sample was taken from the supernatant for determination of viable counts by serial dilution and plating out onto DST agar. For determination of total viable counts of the engulfed bacteria, PMN were lysed with ice cold distilled water following serial dilution as described above (15).

RESULTS

Semiquantitative determination of lectin reacting sites on bacteria and PMN with the Taxonolectin™-system showed different agglutination patterns, especially in case of the lectins DBA, TKA and GS II (Table 2).

Quantitative evaluation of lectins bound to the surfaces of bacteria and PMN expressed as mole lectins/cell is outlined in Table 3. It became obvious that on strain 319014 S DBA is the predominantly bound lectin. In case of strain 319014 R, it is GS II; on the PMN's TKA is bound at the highest amount. Hence the following sequence of bound lectins results: 319014 S, DBA>PNA; 319014 R, GS II>DBA>TKA>PNA; PMN, TKA>PNA>WGA. The results indicate that DGalNac is the widespread sugar on the surface of 319014 S,

Table 2. Agglutination Pattern Carried Out with the Taxonolectin™-System

	PMN	319014 S	319014 R
Con A	-	-	(-)
TKA	++	(+)	+++
PNA	+	+	++
DBA	(+)	+++	++
STA	-	-	+
LFA	-	-	-
UEA I	+	-	+
LCH	+	-	-
GS I	-	-	-
SBA	(+)	-	-
GS II	-	-	+++
WGA	+	-	-
PHA-L	-	-	-
Lotus	-	-	-

Table 3. Mole Lectins Bound Per Cell

	319014 S	319014 R	PMN
PNA	1.9×10^{9}	0.5×10^{9}	1.9×10^{12}
DBA	1.2×10^{10}	0.9×10^{10}	0.5×10^{11}
WGA	Ø	Ø	1.1×10^{12}
STA	3×10^{7}	1.3×10^{9}	Ø
GS II	Ø	1.1×10^{9}	Ø
SBA	0.3×10^{7}	Ø	0.7×10^{12}
UEA	Ø	2.2×10^{9}	2.8×10^{11}
CON A	Ø	0.3×10^{8}	6.1×10^{11}
TKA	Ø	2.3×10^{9}	1.0×10^{13}

on 319014 R it is DGlucNac in terminal position and on PMNs plasma membrane it is DGal.

Indirect evidence of lectins on bacterial outer envelope is given by blocking corresponding lectins which may be responsible for the attachment of PMN according to the scheme outlined in Figure 2. Comparing the phagocytic uptake of the bacteria by the granulocytes with and without preincubating them with PMN lectin specific sugars shows the results summarized in Table 4. It became obvious that the two isogenic strains differ in their surface carbohydrate and sugar residues patterns and their lectin distribution as well. It is of note that specific sugars and corresponding lectins are not localized on the same strain--otherwise the strain would agglutinate itself--and that attachment to PMNs only depends on bacterial lectins, not on sugar residues.

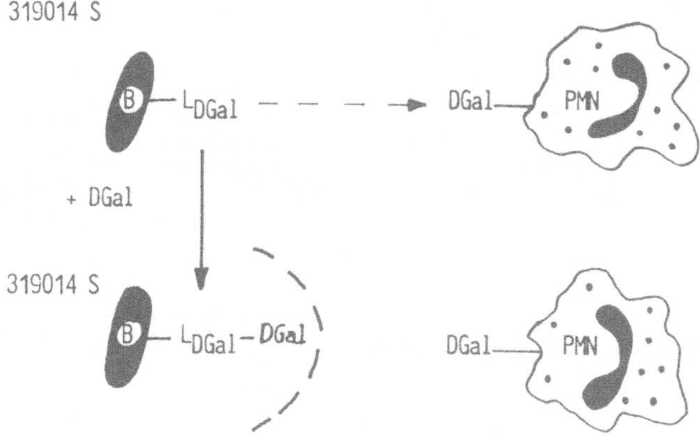

Figure 2. Examples of indirect evidence of lectins on bacterial surface. Strain 319014 S (n DGal on surface) was pretreated with DGal (0.5 m, 10 min), washed twice and then added to the PMNs (DGal on their surfaces). The decrease in phagocytic uptake of about 50% (see Tables 5 and 6) in comparison to the native strain indicates that the strain possesses DGal specific lectins on its surface which were blocked by the pretreatment so that binding to the PMNs was prevented.

Table 4. Effect of Pretreating Bacteria with Sugars Specific to PMN Lectins on Engulfment

	Engulfed bacteria after 15 min.	Intracellular killed bacteria in % of the engulfed
PMN + 319014 S	40	87
+ (319014 S + DGal)	20	81
+ (319014 S + DGalNac)	41.5	86
+ (319014 S + DGluc)	42	93
+ (319014 S + DGlucNac)	6.2	94
+ (319014 S + LFuc)	4	40
+ (319014 S + DMan)	1.5	60
PMN + 319014 R	44	96
+ (319014 R + DGal)	48	98
+ (319014 R + DGalNac)	44	96
+ (319014 R + DGluc)	41	96
+ (319014 R + DGlucNac)	12.8	35
+ (319014 R + LFuc)	48	85
+ (319014 R + DMan)	1.2	68

Engulfed bacteria were calculated as the difference in bacterial counts in the supernatant after 15 min. incubation at 37°C. Intracellular killed bacteria in % of the engulfed are those bacteria viable after lysis of the PMNs.

DISCUSSION

The aim of our investigation was to determine the role of lectins and lectin receptors on bacterial surfaces in phagocytosis by human PMNs. Quantitation of sugar residues on cell surfaces with rhodamin-conjugated

Table 5. Importance of Bacterial Surface Sugar Residues and Lectins for Phagocytic Uptake

Strain	Surface sugar	Corresponding lectin	Attachment to PMN via	Percentual change in engulfment
319014 S	Ø	L_{DGal}	L_{DGal} - DGal	- 50%
	DGalNac	Ø	Ø	no change
	Ø	$L_{DGlucNac}$	$L_{DGlucNac}$ - DGlucNac	- 94%
	Ø	L_{LFuc}	L_{LFuc} - LFuc	- 90%
	Ø	L_{DMan}	L_{DMan} - DMan	- 97%
319014 R	DGal	Ø	Ø	no change
	DGalNac	Ø	Ø	no change
	Ø	$L_{DGlucNac}$	$L_{DGlucNac}$ - DGlucNac	- 71%
	LFuc	Ø	Ø	no change
	Ø	L_{DMan}	L_{DMan} - DMan	- 97%

lectins is possible with the method described by Connelly (4), but there were no methods until now to determine cell-bound lectins quantitatively. Therefore we determined their importance in phagocytosis by blocking them. But we have to consider that lectin binding is affected by many variables, e.g., lectin concentration, number of binding sites, pH and temperature. Scatchard equation experiments to determine the association constants between lectin and receptor sites were not done, because preliminary experiments showed that the concentration of 100 μg/ml was high enough to saturate all binding sites.

As the results mentioned above only the lectins on the surfaces of the particles are important for phagocytosis. This fact corresponds to the investigations done by Rottini (14), who showed that D mannose precoated latex particles in comparison to untreated particles induce no change in ingestion rate by PMN. A further point of discussion is the different pattern of lectin and sugar distribution on the isogenic strains and their different engulfment by the PMN. It may be speculated that change in genetic composition results in different composition of cell wall architecture causing a different rate of phagocytic uptake. Investigations done by Costerton (5), Kenward et al. (11), who showed that acquisition of a plasmid has influence on cell wall composition, point in this direction. Further investigations supporting this assumption are still lacking.

SUMMARY

Two isogenic Pseudomonas aeruginosa strains isolated from clinically proven infection, which only differ in one criterion--the amount of chromosomally mediated β-lactamase production--were investigated in view of their engulfment by human PMNs. It was assumed that differences in phagocytosis are based on different cell wall compositions. To verify this assumption lectin receptors on bacteria and on PMNs were determined directly and the presence or absence of lectins was proven indirectly by blocking them with specific sugar residues. The results obtained showed that attachment of bacteria to PMN does depend only on the lectins, not on the sugars on their surface, and that there are significant differences in carbohydrate and lectin distribution on the strains tested. The resistant strain possesses a lesser amount of lectins on its surface; therefore, its rate of phagocytosis is less effective.

REFERENCES

1. Z. Bar-Shavit, J. Ofek and R. Goldman, Mannose residues on phagocytes as receptors for the attachment of Escherichia coli and Salmonella typhi, Biochem. Biophys. Res. Commun. 78:455 (1977).
2. A. Bøyum, Separation of leukocytes from blood and bone marrow, Scand. J. Clin. Invest. 21(Suppl. 97) (1968).
3. W. A. Collier and J. C. de Miranda, Bakterienhamagglutination I. Versuche mit einem hamagglutinierenden Stamm von E. coli, Antonie von Leeuwenhoek, J. Microbiol. Serol. 21:133 (1955).
4. M. C. Connelly, D. C. Stein, F. E. Young, S. A. More, and P. Z. Allen, Interaction with lectins and differential wheat germ agglutinin binding of pyocin 103 sensitive and resistant Neisseria gonorrhoeae, J. Bacteriol. 148:796 (1981).
5. J. W. Costerton, Pseudomonas aeruginosa in nature and disease, in: "Pseudomonas aeruginosa," C. D. Sabath, ed., Huber, Bern. (1979).
6. R. Goldman and Z. Bar-Shavit, Phagocytosis - modes of particle recognition and stimulation by natural peptides, in:

"Phagocytosis-Past and Future," L. Karnovsky and L. Bolis, eds., Academic Press, New York, London (1982).

7. I. J. Goldstein and C. E. Hayes, The lectins: carbohydrate-binding proteins of plants and animals, in: "Advances in Carbohydrate Chemistry and Biochemistry," R. S. Tipson and D. Horton, eds., Academic Press, New York, San Francisco, London (1978).
8. F. M. Griffin, Mononuclear cell phagocytic mechanisms and host defense, in: "Advances in Host Defense Mechanisms," J. I. Gallin and A. S. Fauci, eds., Raven Press, New York (1982).
9. D. A. Hart, Lectins in biological systems: applications to microbiology, Am. J. Clin. Nutr. 33:2416 (1980).
10. K. Jann, B. Jann, G. Schmidt and K. Vosbeck, Adhesion of Escherichia coli mammalian and yeast cells: role of piliation and hydrophobicity, Infect. Immun. 32:484 (1981).
11. M. A. Kenward, R. W. Brown, S. R. Hesslewood and C. Dillon, Influence of R - plasmid RP_1 of Pseudomonas aeruginosa on cell wall composition, drug resistance and sensitivity to cold shock, Antimicrob. Agents Chemother. 13:446 (1978).
12. H. Lis and N. Sharon, Lectins: Their chemistry and application in immunology, in: "The Antigens," M. Sela, ed., Academic Press, New York (1977).
13. I. Ofek, D. Mirelman and N. Sharon, Adherence of Escherichia coli to human mucosal cells mediated by mannose receptors, Nature (London) 265:623 (1977).
14. G. Rottini, F. Cian, M. R. Sorenzo, R. Albrigo and P. Patriarca, Evidence for the involvement of human polymorphonuclear leucocyte mannose-like receptors in the phagocytosis of Escherichia coli, FEBS Letters 105:307 (1979).
15. G. Stubner and A. Dalhoff, Effect of subinhibitory β-lactam concentrations on intracellular killing of Ps.aeruginosa by human polymorphonuclear granulocytes, 13th International Congress for Chemotherapy, Vienna, Abstract SE 3.2./1-4 (1983).
16. G. Stubner and R. Marre, Use of lectins to characterize surface alterations of β-lactam resistant mutants of Pseudomonas aeruginosa, Symposium: The Influence of Antibiotics on the Host-Parasite Relationship, Munich (1985).
17. G. Uhlenbruck, R. Gross, O. Koch et al., Die Bedeutung von Lektinen fur den Adhasionsmechanismus von Bakterien, Deutsches Arzteblatt 80:27 (1983).
18. D. M. Weir and H. Ogmundsdottir, Non-specific recognition mechanisms by mononuclear phagocytes, Clin. Exp. Immunol. 30:323 (1977).

THE EFFECT OF SUBINHIBITORY CONCENTRATIONS OF CLINDAMYCIN ON THE ADHERENCE AND GLYCOCALYX OF STAPHYLOCOCCUS AUREUS AND BACTEROIDES SPECIES IN VITRO AND IN VIVO

D. W. Lambe, Jr.[1], K. J. Mayberry-Carson[1], W. R. Mayberry[1], B. K. Tober-Meyer[2] and J. W. Costerton[3]

Department of Microbiology[1], Quillen-Dishner College of Medicine, and Division of Laboratory Animal Resources[2], East Tennessee State University, Johnson City, Tennessee
Department of Biology[3], University of Calgary, Calgary Alberta, Canada

INTRODUCTION

The adherence of bacteria to biologically inert surfaces may result in a tenacious and irreversible binding (14). In some systems, this irreversible binding involves the production of bacterial exopolysaccharides which are known also as glycocalyx, or slime. Since the glycocalyx condenses radically during dehydration in preparation for transmission electron microscopy, it has been an elusive structure to demonstrate on bacteria. However, specific antibodies were used by Bayer and Thurow (1) and Mackie et al. (10) to prevent the dehydration collapse of the glycocalyx. This technique gave a true appreciation of the extent of the glycocalyx produced by many genera and species of bacteria.

Glycocalyx production is extensive in bacteria growing in nature and in pathogenic situations. Many organisms may appear to lose the glycocalyx when serially transferred in vitro, but modern staining and stabilization methods have demonstrated extensive glycocalyces on cells of laboratory cultures of *Staphylococcus aureus* (2), group B *Streptococcus* (10), *Escherichia coli* (1), *Pseudomonas aeruginosa* (7), and *Bacteroides* species (8). Marrie and Costerton (12) showed that the glycocalyx of *S. aureus* is of pivotal importance in the adhesion of these cells to plastics. In our own work with osteomyelitis experimentally induced in the rabbit tibia with *S. aureus* (15), we demonstrated, by transmission electron microscopy (TEM), large amounts of glycocalyx produced by the staphylococci.

The effect of subinhibitory concentrations of antibiotics on adherence has been examined by many workers. For example, Vaisanen et al. (18) demonstrated that trimethoprim inhibited the formation of pili in *E. coli*, and Kristiansen et al. (6) showed that lincomycin inhibited the adhesion of *Neisseria meningitidis* by preventing pili formation. Gemmell et al. (5) reported that clindamycin reduced the capsular glycocalyx produced by *Bacteroides fragilis* and increased the susceptibility of *B. fragilis* to phagocytosis by human neutrophils.

Therefore, we developed an in vitro system to study the effect of sub-inhibitory concentrations of clindamycin on the adherence of S. aureus, Bacteroides species and E. coli to bone surface. We established an animal model of experimentally induced osteomyelitis in the rabbit tibia with either S. aureus, or a Bacteroides species and Staphylococcus epidermidis, and studied the effect of clindamycin therapy on osteomyelitis, and we examined human bone from a case of osteomyelitis by scanning electron microscopy (SEM) for the presence of glycocalyx produced by staphylococci and Bacteroides.

MATERIALS AND METHODS

Bacterial Strains

The following bacterial strains, which were isolated from clinical specimens, were used in the in vitro assay for studying bacterial adherence: S. aureus (strain G-24-82); S. epidermidis (G-30-82); Bacteroides thetaiotaomicron (strain 1660-75B); Bacteroides intermedius (strain 704-76A); Bacteroides bivius (strain 573-74A); and E. coli (strain G-25-82). The above strains of staphylococci and B. thetaiotaomicron were used to experimentally induce osteomyelitis in the rabbit tibia. The strains were cultured in brain heart infusion broth supplemented (BHIS) with 5 µg hemin (Sigma) and 0.5 µg/ml menadione (Sigma) at 35°C for 48 hrs.

Minimal Inhibitory Concentration (MIC) Determination

The MIC value of clindamycin hydrochloride (The Upjohn Co., Kalamazoo, Mich.) for all bacterial strains was determined by using the 2-3-7 antibiotic dilution method in BHIS broth; the antibiotic concentrations ranged from 0.0078 µg/ml to 256 µg/ml. The inoculum for the antibiotic dilutions was a BHIS broth culture of the test strain grown for 24 hrs at 35°C. The inoculum was adjusted to the turbidity of one-half of a no. 1 McFarland nephelometer standard. One ml of this inoculum was added to 9 ml of BHIS broth containing a certain concentration of clindamycin. The inoculated tubes were incubated at 35°C for 48 hrs. The MIC was recorded as the lowest concentration of clindamycin which completely inhibited the macroscopic growth of the organism. Since many anaerobes grow in BHIS broth but not in Mueller-Hinton broth, BHIS broth was used to compare the bacterial adherence of test strains to bone. The MIC's of clindamycin for the strains tested were: S. aureus, 0.25 µg/ml; S. epidermidis, 0.25 µg/ml; B. intermedius, 0.0039 µg/ml; B. thetaiotaomicron, 0.125 µg/ml; B. bivius, 0.0078 µg/ml; and E. coli, 256 µg/ml.

In Vitro System for Bacterial Adherence

Rabbit tibiae discs approximately 5 mm in thickness were cleaned and sterilized at 121°C for 30 min. Five discs were added to 9.9 ml of BHIS per tube with one of the following antibiotic concentrations: 0.1 MIC, 0.25 MIC, 0.5 MIC or 1.0 MIC of each strain. A control tube had no clindamycin. An inoculum of 0.1 ml of the test strain, containing approximately 1×10^7 cells, was added to each tube. The tubes were incubated at 37°C for 48 hrs. Then the bone discs were removed and processed for SEM (15). Quantitative plate counts of cells remaining in the broth were performed. Sedimented cells from the broth and cells scraped from the bone discs were processed for TEM (15).

Induction of Osteomyelitis in the Rabbit Tibia

Osteomyelitis was induced in the rabbit tibia as described previously (15). Briefly, a duct was drilled into the medullary cavity of the rabbit tibia with a sterile dentist's drill. 0.1 ml of a sclerosing agent, sodium morrhuate (Torigian Laboratories, Inc.), bacterial cells (10^6), 0.1 ml of sterile saline, and a 4.5 cm piece of sterile catheter were inserted into the medullary cavity. The drill hole was sealed with sterile bone wax and the incision was closed. The rabbits were observed for weight loss, swelling at the injection site and discomfort. The tibiae, were examined periodically by roentgenography and graded visually.

Samples of infected bone marrow, bone scrapings and catheter were cultured for bacteria and examined by three procedures: SEM, TEM, and the indirect fluorescent antibody (IFA) technique (8). Hematoxylin and eosin-stained sections of bone were examined for histopathological lesions.

Treatment of Experimental Osteomyelitis with Clindamycin Phosphate and Examination of Specimens

After rabbits developed acute osteomyelitis, within three to four weeks after injection of the test organisms, they were treated with clindamycin phosphate (The Upjohn Co.) for one, two or three weeks. Clindamycin phosphate injectable solution was injected subcutaneously into the scruff of the neck three times a day. The dosage of clindamycin for each rabbit was 280 mg/kg/day. Control groups were not treated with antibiotic. The tibiae were harvested from each animal after the treatment period. Bone tissue and bone marrow samples were processed as described above.

RESULTS

Demonstration of Glycocalyx

The staphylococci (*S. aureus*; *S. epidermidis*) and the *Bacteroides* species (*B. intermedius*; *B. thetaiotaomicron*) used in these studies produced large amounts of glycocalyx as demonstrated by TEM and the indirect FA procedure (8,15). In addition, test strains of *S. epidermidis*, *B. bivius*, and *E. coli* examined by the in vitro procedures produced large amounts of glycocalyx. Although these strains had been transferred in culture innumerable times, all of these species produced an observable glycocalyx which was fully retained as an integral capsule, as well as slime which surrounded a cell or a microcolony or was detached from cells as peripheral slime.

Effect of Subinhibitory Concentrations of Clindamycin on Bacterial Adherence to Bone Surface In Vitro

In the absence of clindamycin, bone surfaces exposed to *S. aureus* for 48 hrs were heavily colonized with *S. aureus* cells which formed large aggregates of microcolonies on the bone surface (Figure 1a). When the dehydrative collapse of the glycocalyx was prevented by stabilization with homologous antibodies to *S. aureus*, TEM of the staphylococcal cells on the colonized bone surface showed gram-positive cell walls (2) enmeshed in a very extensive and continuous matrix of exopolysaccharide glycocalyx (Figure 1b) which stained with ruthenium red. A concentration of 0.1 MIC of clindamycin (0.025 μg/ml) in the medium had no discernible effect on bacterial growth (5.9×10^8 cells/ml), but it reduced colonization of the bone by approximately 80% relative to the control system (Figure 1c). Bacterial cells within microcolonies were surrounded by glycocalyx which had been condensed into fibrous strands due to dehydration. TEM of antibody-stabilized material from the bone scraping showed a reduction in the amount of glycocalyx at the cell surfaces and in the intercellular spaces. In the presence of 0.25 MIC (0.0625 μg/ml) of clindamycin, the extent of exopolysaccharide was sharply diminished as was the amount of adhesion to bone surface. The presence of 0.5 MIC (0.125 μg/ml) and 1.0 MIC (0.25 μg/ml) suppressed growth in BHIS broth, but these concentrations of clindamycin totally inhibited adhesion of the staphylococci to the bone surface. TEM showed a further diminution of the exopolysaccharide glycocalyx produced by the cocci. In the presence of 1.0 MIC of clindamycin the external bone surface appears the same as

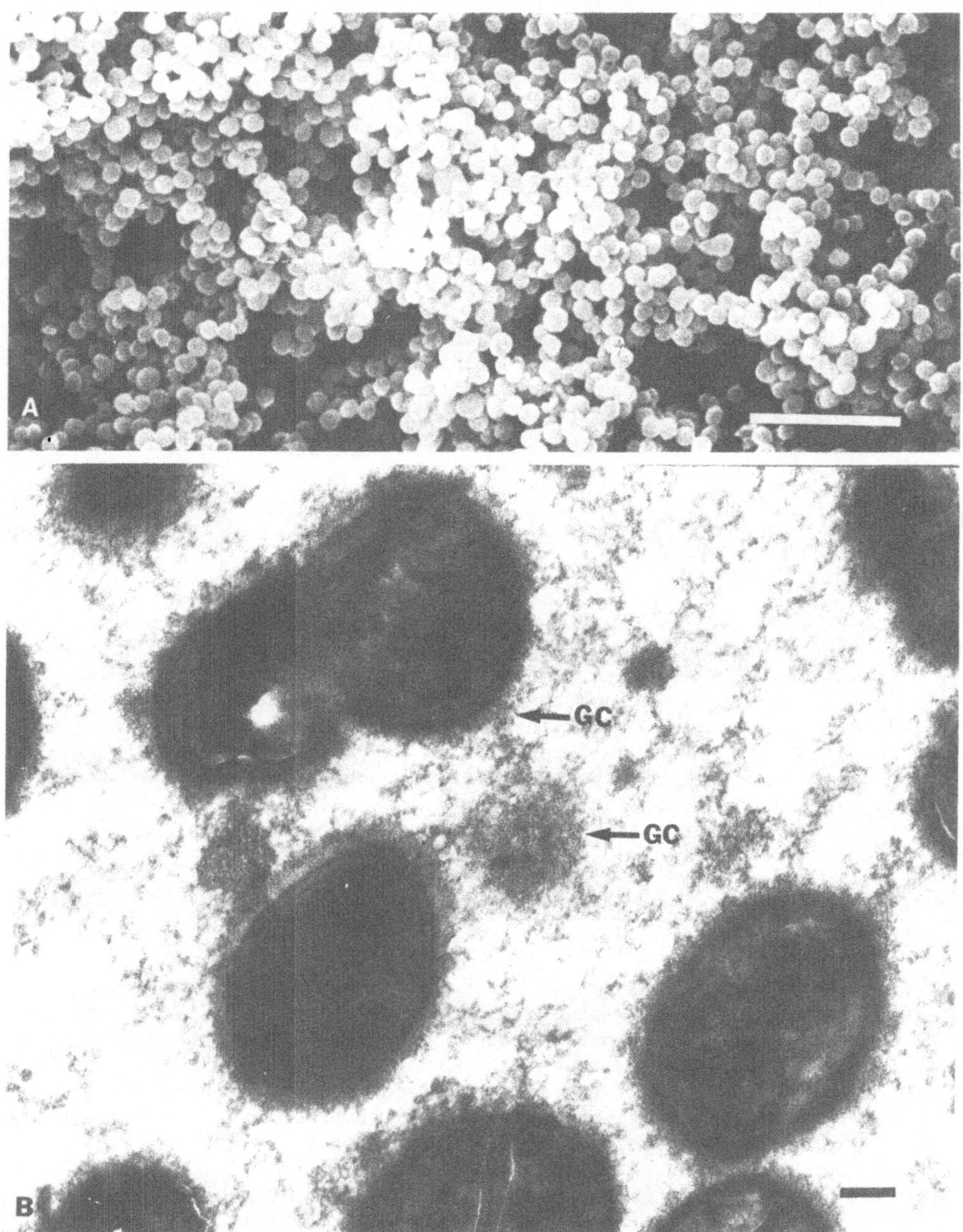

Figure 1. In vitro colonization of rabbit bone by Staphylococcus aureus at 48 hrs. (A) In absence of clindamycin, large aggregates of microcolonies formed on the bone surface. Bar = 5 μm; (B) TEM of material scraped from bone surface stabilized with S. aureus antiserum and stained with ruthenium red. Gram-positive cocci were surrounded by extensive glycocalyx (arrows GC). Bar = 5 μm

control bone as shown in Figure 1d. The haversian canals were visible and bacterial masses were absent.

The same series of in vitro experiments as described above for S. aureus were performed for B. intermedius, B. thetaiotaomicron and B. bivius. The

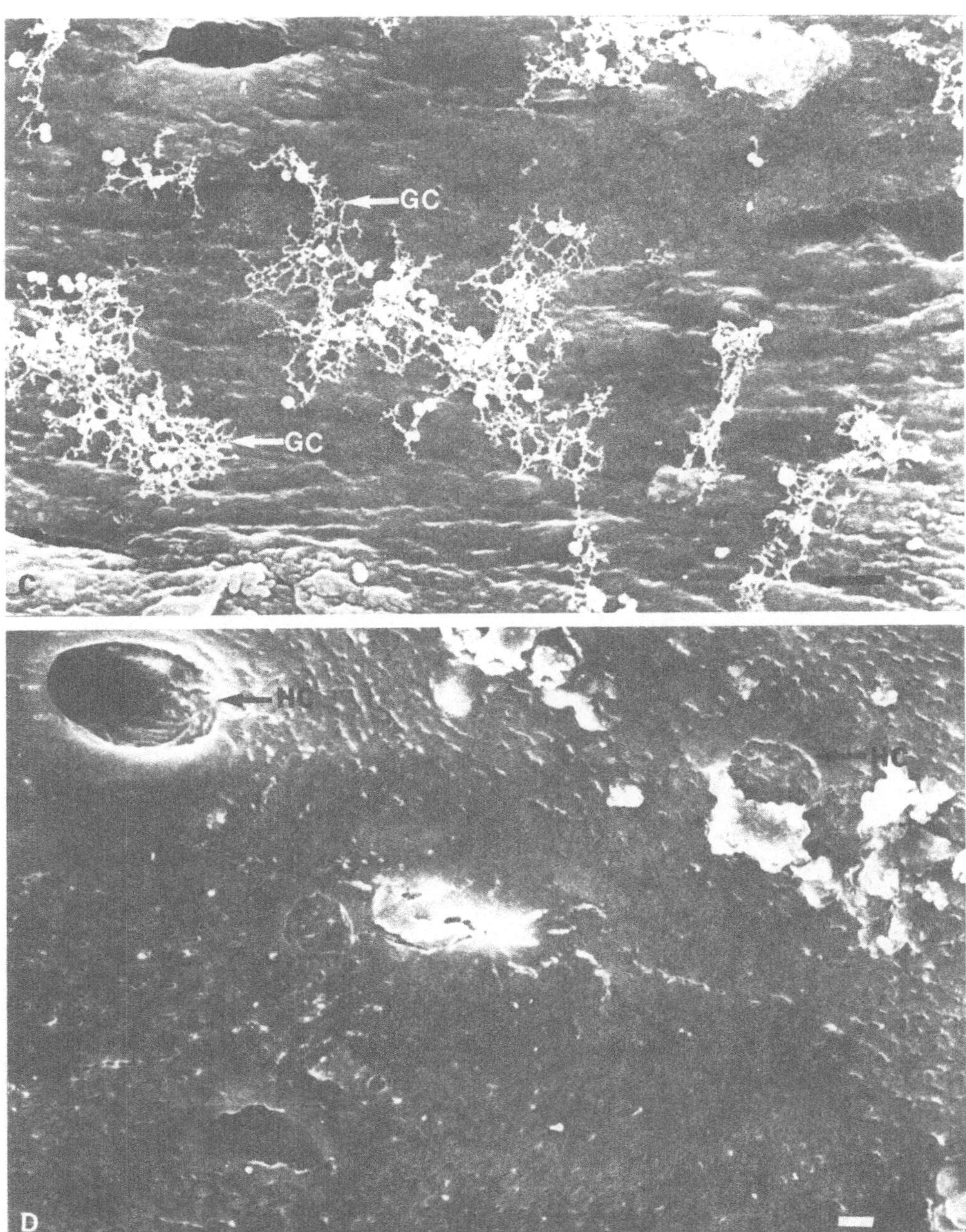

Figure 1. (C) 0.1 MIC (0.0025 μg/ml) of clindamycin decreased bacterial adherence 80% as shown by SEM. Condensed glycocalyx strands (arrows GS) appeared to attach cells to bone. Bar = 5 μm; (D) SEM of the smooth external surface of a bone disc exposed to uninoculated BHIS broth for 48 hr. Haversian canals (arrows HC) were visible. Bar = 5 μm.

results for *B. intermedius* were typical of all three species, thus, *B. intermedius* illustrations will serve as an example. In the absence of clindamycin or in the presence of 0.1 MIC (0.00039 μg/ml), *B. intermedius* cells colonized the bone surface heavily (Figure 2a). In the absence of clindamycin and in the presence of 0.1 MIC of clindamycin the bacterial count was approximately 10^8 cells/ml. Multiple condensed strands of glycocalyx were wrapped around

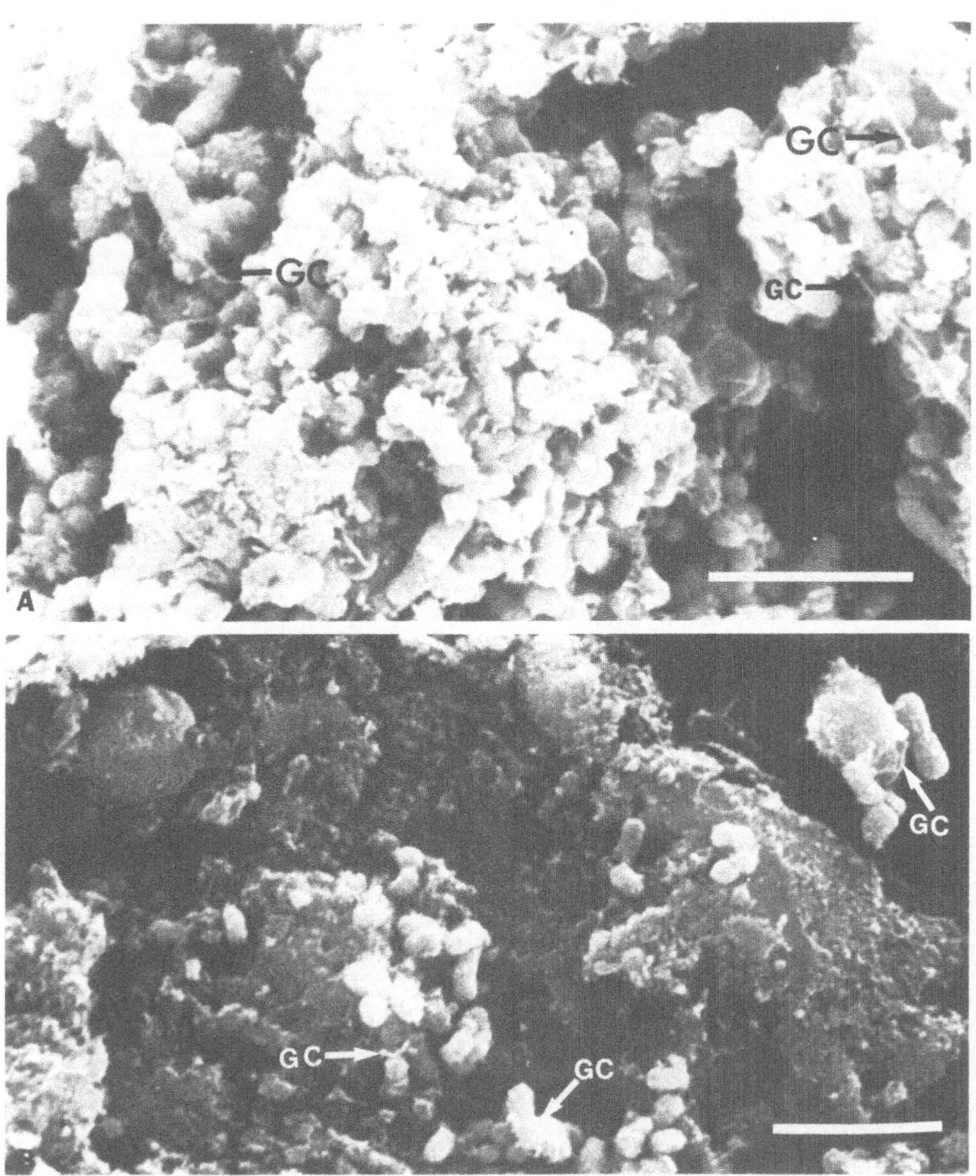

Figure 2. In vitro colonization of rabbit bone by *Bacteroides intermedius* at 48 hr. (A) In the absence or presence of 0.1 MIC (0.00039 μg/ml) of clindamycin, large aggreates of bacilli adhered to one another and to bone surface. Condensed strands of glycocalyx (arrows GC) were evident. Bar = 5 μm; (B) 0.25 MIC (0.00097 μg/ml) of clindamycin significantly decreased colonization of bacilli to bone. Condensed strands of glycocalyx (arrow GC) attached to bacilli were still visible. Bar = 5 μm.

the bacterial cells. Bacilli, coccobacilli, and coccoid forms--all typical of B. intermedius cell morphology--were present. In the presence of 0.25 MIC (0.0097 μg/ml) of clindamycin, colonization decreased from heavy to moderate (Figure 2b). 0.5 MIC (0.00195 μg/ml) of clindamycin further decreased colonization of the bacilli from moderate to light, only occasionally

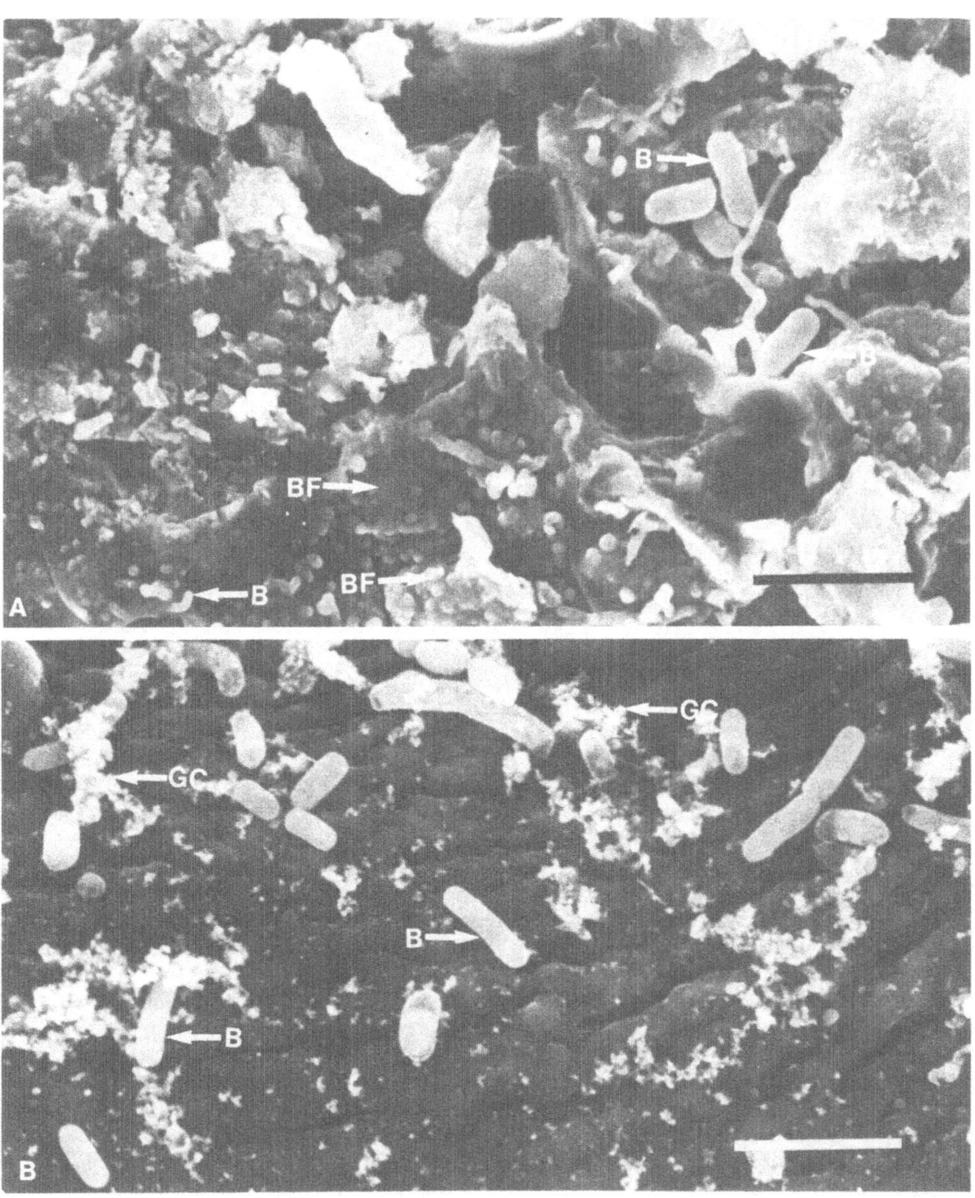

Figure 3. Adherence of Escherichia coli to rabbit bone surface in vitro at 48 hr. (A) In the absence of or in the presence of 0.1 MIC (25.6 μg/ml) of clindamycin, most bone surface was coated with a thick biofilm (arrow BF) with bacilli (arrows B) protruding through the biofilm. A few large bacilli (arrows B) were seen on top of the biofilm. Bar = 5 μm; (B) 0.25 MIC (64 μg/ml) of clindamycin decreased adherence to sparse colonization. Bacilli (arrows B) and some glycocalyx (arrows GC) were visible. Bar = 5 μm.

organisms adhered to the bone. Condensed strands of glycocalyx attached to the bacteria and the bone surface were clearly visible. In the presence of 1.0 MIC (0.0039 μg/ml) of clindamycin, there was no colonization of the bone by B. intermedius although the viable count was approximately 10^3 organisms/ml BHIS broth. Similar results were obtained with B. thetaiotaomicron and B. bivius.

A clindamycin-resistant strain of E. coli was cultured in varying concentrations of clindamycin. In the absence of clindamycin or in the presence of 0.1 MIC of clindamycin (25.6 μg/ml), most of the bone surface was heavily colonized (Figure 3a). In the heavily colonized area a biofilm covered the bone surface with bacilli protruding through the biofilm. In other areas of slightly less colonization, individual bacilli were more easily discernible. In the presence of 0.25 MIC (64 μg/ml), the adherence decreased significantly so that only a few bacilli and scant glycocalyx were present on the bone surface (Figure 3b). At 0.5 MIC (128 μg/ml) of clindamycin there was sparse colonization of the bone. There was no adherence of E. coli cells to the bone in the presence of 1.0 MIC (256 μg/ml) of clindamycin.

Clindamycin Treatment of Rabbits with S. aureus Induced Osteomyelitis

Infected, untreated control animals were sacrificed at intervals of two, three, five and six weeks after infection. After three to four weeks, 80% of the animals developed radiological changes consistent with osteomyelitis. S. aureus was cultured from the bone marrow, and bone scrapings from the infected tibia of these animals. Histological examination was compatible with acute osteomyelitis. SEM of these bones showed extensive coverage of the bone surface with an exopolysaccharide matrix filled with masses of coccoid profiles (Figure 4a). TEM revealed microcolonies of gram-positive cocci enclosed in large amounts of ruthenium red-stained glycocalyx.

After induction of acute osteomyelitis with S. aureus in the rabbits, clindamycin was used to treat the infected animals for one, two or three week periods. At the end of one week of treatment with clindamycin, SEM of samples of infected bone tissue revealed masses of coccoid profiles embedded in a thick matrix of condensed exopolysaccharide material that covered the bone tissue. TEM showed Gram-positive cocci surrounded by ruthenium red-stained extracellular fibrillar material. Radiology, appearance at necropsy and histological samples of animals treated for one week were consistent with a diagnosis of osteomyelitis. Recovery of S. aureus from all microbiological samples from these animals paralleled the electron microscopic results.

After two weeks of treatment with clindamycin, SEM of samples of bone tissue taken at necropsy revealed very few coccoid profiles in exopolysaccharide adhering to the bone and marrow. Bacterial cells were so reduced in number after two weeks of clindamycin treatment that TEM was not useful. Radiological results did not change significantly in the two week clindamycin-treated animals; however, the clinical appearance of the bone at necropsy was more normal and there was definite evidence of bone repair in these animals. No bacteria were cultured from any of the sampling sites and Gram stains of the samples were negative.

After three weeks of clindamycin therapy, SEM of tissue samples showed very few coccoid profiles, as was seen with the animals treated for two weeks. Bone chips showed only slight remnants of a biofilm (Figure 4b). Radiological results did change somewhat, showing a decrease in severity of the disease in the animals treated with clindamycin for three weeks. The clinical appearance of the tibiae at necropsy was almost normal with evidence of bone repair. A few gram-positive cocci were seen in the gram stains of only two marrow samples and one bone scraping sample. However, microbiological culture results were negative. Histological examination of tissues was negative for osteomyelitis.

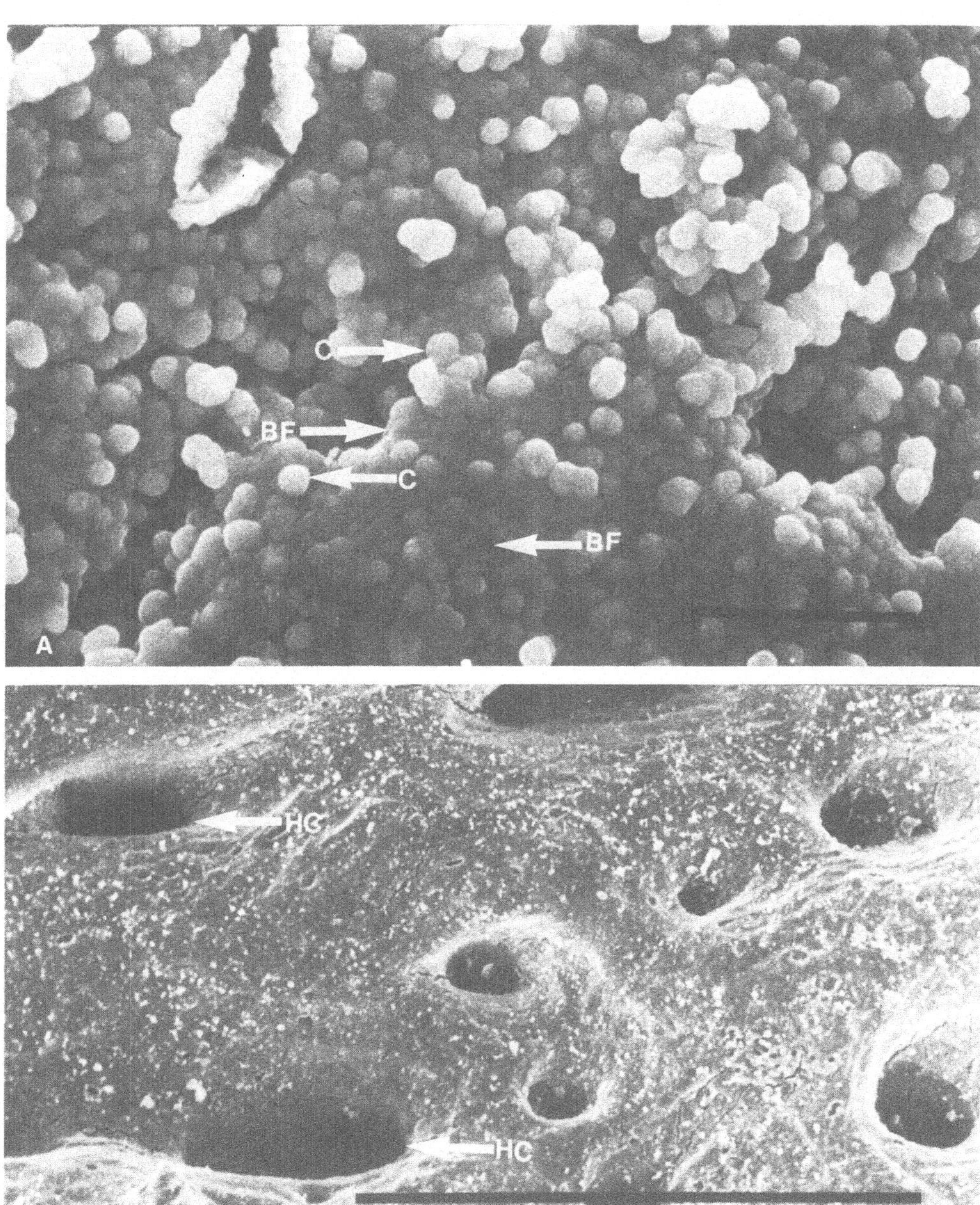

Figure 4. SEM of infected rabbit tibia with and without clindamycin treatment. (A) Bone surface showed coddoid profiles (arrows C) buried in a confluent biofilm (arrows BF) of glycocalyx typical of untreated animals and animals treated for one week with clindamycin. Bar = 5μm; (B) after three weeks of clindamycin treatment bone surfaces showed only slight remnants of a biofilm. The haversian canals (arrows HC) were visible again. Bar = 500 μm.

Bacterial Adherence and Glycocalyx Production in Human Osteomyelitis

Several bones from human patients with osteomyelitis were examined in our laboratory with SEM, TEM and the indirect FA technique. A 69 year old

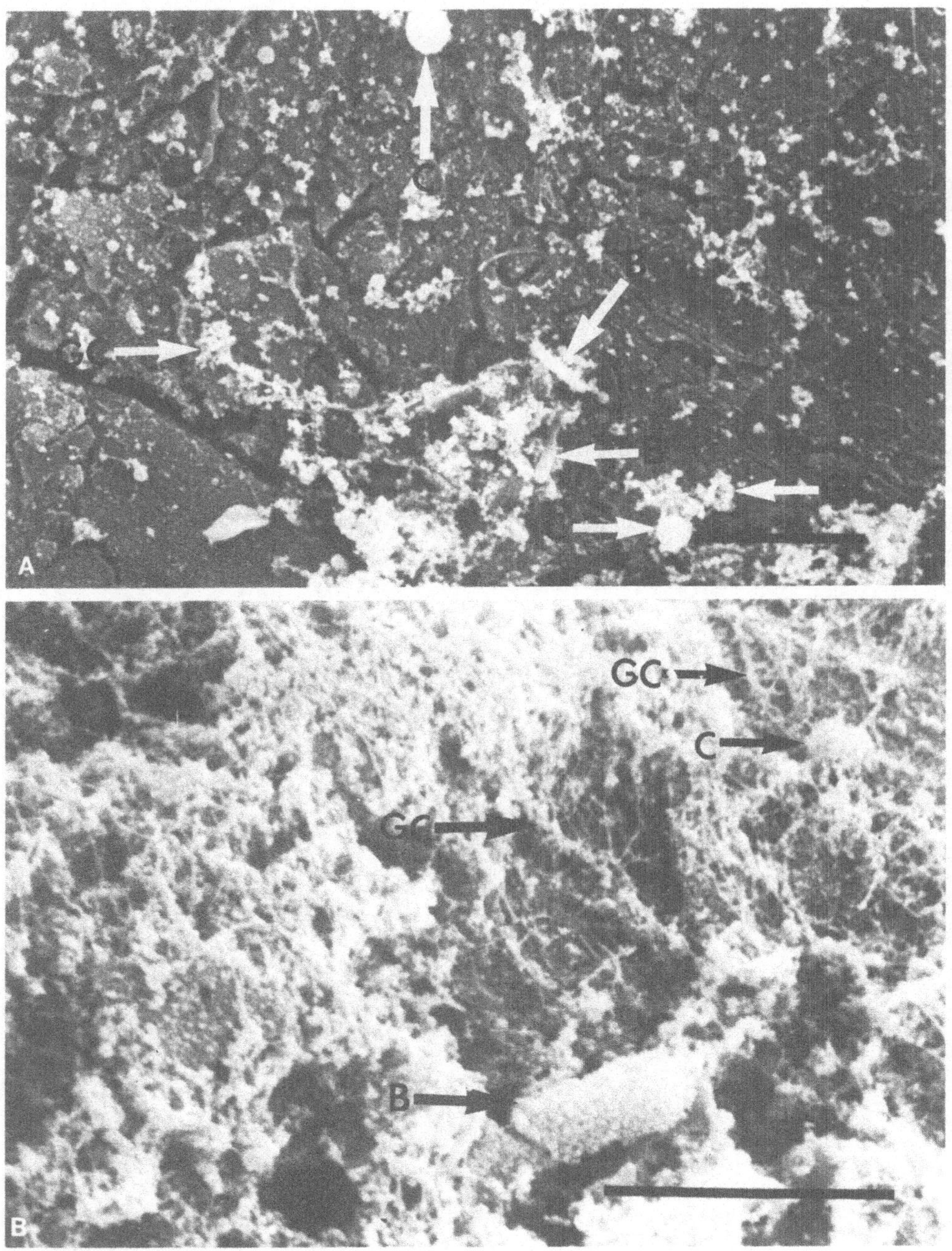

Figure 5. SEM of bone chips from a patient with osteomyelitis. (A) Bacilli (arrows B), cocci (arrows C) and glycocalyx (arrows GC) were visible. Bar = 5 μm; (B) A bacillus (arrow B), cocci (arrows C), and tangled masses of glycocalyx fibers (arrows GC) attached to the bone surface. Bar = 5 μm.

diabetic, male with a foot ulcer developed osteomyelitis in the toe which was amputated; this case will illustrate the glycocalyx in human osteomyelitis.

The hospital clinical laboratory cultured beta-hemolytic *Streptococcus* and *Staphylococcus* from a pre-surgical specimen. When the toe was removed, a portion of the bone cultured in the hospital laboratory was negative for aerobes and anaerobes. Another portion of the bone was placed in a sterile Petri plate in an anaerobe jar. The bone was in the anaerobe chamber in our laboratory within 20 minutes after it was removed from the patient. The aerobe culture was negative, but the anaerobe culture yielded: *B. fragilis*, *Bacteroides asaccharolyticus*, *Peptostreptococcus anaerobius*, *Peptostreptococcus magnus*, and *Propionibacterium acnes*.

The gram stain of the infected bone tissue in our laboratory showed: gram-negative bacilli morphologically compatible with *B. fragilis* and *B. asaccharolyticus*. The large capsules of bacilli were very evident in the gram stain. Some of the gram-positive cocci had a diameter of about 1 to 2 microns which is compatible with the size of *P. anaerobius*; other cocci were approximately 5 microns in diameter which is compatible with the size of *P. magnus*. The cocci had capsules that were smaller than those of the gram-negative rods.

SEM of the bone surface showed bacilli and cocci with glycocalyx linking the organisms and the bone surface (Figure 5a). An enlargement of another bone surface showed a bacillus covered with accretions of exopolysaccharides and cocci. Tangled masses of condensed glycocalyx strands covered large areas of the bone surface (Figure 5b). On another area of bone surface, a clump of large and small cocci was attached to the bone surface by strands of glycocalyx (Figure 6a). In Figure 6b the large cocci of 1.8 to 5 μm in diameter were compatible with the size of *P. magnus*, and the smaller cocci with a diameter of approximately 0.8 to 1 μm in diameter were of a size compatible with *P. anaerobius*. The bacilli and cocci embedded in large amounts of glycocalyx seen in this piece of infected bone from a patient with osteomyelitis were similar to the biofilm demonstrated on the bone surfaces of rabbit tibiae experimentally infected in our laboratory with *Bacteroides* and staphylococci (unpublished results).

DISCUSSION

Various aerobic bacteria, including staphylococci and *P. aeruginosa*, are frequently cultured form human osteomyelitis specimens, although the isolation of anaerobic bacteria vary from 5% to 39% depending on the study. However, when proper anaerobe culture techniques are used, and when anaerobe plate cultures are incubated for seven to 10 days, anaerobes are more frequently isolated from osteomyelitis specimens. The anaerobes may play a more important role in osteomyelitis than known previously.

The glycocalyx is a universal structure of bacteria which we have demonstrated on all strains of anaerobic bacteria examined (8). The glycocalyx consists of a capsule and exopolysaccharides, or slime, which may be attached to the bacterial cell, or detached into the surrounding milieu. Cells of both *S. aureus* (11) and *S. epidermidis* (3) produce glycocalyx. Glycocalyx-enclosed microcolonies are formed on smooth, and irregular, surfaces (9); the microcolonies may develop into solid biofilms (11,12,13).

Chronic osteomyelitis is noted for its resistance to both medical and surgical forms of treatment. Information regarding host resistance and bacterial virulence factors which permit the initiation and persistence of human osteomyelitis is lacking. Therefore, therapy is often based on anecdotal experience or uncontrolled clinical studies.

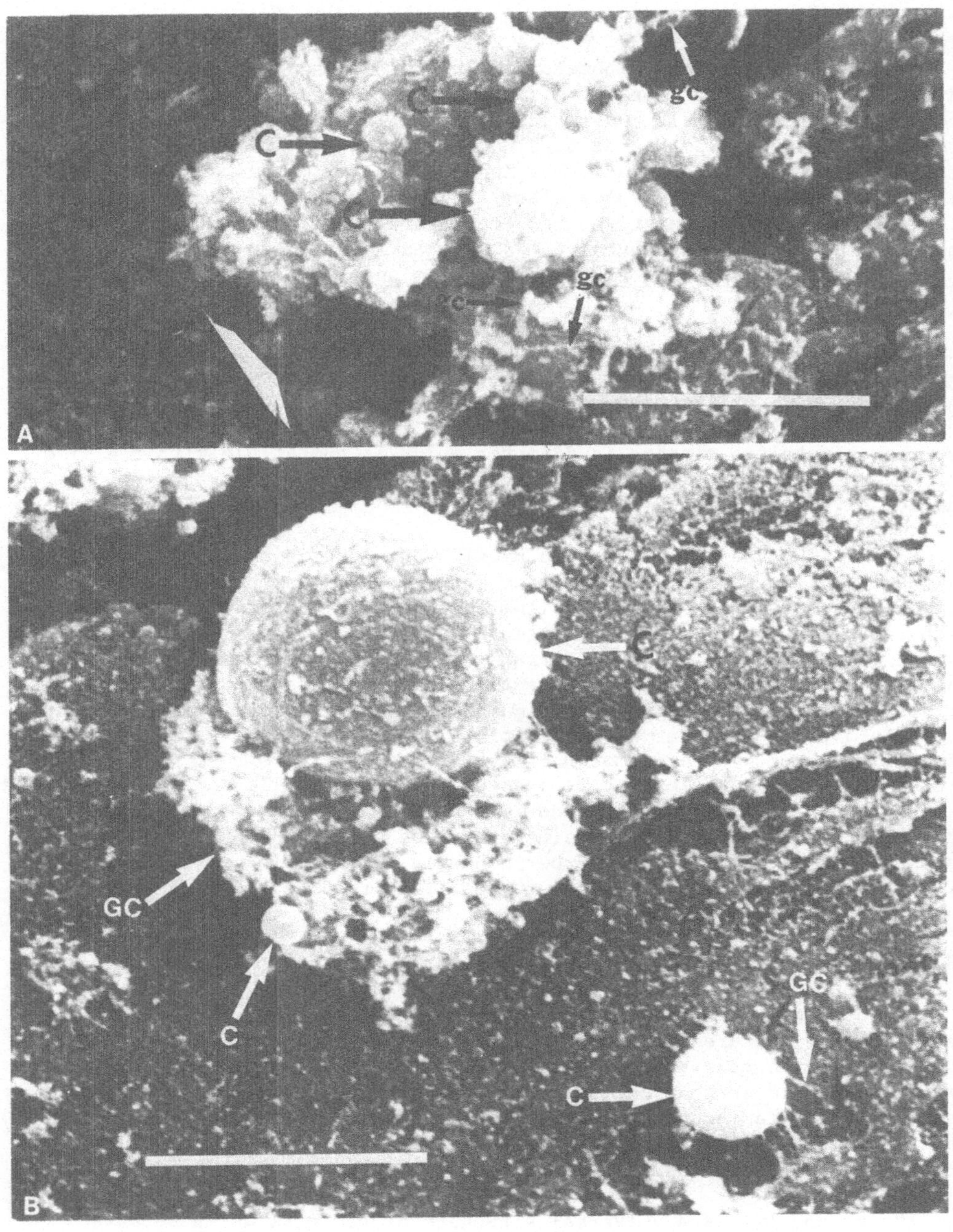

Figure 6. SEM of bone surface from a patient with osteomyelitis. (A) A clump of small and large cocci (arrows C) was present and glycocalyx strands (arrows GC) attached cocci to bone surface. Bar = 5 µm; (B) An SEM enlargement showed cocci 1.8 to 5 µm in diameter, the size of P. magnus; and cocci 0.8 to 1 µm in diameter, the size of P. anaerobius. Glycocalyx strands (arrows GC) connected cocci to (arrows C) bone surface. Bar = 5 µm.

To determine if glycocalyx was present in osteomyelitis, we induced S. aureus osteomyelitis in the rabbit tibia and inserted a catheter which served as a foreign body. SEM and TEM showed gram-positive cocci surrounded by glycocalyx. Glycocalyx detached from the bacterial cells and adhered to structures in the bone marrow and to bone surface. With such large masses of staphylococci encased in copious quantities of glycocalyx, it becomes more obvious why osteomyelitis is recalcitrant to treatment. Similar microcolony formation occurs with P. aeruginosa in patients with cystic fibrosis (7). Some antibiotics may not penetrate the glycocalyx (4), phagocytosis by neutrophils would be inhibited by large microcolonies of staphylococci, and antibody action would be impeded. Other workers proposed that the glycocalyces of S. aureus serve a protective mechanism for the bacterial cells (2). Glycocalyx interferes with phagocytosis by masking peptidoglycan (16,17), envelops teichoic acid which enhances opsonization (19), and consumes complement (20).

In our rabbit model of osteomyelitis, the normal bone surface was significantly altered by copious glycocalyx that adhered to bone with the appearance of caked-on accretions. The S. aureus grew in the rabbit tibia within thick, adherent, glycocalyx-enclosed biofilms which presented problems for the host defense mechanisms to function properly. When experimentally induced osteomyelitis was treated for three weeks with a therapeutic regimen of clindamycin, the bacteriological cultures of the bone marrow and bone were negative, histological examination of tissues were negative for osteomyelitis, and the bone surfaces was clear except for slight remnants of a biofilm.

One of several Bacteroides species, or S. epidermidis alone, failed to produce osteomyelitis in our rabbit model (unpublished results). However, when any one Bacteroides species was injected simultaneously with S. epidermidis into the rabbit tibia, acute osteomyelitis developed. A thick, viscous glycocalyx was formed by this bacterial combination, and a thick, smooth, velvet-like glycocalyx enclosed innumerable microcolonies as well as covered bone surfaces. When these animals were treated for three weeks with clindamycin, SEM showed only a few cocci, although the gram stains and cultures were negative. This provided evidence that organisms may persist in the bone marrow with negative cultures. Also, this study indicated that osteomyelitis caused by a mixed aerobic and anaerobic infection may take longer to resolve with antibiotics than osteomyelitis caused by S. aureus alone.

Subinhibitory concentrations of clindamycin inhibited adherence of S. aureus, B. intermedius, B. thetaiotaomicron, B. bivius and E. coli to bone surfaces in vitro. A lower concentration of clindamycin was required to inhibit the adherence of S. aureus than any other genus tested which indicated possible differences in the glycocalyx of various organisms. At present, it is unknown if the glycocalyx of staphylococci and Bacteroides is the adhesin, but it is obvious that the glycocalyx of these bacteria is important in adherence to bone.

Clindamycin appears to have several advantages in treating chronic infections in which the bacterial glycocalyx plays a major role in the infectious process. Clindamycin has a slight positive charge which may explain, in part, why it penetrates the bacterial glycocalyx which is negatively charged. Clindamycin administered prophylactically prevented S. aureus osteomyelitis even in the presence of a foreign body which indicated the potential of clindamycin as a prophylactic agent in bone surgery with high risk infections. Finally, clindamycin cured acute osteomyelitis in our rabbit model within three weeks after treatment was initiated.

ACKNOWLEDGMENTS

This research was supported by The Upjohn Co., and grant A5731 of the Natural Research Council of Canada. We thank K. Fortner, J. Nelligan, and R. Costerton for expert technical assistance and J. Taylor for typing the manuscript.

REFERENCES

1. M. E. Bayer and H. Thurow, Polysaccharide capsule of Escherichia coli: microscopic study of its size, structure, and sites of synthesis, J. Bacteriol. 130:911 (1977).
2. G. G. Caputy and J. W. Costerton, Morphological examination of the glycocalyces of Staphylococcus aureus strains Wiley and Smith, Infect. Immun. 36:759 (1982).
3. G. D. Christensen, W. A. Simpson, A. L. Bisno and E. H. Beachey, Adherence of slime-producing strains of Staphylococcus epidermidis to smooth surfaces, Infect. Immun. 37:318 (1982).
4. J. W. Costerton, Cell envelope as a barrier to antibiotics, in: "Microbiology," D. Schlessinger, ed., American Society for Microbiology, Washington, D.C. (1977).
5. C. G. Gemmell, P. K. Peterson, D. Schmeling, J. Mathews and P. G. Quie, Antibiotic-induced modification of Bacteroides fragilis and its susceptibility to phagocytosis by human polymorphonuclear leucocytes, Eur. J. Clin. Microbiol. 2:327 (1983).
6. B. -E. Kristiansen, L. Rustad, O. Spanne and B. Bjorvatn, Effect of subminimal inhibitory concentrations of antimicrobial agents on the piliation and adherence of Neisseria meningitidis, Antimicrob. Agents Chemother. 24:731 (1983).
7. J. Lam, R. Chan, K. Lam and J. W. Costerton, Production of mucoid microcolonies by Pseudomonas aeruginosa within infected lungs in cystic fibrosis, Infect. Immun. 28:546 (1980).
8. D. W. Lambe, Jr., K. J. Mayberry-Carson, K. P. Ferguson and J. W. Costerton, Morphological stabilization of the glycocalyces in 23 strains of five Bacteroides species using specific antisera, Can. J. Microbiol. 30:809 (1984).
9. R. Locci, G. Peters and G. Pulverer, Microbial colonization of prosthetic devices. I. Microtopographical characteristics of intravenous catheters as detected by scanning electron microscopy, Zbl. Bakt. Hyg. I. Abt. Orig. B 175:285 (1981).
10. E. G. Mackie, K. N. Brown, J. Lam and J. W. Costerton, Morphological stabilization of capsules of group B streptococci, types Ia, Ib, II and III with specific antibody, J. Bacteriol. 138:609 (1979).
11. T. J. Marrie and J. W. Costerton, A scanning and transmission electron microscopic study of an infected endocardial pacemaker lead, Circulation 66:1339 (1982).
12. T. J. Marrie and J. W. Costerton, Scanning electron microscopic study of uropathogen adherence to a plastic surface, Appl. Environ. Microbiol. 45:1018 (1983).
13. T. J. Marrie, M. A. Noble and J. W. Costerton, Examination of the morphology of bacteria adhering to peritoneal dialysis catheters by scanning and transmission electron microscopy, J. Clin. Microbiol. 18:1388 (1983).
14. K. C. Marshall, R. Stout and R. Mitchell, Mechanism of the initial events in the sorption of marine bacteria to surfaces, J. Gen. Microbiol. 68:337 (1971).
15. K. J. Mayberry-Carson, B. Tober-Meyer, J. K. Smith, D. W. Lambe, Jr. and J. W. Costerton, Bacterial adherence and glycocalyx formation in osteomyelitis experimentally induced with Staphylococcus aureus, Infect. Immun. 43:825 (1984).

16. P. K. Peterson, Y. Kim, B. J. Wilkinson, D. Schmeling, A. F. Michael and P. G. Quie, Dichotomy between opsonization and serum complement activation by encapsulated staphylococci, Infect. Immun. 20:770 (1978).
17. P. K. Peterson, B. J. Wilkinson, Y. Kim, D. Schmeling and P. G. Quie, Influence of encapsulation on staphylococcal opsonization and phagocytosis by human polymorphonuclear leukocytes, Infect. Immun. 19:943 (1978).
18. V. Vaisánen, K. Lounatmaa and T. K. Korhonen, Effects of sublethal concentrations of antimicrobial agents on the hemagglutination, adhesion, and ultrastructure of pyelonephritogenic Escherichia coli strains, Antimicrob. Agents Chemother. 22:120 (1982).
19. B. J. Wilkinson, Y. Kim, P. K. Peterson, P. G. Quie and A. F. Michael, Activation of complement by cell surface components of Staphylococcus aureus, Infect. Immun. 20:388 (1978).
20. B. J. Wilkinson, Y. Kim and P. K. Peterson, Factors affecting complement activation by Staphylococcus aureus cell walls, their components, and mutants altered in teichoic acid, Infect. Immun. 32:216 (1981).

IN VITRO EFFECTS OF SUB-MIC'S OF ANTIBIOTICS ON THE ANTIGENICITY AND IMMUNOGENICITY OF PSEUDOMONAS AERUGINOSA

Philippe H. Lagrange, Herve Richet and
Marie Christine Escande

Laboratoire Central de Microbiologie
Paris, France

INTRODUCTION

In addition to the studies on direct or indirect effects of antibiotics (AB) on the host immune responses of normal or infected hosts, some researchers have recently directed their activity toward the pathogenic bacteria themselves (1). Clearly, the aim of research on AB is to determine how such drugs can be used in the therapy of infectious diseases to eradicate bacteria from the site of infection. Yet, most research on these drugs and their effects on bacteria has been carried out at AB concentrations equal to or greater than the minimum inhibitory concentrations (MIC's) or the minimum bactericidal concentrations (MBC's). At concentrations lower than the MIC, AB produce effects which are not milder than those seen at the MIC, but which are different in kind. At this point, the AB actions are not considered any further on the multiplication mechanisms but rather on the modification of bacterial morphology and ultrastructure and on their ultimate influences upon the host's anti-infectious mechanisms.

In the past years the observations of the effects of sub MIC's of AB on bacteria in vitro, have gathered momentum and showed bacterial modifications of cellular morphology, serological properties associated with changes in their susceptibility to phagocytosis, and killing by polymorphonuclear phagocytes (11). These authors investigated in vitro the bactericidal and phagocytic ability of rabbit leucocytes on Pseudomonas aeruginosa in the presence or absence of different AB, at several concentrations, in a medium containing no serum. Only inhibitors of cell wall biosynthesis, at sub MIC, could enhance phagocytosis and polymorphonuclear bactericidal activity. Probably the bacteria became weaker and more susceptible to the leucocyte bactericidal system. Similarly several studies did demonstrate the in vivo potentiation of defense mechanisms by sub MIC's of AB. Such doses may have complementary activities on bacteria beside a curbing effect, like a decrease in the formation of pathogenicity or virulence factors and alterations of immunogenic determinants as shown recently (10). The possibility that antibiotic exposure of Ps. aeruginosa, one of the most common causes of severe and lethal nosocomial infections in the immunocompromised patients in our hospital (3), might have similar effects, has been evaluated in this study in which morphological alterations associated with changes in antigenicity and immunogenicity of in vitro AB treated Ps. aeruginosa were compared to those of normal non-treated bacteria.

MATERIALS AND METHODS

Animals

All studies were performed using female specific pathogen-free outbred Swiss (OF1) mice, weighing 20-24 g, 6 to 8 weeks old. Animals were housed in plastic cages, maintained in a protected environment under filtered air flow in positive pressure incubators (ESI, Cachan, France). They were fed with a sterilized, vitamin supplemented diet and sterile water (pH 3) at libitum.

Bacteria

Two strains of *Ps. aeruginosa*, strain 011 and 016, were used in this study. Both strains were isolated from infected patients and are all part of our stock culture collection. After biochemical and serological identification, they were maintained in Trypticase Soy Agar (TSA). They were grown usually overnight at 37°C on Trypticase Soy Agar (TSA) containing various concentrations of the antibiotic tested. A control was cultured without antibiotics. The bacteria were washed three times in phosphate buffered sterile saline (PBS), pH 7.4 and adjusted photometrically to a final concentration of 2 x 10^8 CFU/ml according to previously established standard curves. Semi-dry weight and protein contents from aliquots were measured on pellet after one centrifugation at 4000 g during 15 min at 4°C. The bacteria were further characterized by Gram stain, biochemical criteria and serological agglutination test. Suspensions were heated for two hours at 60°C, washed again and stored in aliquots at 80°C until use. Tests of bacterial viability yielded negative results. The one-step fixation, inblock staining method was used in processing for election microscopy, using a Philips 300 electron microscope operated at 80 KV and provided a 200 µm condenser aperture and a 30 µm objective aperture. Multiple sections were examined at final magnification of 4,000 - 100,000 x.

Antibiotics

Carbenicillin, Ticarcillin, Amoxicillin (Beecham), Fosfomycin (Boehringer) and Chloramphenicol (Roussel) were used. Minimum inhibitory concentration (MIC's) were determined by the microdilution method using TS broth with 1% glucose and 0.004% phenol red added. The inoculum was adjusted to 10^5 colony forming units (CFU)/ml. The results were read after incubation for 18 hrs. at 37°C. The MIC's were for Carbenicillin 32 mg/l, Ticarcillin 16 mg/l, amoxicillin >64 mg/l, fosfomycin 64 µg/l and Chloramphenicol 8 mg/l.

Absorption Studies

The commercially available monospecific anti 011 and anti 016 sera (Institut Pasteur Production, Marnes la Coquette, France) were used in this study. In some experiments, one ml of homologous or heterologous serum was incubated and shaken for 1 hr at 4°C with the same amount of untreated and AB treated bacteria, respectively, to remove type specific antibodies. After centrifugation at 4000 g for 15 min the supernatant was removed and the agglutination test was performed with normal non-treated homologous or heterologous type bacteria. Such supernatants or normal immune serum were titrated in a quantitative agglutination test on slides by mixing carefully the normal non-treated homologous cells in one or two drops of undiluted or serially diluted serum, to determine the levels of antibody to the total 0 antigen.

Immunization

Mice were inoculated either subcutaneously (SC) or intraperitoneally (IP) with each type of sub MIC's AB treated or non-treated bacteria, in a volume of 0.5 ml. Control mice received 0.5 ml of saline by the same route. For each group, the injected mice were randomized into three cages with eight mice, in order to detect a possible cage effect. At varying time intervals, the vaccinated and control mice were bled by retro-orbital puncture, and the individual immune serum stored in aliquots at 20°C until use.

Animal Challenge

The bacterial suspensions (0.5 ml), diluted in saline, were inoculated intravenously (IV) or IP. The normal or AB treated bacteria were obtained from a log-phase culture in shaken TS broth after 5-6 hours incubation at 37°C. The 50% lethal doses were graphically estimated after the IV injection, using the cumulative percentage of mortality after three days by the probits method (log dose/probit of the mortality percentage) in groups of 15 mice each. In addition, the number of bacteria present in the blood and in minced spleen and liver suspensions from infected mice were determined by standard bacterial plating assays with nutrient agar and ten-fold serial dilutions of the test suspension. The organs were obtained at autopsy, washed in saline and then individually homogenized with a teflon-tipped Tri R homogenized in the cold. 0.1 ml aliquots were tested for number of CFU/ml, counted after 24 hours incubation at 37°C. Blood clearance tests were performed by measuring the number of bacteria/ml of blood according to the time after the IP injection of the challenge inoculum (15 min to 4 hours), as described elsewhere (4). In brief, 5 µl of blood from individual mice were harvested at the extremity of the tail with an Eppendorf micropipette and immediately diluted in 0.5 ml of distilled water, and the number of bacteria were determined after plating ten-fold serial dilutions on agar. For each dilution, the number of bacteria were estimated in triplicate. The threshold of sensitivity of this method was $10^{2.52}$ bacteria per ml of blood (around 300 bacteria/ml).

Statistical Test

The statistical comparison was carried out by student's *t* test for non-paired data.

RESULTS

Morphological Alterations

Exposure of *Pseudomonas aeruginosa* 011 to 1/4 or 1/2 of the MIC of carbenicillin induced obvious morphological alterations compared with the control (Figure 1a); the β-lactam treated bacterial cells appeared filamentous on microscopic examination (Figure 1c, 1d). Fosfomycin induced pleomorphic forms and chloramphenicol was never able to induce alterations of cultured bacteria (results not shown). After relatively short exposure (5 hrs) of susceptible *Ps. aeruginosa* 011 to concentrations at or above MIC, the septa became irregularly shaped and showed a loss in density and the peripheral cell wall became markedly thin (Figure 2b, 2d). The filaments tend to lyse at both ends. Apparent reduced numbers of ribosomes were not observed in the carbenicillin treated bacteria compared to normal (Figure 2d). The reversibility of these morphological alterations was observed when *Ps. aeruginosa*, exposed to 1/2 - 1/3 MIC of carbenicillin, transferred to drug-free agar and incubated 4 hours at 37°C, showed a significant increase in the number of CFU and returned to rod-like morphology. The same findings were also observed when such filamentation in vitro AB treated

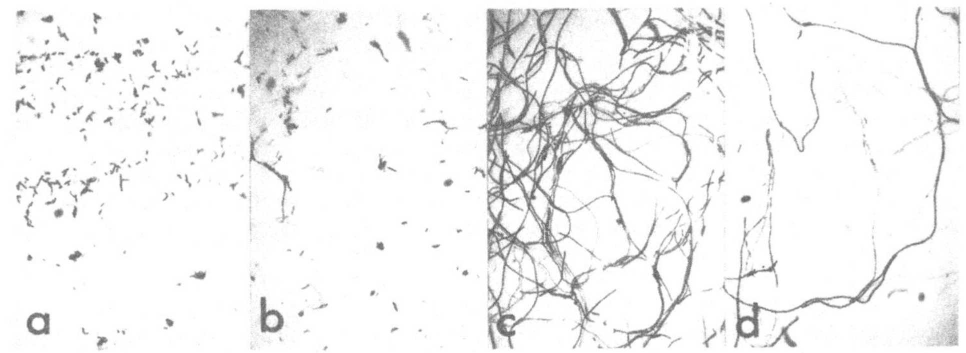

Figure 1. Pseudomonas aeruginosa grown on drug-free agar (a) or in the presence of varying concentrations of Carbenicillin, 8 μg/l (b), 16 μg/l (c) and 32 μg/l (d) Gramm stain, 3000x.

bacteria were IP inoculated in mice. Thus, the increase in CFU of in vivo or in vitro growth on drug-free agar and in normal mice clearly demonstrated that these bacteria were not dying cells. It is possible that these paired membranes herald the growth initiation of aberrant cross walls.

Antigenicity of AB Treated Ps. aeruginosa

Some bacteria exposed to sub MIC of AB have shown increased vulnerability to immunodefense mechanisms. For instance, Ps. aeruginosa grown in

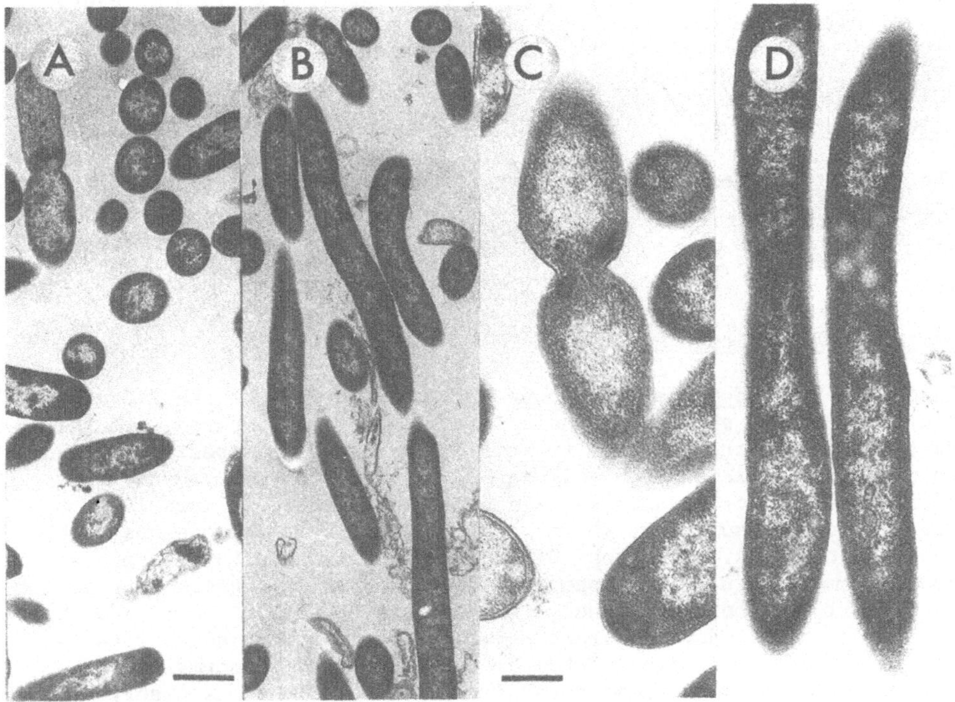

Figure 2. Pseudomonas aeruginosa grown in TS broth for 5 hrs without (A,C) or with (B,D) 32 μg/ml of carbenicillin (A,B: bar = 1 μm, 4000x; C,D: bar = 1 μm, 10000x).

Table 1. Different Characteristics of *Ps. aeruginosa* 011 Cultivated in Presence of sub-MIC's of Carbenicillin[a]

	C16	N
OD	0.200	0.200
cfu/ml	5×10^8	7×10^8
Semi-dry weight/ml	0.385 mg	0.456 mg
Protein content/ml	0.175 mg	0.160 mg
Residual agglutination		
before heating	dilution 1/2	total
60°C (2 hrs)	dilution 1/2	total
100°C (2 hrs)	1/2	1/2

[a]*Ps. aeruginosa* 011 was cultivated during 24 hrs at 37°C by the membrane technique on solid agar medium containing 16 μg/ml of carbenicillin. Colonies were harvested, washed twice with sterile non-pyrogenic 0.15 M NaCl and resuspended to the desired optical density.

the presence of 1/16 carbenicillin (11) showed increased susceptibility to phagocytosis. Moreover, recently it has been shown (10) that uptake rates of untreated and antibiotic treated bacteria did not differ when normal serum was used for opsonization. However, in the presence of rabbit immune serum, untreated bacteria still required the participation of the complement system for optimal opsonization, whereas bacteria treated with β-lactam antibiotics did not. Antibacterial agents that affect peptidoglycan and cause morphological and biochemical changes in the cell wall could also produce change in the antigenic structure of Gram (-ve) bacilli, since it has been shown that surface antigenic constituents of these cells are attached to peptidoglycan principally by covalent linkages. For instance,

Table 2. Residual Agglutination of Immune Serum After Absorption by *Ps. aeruginosa* 011 Strain, Cultivated in Presence of sub-MIC's of Different Antibiotics

Antibiotic	sub-MIC's	Treatment	Residual agglutination (dilution of the absorbed serum) undiluted	1/2	1/4
Carbenicillin	16 μg/ml	+	-	-	-
		-	+	+	-
Ticarcillin	8 μg/ml	+	-	-	-
		-	+	-	-
Amoxicillin	32 μg/ml	+	-	-	-
		-	+	-	-
Chloramphenicol	16 μg/ml	+	+	+	-
		-	+	+	-
Carbenicillin	16 μg/ml	+	+	+	-
Chloramphenicol	0.12 μg/ml	-	+	+	-
Fosfomycin	8 μg/ml	+	+	-	-
		-	+	+	-

Table 3. Specific Residual Agglutination of Immune Serum after Absorption by Ps. aeruginosa 011 Cultivated with or without Carbenicillin

Immune Serum	Bacteria	Residual agglutination (dilution of the absorbed serum) undiluted	1/2	1/4
anti 011[a]	C16	-	-	-
	N	+	+	-
anti 016[b]	C16	+	+	-
	N	+	+	-

(a) Immune serum anti 011 has been in contact with the same amount of treated and non-treated bacteria during one hour at 20°C, and after centrifugation the supernatant was diluted and tested for the residual agglutination with a normal non-treated homologous strain.
(b) Immune serum anti 016 was absorbed with the same amount of treated and non-treated Ps. aeruginosa 011 during one hour at 20°C and after centrifugation, the supernatant was tested for the residual agglutination with a normal non-treated Ps. aeruginosa 016 strain.

evidence was presented that bacteria grown in presence of sub-MIC's AB altered the agglutination properties of normal bacteria (7), compared to those exposed to the same concentration of bacteria (Table 1) as evidenced by optical density (OD), CFU/ml, semi-dry weight, and protein contents. Residual agglutination was shown to disappear totally when immune specific serum was absorbed with the AB treated bacteria. Absorption was only partial when normal non-treated bacteria were used. Moreover, this augmented absorption capacity of the same amount of bacteria was retained in AB treated bacteria heated for 2 hours at 60°C but not if treated at 100°C for 2 hours.

This increased antigenicity of AB treated Ps. aeruginosa was also evidenced when all three β-lactam AB (Carbenicillin, Ticarcillin and Amoxicillin) were used (Table 2). In contrast, no such alterations were observed when Chloramphenicol alone was used. Moreover, bacteria grown in presence of Carbenicillin (16 μg/ml) lost their increased antigenicity when they were added as low as 0.12 μg/ml of Chloramphenicol. Fosfomycin (8 μg/ml) was shown to give intermediate results. Specificity of such increased antigenicity was next tested, using absorption of anti 016 serum with non-treated or Carbenicillin treated Ps. aeruginosa 011 serogroup. Residual agglutination of this serum was tested next with Ps. aeruginosa 016 serogroup. As shown in Table 3, alterations of antigenicity was specific since 011 serogroup Ps. aeruginosa treated by Carbenicillin was able to totally absorb the specific anti-serum.

Immunogenicity of AB-Treated Ps. aeruginosa

Since host immune factors appear important for the elimination of micro organisms and effectiveness of some semi-synthetic penicillins have shown to be higher against gram negative micro-organisms in vivo than in vitro (13), evidence was given by the same authors (5) that increased immunogenicity, as tested by higher blood clearance and higher killing in the spleen and liver, occurred in mice treated in vivo with Cyclacillin. Furthermore, a significantly higher antibody plaque response against E. coli developed in AB-treated mice than in untreated mice. Since AB treated Ps. aeruginosa were shown to exhibit higher surface antigenicity, the next experiments were done to study the relative immunogenicity of such bacteria when inoculated in mice. The results of such experiments demonstrated that mice immunized by one IP injection (Figure 3, left) or by one SC inoculation (Figure 3, right) developed higher antibody titers when inoculated with sub-MIC's AB treated bacteria than with the same amount of non-treated bacteria, both having an apparent peak 14 days after immunization. At that day, other groups of mice, IP immunized, were challenged IV, with 1.8×10^8 live Ps. aeruginosa 011 serogroup. Significant protection was observed in both immunized groups compared to normal control (Figure 4). Nevertheless, there was an inverse relationship between the level of antibodies and the number of bacteria found in liver, three days after challenge in the survivors. When antibody titers were measured in other groups of mice, which have survived after a similar challenge, it was shown that significantly higher titers developed in mice immunized with in vitro AB treated bacteria than in mice treated with non-treated bacteria (Figure 5). Since it was shown that the major effect of specific antibody in Pseudomonas infection results in clearing bacteria from the blood, mice were SC immunized as already described, and twenty-one days they were challenged with 1×10^5 live normal bacteria. Clearance of blood from Ps. aeruginosa was increased in immune mice, and a higher clearance rate was noticed during the first hour when mice were immunized with AB treated bacteria compared to those immunized with non-treated bacteria (Figure 6).

All the preceding experiments have been done using bacteria grown on agar with sub-MIC's AB. Since it was reported that if MIC defines antibacterial activity at high drug concentrations, the minimum antibiotic concentration (MAC) inhibition describes antibacterial activity at low concentrations (9). MAC was determined according to the broth technique and MIC/MAC

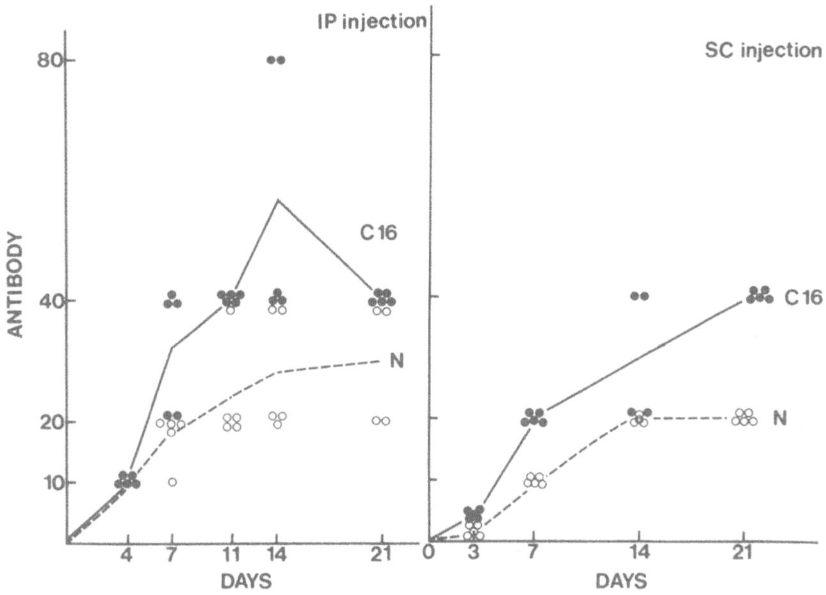

Figure 3. Left: Specific agglutination titers in sera harvested at varying time intervals in mice injected intraperitoneally with 0.5 ml of 1/2 MIC of Carbenicillin (C16) treated or non-treated (N) Ps. aeruginosa, 011 serogroup. Right: specific agglutination titers in mice immunized subcutaneously with the same treated or non-treated bacteria.

ratios for Carbenicillin with Ps. aeruginosa were calculated using a photometric method. The results of such experiments showed a MIC/MAC ratio of 3, determined over a 5 hour period. Filamentous forms of bacteria did appear with MIC's AB (32 μg/ml) and above as soon as three hours after, became visible after 5 hours with 1/2 MIC's (16 μg/ml) and persit thereafter. When absorption studies were performed with bacteria treated with 16 μg/ml and 32 μg/ml Carbenicillin, and harvested 5 and 18 hrs after inoculation of the broth, only the bacteria treated during 5 hrs with the 1/2 MIC were able to totally absorb the immune serum. Thus, we then compared the immunogenicity of such treated bacteria. The results of an experiment are shown in Figure 7. Once again 1/2 sub-MIC's Carbenicillin treated bacteria, harvested after 5 hrs, gave the highest antibody levels, and were associated with the better clearance rate against virulent challenge with 0.5×10^6 live normal Ps. aeruginosa 011 serogroup.

Virulence of AB Treated Ps. aeruginosa

The next experiment was done to explore the residual virulence of sub-MIC's AB treated bacteria harvested at 5 hrs as described previously. Determinations of LD50 were performed using IV inoculation of ten-fold serial dilutions of treated and non-treated bacteria in separate groups of 15 mice each. The results of such an experiment are shown in Figure 8 and it was

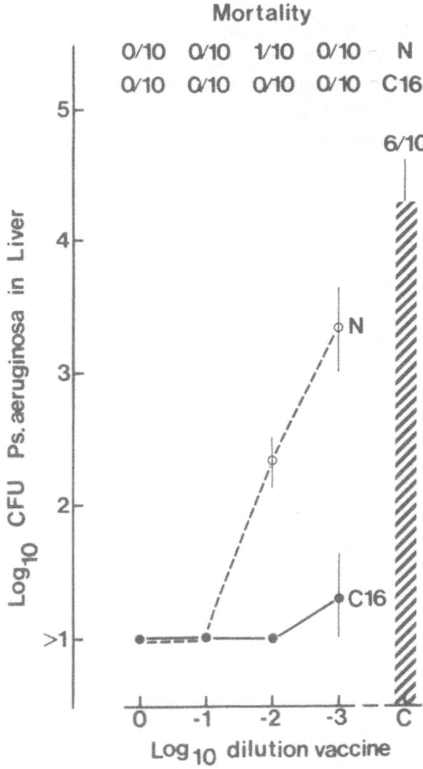

Figure 4. Numbers of viable Ps. aeruginosa (011_8 serogroup) found in liver 3 days after 1 IV challenge (1.8×10^8 live non-treated bacteria per mouse) of normal mice (C) and of mice immunized IP with 0.5 ml of serial ten-fold dilutions of C16 vaccine (C16) or non-treated (N) heat-killed bacteria given 14 days prior to challenge. Mean of 5 mice ± SEM. Mortality rates are given on the top of the graph.

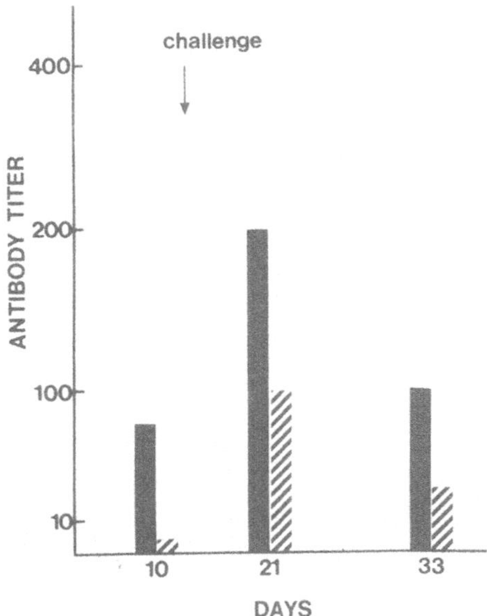

Figure 5. Specific agglutination titers in mice immunized ip with undi-undiluted C16 vaccine (black br) or with non-AB treated Ps aeruginosa (hatched bar) before and after one IV challenge of 1.8 x 10^8 Ps aeruginosa 0.11/mouse. Mean of 6 mice per group.

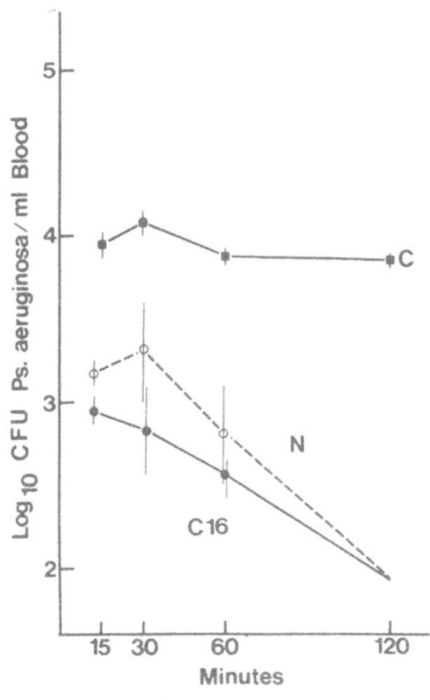

Figure 6. Blood clearance of normal non-antibiotic treated Ps aeruginosa in normal mice (C) and in mice immunized subcutaneously with 0.5 ml of undiluted non-treated (N) and carbenicillin treated (C16) Ps aeruginosa, given 21 days prior the IV challenge (1 x 10^5 live bacteria/mouse) Mean of 6 mice ± SEM.

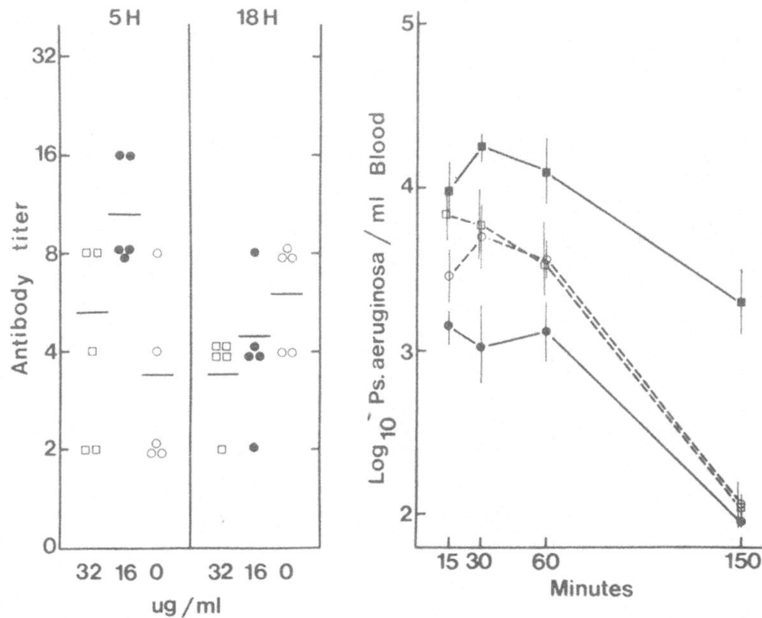

Figure 7. Left: specific agglutination titers in serum of mice harvested 14 days after one SC injection of 0.5 ml of same concentration of Ps aeruginosa 011 grown for 5 or 18 hr in TS broth containing non-antibiotic (0), 16 µg/ml (●), or 32 µg/ml (□) of carbenicillin. Right: blood clearance of normal non-treated Ps aeruginosa after one IV challenge (5 x 10^5 bacteria/mouse) in separate groups of normal or immunized mice (same symbols). Mean of 6 mice ± SEM.

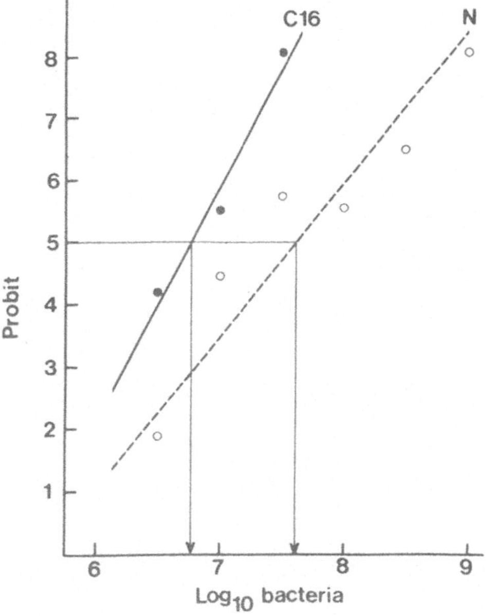

Figure 8. Cumulative percentage of mortality after 3 days expressed with probit method (log10 inoculum dose/probit of mortality percentage) in separate groups of 15 mice inoculated IV with Ps. aeruginosa 011 grown for 5 hr in TS broth containing no antibiotic (0) or 16 µg/ml (1/2 MIC) of Carbenicillin (●). Groups of 15 mice.

concluded that C16 treated bacteria were more virulent than non-treated bacteria since the respective measured LD50 were $10^{6.75}$ and $10^{7.62}$. However, such apparent surprising results may be explained by the fact that sub-MIC's AB treated bacteria, grown in broth, were able to increase in the number of CFU, and return to rod-like morphology when transferred to drug-free medium or inoculated in mice; the challenge inoculum being already diluted and tested for CFU, without regrowth in drug-free medium.

DISCUSSION

Our study has shown that pretreatment of Ps. aeruginosa with 1/2 or 1/4 of the MIC of Carbenicillin, Ticarcillin, Amoxicillin, changed the morphologic and ultrastructure of the bacteria. Their significant cellular alterations were accompanied by changes of surface characteristics of the bacteria, the AB treated bacteria being more able to absorb specific antibodies in a residual agglutination test. This increased expression of antigenicity was already described with Salmonella typhimurium treated by Ampicillin (7) and recently with Cefoperazone treated Ps. aeruginosa (10). This author showed that absorbed heated immune serum by those AB treated bacteria was less efficient in inducing opsonizing activity than heated immune serum absorbed with the same amount of non-treated bacteria. It was also shown to be specific since absorption with other bacterial species did not abrogate the opsonizing capacity of the heated serum. Increased antigenicity was also associated with higher immunogenicity since immunized mice always showed higher levels of specific antibodies; a similar finding has already been described (12). These results were also associated with a better blood clearance rate in such immunized mice, against normal non-treated bacteria, followed by a lower multiplication of the challenge inoculum in the target organ. Preliminary results have also evidenced that the same amount of culture filtration of sub-MIC's treated bacteria were also more able to protect mice and gave higher agglutinin antibody levels than culture filtrate from non-AB treated bacteria (results not shown), protection being based on opsonic and antitoxic activities (6). Moreover, enhanced leukocyte phagocytosis and killing of opsonized Ps. aeruginosa cultivated in presence of β-lactam antibiotics, without the need of heat labile serum component, might influence markedly the outcome of the infectious process locally, in presence of sub-MIC of antibiotics and might prove important in a patient with complement deficiencies. However, in our study, in contrast with results obtained by others (2,11), AB treated bacteria were shown to be more virulent, in our protocol, than did non-treated bacteria. These results might be explained by the fact that sub-MIC's AB treated bacteria are not dying cells, but are inhibited not in cell wall synthesis but in the septum formation which could lengthen the filamentous forms produced by β-lactam antibiotics, as reviewed recently (9). Moreover, it might also be important to consider that the morphological structural changes produced by sub-MIC of antibiotics are different from those produced by antibiotics at concentrations equal to or higher than the MIC (Figure 6). These might involve different mechanisms induced by different concentrations of antibiotics.

These results suggest that the modifications induced in bacterial forms by sub-MIC's of AB have different effects on antibody formation and antigen antibody reactions, in helping the host to break the chain of events produced by pathogenic bacteria. Since the defense system and the drugs are acting synergistically against many infective strains, their effect may occur in presence of minute doses of the drugs which could be reached by less frequent administration of antibiotics. Such procedures might be useful in expressing specific epitopes of genetically manipulated bacteria in order to increase the yield of specific antigen produced in vitro.

In conclusion, cell-wall alteration induced by sub-MIC's of β-lactam AB seems to be associated with an increase in the expression of specific epitopes at the bacterial surface, which may increase the clearance of such bacteria and produce a more efficient immune response. Further in vivo and in vitro studies are needed to analyze the validity of such conclusions.

REFERENCES

1. S. Åhlstedt, The antibacterial effects of low concentrations of antibiotics and host defense factors: a review, J. Antimicrob. Chemother. 8(Suppl. C):59 (1981).
2. S. Ahlstedt and B. Kaiser, Synergistic protective effects of antibodies and ampicillin in mice infected intraperitoneally with Escherichia coli, Infection 6(Suppl. 1):86 (1978).
3. B. Campillo, H. Richet, B. Rio, J. P. Marie, J. P. Arago, P. H. LaGrange and R. Zittoun, Septicemies à Pseudomonas aeruginosa de serotype 016 dans un service d'hèmato-oncologie: revue de 17 cas, Ann. Med. Int. (in press) (1985).
4. F. Daoulas-le Bourdelles, P. Berche and M. Veron, Vaccin acellulaire de Pseudomonas aeruginosa: II. Estimation du pouvoir protecteur d'un immun-serum par une mesure de la clairance bacterienne, Ann. Microbiol. (Inst. Pasteur) 128 B:61 (1977).
5. H. Friedman and G. H. Warren, Cyclacillin induced potentiation of Escherichia coli immunogenicity in vivo and in vitro, Chemotherapy 23:324 (1977).
6. A. A. I. Kostiala, Pseudomonas aeruginosa infection and vaccination in the rat, J. Med. Microbiol. 13:201 (1980).
7. V. Lorian, B. Atkinson and W. H. Ewing, Agglutination with 0 sera of Salmonella exposed to antibiotics Amer. J. Clin. Pathol. 66:1004 (1976).
8. V. Lorian, M. Koike, O. Zak, V. Zanon, L. D. Sabath, C. G. Grassi and W. Stille, Effect of subinhibitory concentrations of antibiotics on bacteria, in: "Current Chemotherapy," Volume 1, W. Siegenthaler and R. Luthy, eds., A. S. M., Washington (1978).
9. V. Lorian, Effects of subminimum inhibitory concentrations of antibiotics on bacteria, in: "Antibiotics in Laboratory Medicine," V. Lorian, ed., Williams and Wilkins Co., Baltimore (1980).
10. D. Milatovic, Influence of subinhibitory concentrations of antibiotics on opsonization and phagocytosis of Pseudomonas aeruginosa by human polymorphonuclear leukocytes, Eur. J. Clin. Microbiol. 3:288 (1984).
11. M. Nishida, Y. Mine, S. Nonoyama and Y. Yokota, Effect of antibiotics on the phagocytosis and killing of Pseudomonas aeruginosa by rabbit polymorphonuclear leukocytes, Chemotherapy 22:203 (1976).
12. I. Viano, P. Martinetto, A. Valtz, M. Santiano and S. Barbaro, Variability of immune response induced by bacteria treated with subminimal inhibitory concentrations of fosfomycin, Rev. Infect. Dis. 1:858 (1979).
13. J. A. Yurchenco, M. W. Hopper, T. D. Vince and G. H. Warren, Cyclacillin, a semi-synthetic aminoalicyclic penicillin. I. Antibacterial activity in vitro and in vivo compared with ampicillin and cephaloxin, Chemotherapy 15:209 (1970).

ANTIBIOTIC SUSCEPTIBILITY OF BACTERIA AS RELATED TO IMMUNOGENICITY

Nicola Siegmund-Schultze, Sigrid Schell and Kathryn Nixdorff

Institut für Mikrobiologie
Technische Hochschule Darmstadt
Darmstadt, F.R.G.

INTRODUCTION

Over the past several years we have been investigating the characteristics of the immune responses to antigens from the outer membrane of gram-negative bacteria, and how these responses can be modulated by complexing the antigens with other components of the outer membrane. As a model for these studies, we have been using defined complexes produced from isolated, purified components of the outer membrane of *Proteus mirabilis*. In these complexes, the isolated components serve as immunogens and as modulators alike.

In the course of these studies, we found that outer membrane components have a profound effect in modulating both the strength and the character of the antibody-producing cell responses in mice to lipopolysaccharide (LPS). In this regard, the specific responses to LPS were altered from relatively weak responses that were predominantly IgM in character with very little production of IgG to much stronger responses that were mainly IgG in character when LPS was complexed with bacterial membrane phospholipids (16) or with outer membrane proteins (3,5). Depending upon the outer membrane component used as a modulator, a selective, enhanced induction of either IgG1 or IgG2 antibody-producing cells specific for LPS was observed (3,6).

Since these studies form the basis of our present investigations into the characteristics of the immune responses to surface components of antibiotic-treated bacteria, we have summarized some of the results of these earlier investigations in Table 1 for greater clarity. We immunized mice with either LPS alone, LPS mixed with phospholipids, LPS mixed with an outer membrane protein with an apparent molecular weight of 39,000 (39 K protein) or LPS mixed with the outer membrane lipoprotein from *P. mirabilis*. Components were mixed by sonication. The IgM and the IgG subclasses of plaque-forming cells (PFC) were measured against LPS coupled to sheep red blood cells (SRBC) on day 19, the height of the secondary responses when modulating effects are most pronounced.

As can be seen from the data in Table 1, the IgG responses to LPS alone were relatively weak, and the number of PFC were distributed mainly in the IgG1 (40% of total IgG) and the IgG2 (44% of total IgG) subclasses. When LPS was complexed with phospholipids, both the strength and the subclass distribution of the IgG responses were altered. In this case, the predominant subclass of PFC was IgG1. When LPS was complexed with the 39 K

Table 1. Secondary IgM and IgG Subclass Responses in Mice to P. mirabilis D52 LPS Alone and in Combination with Phospholipids, 39 K Protein and Lipoprotein[a]

Immunogen[b]	Antibody type	PFC/10^6 spleen cells[c] on day 19	% IgG subclass of total IgG
LPS	IgM	10 ± 1	-
"	IgG1	17 ± 3	40
"	IgG2	19 ± 5	44
"	IgG3	7 ± 1	16
LPS + Phospholipids	IgM	26 ± 15	-
"	IgG1	1793 ± 507	82
"	IgG2	248 ± 12	11
"	IgG3	147 ± 21	7
LPS + K Protein	IgM	31 ± 5	-
"	IgG1	337 ± 75	25
"	IgG2	818 ± 133	62
"	IgG3	168 ± 49	13
LPS + Lipoprotein	IgM	12 ± 1	-
"	IgG1	369 ± 64	59
"	IgG2	143 ± 21	23
"	IgG3	113 ± 24	18

[a]Data from Karch, Gmeiner and Nixdorff (3).
[b]Dosages per injection were 25 μg LPS, 300 μg phospholipids and 12.5 μg proteins. Mice received a primary injection on day 0 and a secondary injection on day 14.
[c]Geometric means ± standard errors of PFC. Values are the results of 3-5 separate experiments. Responses were measured against P. mirabilis D52 LPS coupled to SRBC.

protein, a selective enhancement of the IgG2 subclass of PFC was observed. With lipoprotein as modulator, mainly IgG1 PFC were induced.

These results illustrate that various combinations of outer membrane components can effect the induction of quantitatively and qualitatively different types of responses. It should be mentioned that the IgG responses are highly specific for the particular serotype of LPS used as immunogen (5,6,16) and are T cell dependent (Schell and Nixdorff, unpublished results).

In a recent investigation (14), we reported certain changes in outer membrane composition of P. mirabilis after treatment of this organism with beta-lactam antibiotics. For the present investigation, we have employed the sensitive assay system described above to determine if these changes in outer membrane composition affect the characteristics of the immune responses to LPS as antigen, complexed with other components in the cell surface structure.

We have used a model system consisting of the bacterial form of P. mirabilis strain VI and various forms of this strain with progressive cell wall defects (filament form, unstable spheroplast L-form and stable protoplast L-form) induced by beta-lactam antibiotics. Cell walls or protoplast membranes isolated from these forms were injected intraperitoneally into mice and the secondary IgM and IgG subclass responses to LPS were measured in the hemolytic plaque assay.

MATERIALS AND METHODS

Bacteria

P. mirabilis IV and its stable protoplast L-form were obtained from Dr. H. H. Martin, Institut für Mikrobiologie, Technische Hochschule Darmstadt, F.R.G. The stable protoplast L-form was originally obtained from Dr. U. Taubeneck (Jena, G.D.R.).

Antibiotics

The beta-lactam antibiotic cefuroxime (Hoechst AG, Frankfurt/Main, F.R.G.) was used for the induction of the filament form of *P. mirabilis* VI. This antibiotic was chosen because of its ability to specifically induce filament formation (11). The beta-lactam antibiotic cefoxitin (MSD-Sharp & Dohme GmbH, Munich, F.R.G.) was used to induce spheroplast formation in *P. mirabilis* VI.

Cultivation of the Various Cell Forms of P. mirabilis VI

For cultivation of the bacterial form in large amounts, an overnight culture of *P. mirabilis* VI at 37°C in L-medium (10) was added to eight flasks containing 400 ml L-medium to an optical density at 578 nm (O.D.) of 0.1-0.2 (Eppendorf Photometer, Netheler & Hinz GmbH, Hamburg, F.R.G.). This culture was incubated at 37°C with shaking at 120 rpm until an O.D. of 1.0 was reached (mid-logarithmic phase of growth). The culture was then rapidly cooled in an ice bath and the cells were harvested by centrifugation at 4°C.

For cultivation of the filament form in large amounts, 1.0 ml of an overnight culture of the bacterial form was added to each of several flasks containing 50 ml L-medium plus 0.1 μg cefuroxime/ml and incubated overnight at 37°C with shaking at 120 rpm. From this culture, eight flasks containing 400 ml L-medium plus 0.1 μg cefuroxime/ml were inoculated to an O.D. of 0.1-0.2. This culture was incubated at 37°C with shaking at 120 rpm until an O.D. of 1.0 was reached (mid-logarithmic phase of growth). The cells were harvested as above.

P. mirabilis VI was induced to spheroplast formation two to three days before cultivation in large amounts by addition of 60 μg cefoxitin/ml L-medium. On the first day of induction, the culture was incubated overnight at 37°C without shaking. On the second day, 1.0 ml of the culture from the first day was inoculated into each of several flasks containing 50 ml L-medium plus 60 μg cefoxitin/ml. This culture was incubated at 37°C with increasing degrees of shaking during the day (70 rpm, 90 rpm) and finally with shaking at 120 rpm overnight. On the third day, the overnight culture from the second day was added to eight flasks containing 400 ml L-medium plus 60 μg cefoxitin/ml to an O.D. of 0.1-0.2 and incubated at 37°C with shaking (120 rpm) to an O.D. of 0.9 (mid-logarithmic phase of growth). Cells were harvested as above.

The stable protoplast L-form of *P. mirabilis* VI was originally induced by penicillin G (19). This form is completely devoid of cell wall components except for small amounts of LPS contained in the cytoplasmic membrane (1) and grows well and maintains its defect in the absence of antibiotics. Cultivation of the stable protoplast L-form began three to four days before cultivation in large amounts. Each day a fresh culture was initiated from the culture of the previous day and incubated at 37°C with shaking at 120 rpm. Cultivation in large amounts to the mid-logarithmic phase of growth (O.D. of 0.8) was carried out as described above for the bacterial form.

Isolation of Cell Walls

Cell walls of *P. mirabilis* VI free of cytoplasmic membranes and cell contents were obtained by shaking aqueous suspensions of bacteria with glass beads (0.17 mm diameter) in a cooled cell mill (E. Bühler, Tubingen, F.R.G.) for 20 min. in the presence of 0.4% sodium dodecyl sulfate (SDS) as described by Martin (1964). Approximately 10 g bacteria (wet weight) were mixed with 90 ml of 0.4% SDS, pH 7.0, and 150µg of glass beads. To obtain cell walls of the filament form, treatment for 5 min in the cell mill was sufficient. The spheroplast L-form was treated for only 5 sec in the cell mill. Cell walls were washed thoroughly and harvested by centrifugation.

Isolation of Protoplast Membranes

Membranes of the protoplast L-form of *P. mirabilis* VI were obtained by osmotic lysis according to Kroll, Gmeiner and Martin (1980).

SDS-Polyacrylamide Gel Electrophoresis

SDS-polyacrylamide gel electrophoresis of proteins in cell walls was carried out in a slab gel apparatus GE4 (Deutsche Pharmacia, Freiburg, F.R.G.) according to Lugtenberg et al. (8) as previously described (13).

Analytical Methods

Protein content of cell walls was determined by a modification of the Lowry procedure (9). Amounts of phospholipids and LPS were determined by gas-liquid chromatography of fatty acids as described by Gmeiner and Martin (1).

Experimental Animals

Specific pathogen-free female NMRI mice were obtained from Charles River Wiga, Sulzfeld, F.R.G. All mice were seven weeks old at the time of primary immunization.

Immunization of Mice

Mice were injected intraperitoneally with 0.25 mg (dry weight) per injection of cell walls or protoplast membranes contained in 0.2 ml 0.9% NaCl. A primary injection was given on day 0 and a secondary injection on day 14.

Assay of Antibody-Producing Cells

The IgM and the IgG antibody-producing cell responses to LPS were measured in the hemolytic plaque test (2), using a modification of the microscope slide assay (12) with SRBC sensitized with alkali-treated LPS (17) as previously described (3). For the measurement of IgG subclass responses, indirect plaques were developed with specific rabbit anti-mouse IgG1, $IgG2_{ab}$ or IgG3 sera (Nordic Laboratories, Tilburg, NL). The specificities of these subclass antisera have been documented (3).

Table 2. Amounts of Protein, Phospholipids and LPS Contained in 0.25 mg (dry weight) Cell Walls of the Bacterial Form, the Filament Form and the Spheroplast L-Form, or in 0.25 mg Cytoplasmic Membranes of the Protoplast L-Form of P. mirabilis VI[a]

Cell type	Protein (μg)	Phospholipids (nmol C_{16})[b]	LPS (nmol $C_{14\text{-OH}}$)[c]
Bacterial form	137.50	24.01	31.51
Filament form	132.50	16.67	30.35
Spheroplast L-form	165.00	46.96	42.27
Protoplast L-form	110.00	44.77	6.00

[a]Values in the table represent the means taken from two determinations each on two separate samples, calculated from results presented in Nixdorff, Martin and Siegmund-Schultze (14) and in Karch and Nixdorff (4)
[b]C_{16} = palmitic acid
[c]$C_{14\text{-OH}}$ = beta-hydroxy myristic acid

RESULTS AND DISCUSSION

Composition of Cell Walls and Protoplast Membranes Injected into Mice

We recently presented the results of quantitative analyses of protein, phospholipids and LPS in cell walls of the bacterial form, the filament form and the spheroplast L-form of P. mirabilis VI (14). In this same report, we also included data on the analyses of the cytoplasmic membranes of the protoplast L-form obtained previously (4). The data presented in Table 2 were calculated from these results for 0.25 mg cell walls or protoplast

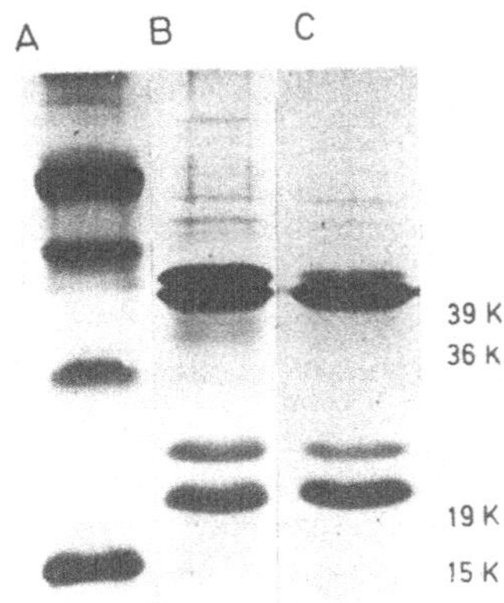

Figure 1. SDS-polyacrylamide gel electrophoresis of proteins from cell walls of the bacterial form and the filament form of P. mirabilis VI. In each case, samples of cell walls containing the same amounts of protein were extracted with 2% SDS for 5 min at 100° C. A, standard proteins: bovine serum albumin (67 K), egg albumin (45 K), chymotrypsinogen (25 K) and cytochrome C (12.5 K). B, 45 μg protein from cell walls of the bacterial form. C, 45 μg protein from cell walls of filament form. Results were reported previously in (14).

membranes, which represent the amounts of the various components that mice received per injection.

Based on these analyses, certain changes in the quantitative composition of the various cell surface components after treatment of P. mirabilis VI with antibiotics can be observed. Significant differences in comparison with the amounts of these components determined in the bacterial form cell walls include an increase in the amounts of phospholipids in the spheroplast cell walls and in the protoplast membranes, as well as a decrease in the amount of LPS in protoplast membranes.

Although the filament form showed no significant quantitative differences, a qualitative change in the outer membrane protein pattern was observed (Figure 1). In cell walls of the bacterial form, four major outer membrane proteins with apparent molecular weights of 39 K, 36 K, 19 K and 15 K can be detected. The outer membrane protein pattern of the filament form showed an apparent decrease in the amount of the 39 K protein, which was consistent from batch to batch of isolated cell walls. Further work will have to be carried out in order to determine if this is a true decrease or an alteration in the sensitivity of the 39 K protein to heat modification. In this regard, it was recently reported (18) that treatment of opaque clones of Neisseria gonorrhoeae with subinhibitory concentrations of antibiotics led to incomplete heat modification of an outer membrane protein. Thus, the possibility exists that the 39 K protein of P. mirabilis, which is heat modifiable (Bub, Bieker and Nixdorff, unpublished observations), was altered in this respect by treatment of the bacterium with subinhibitory concentrations of cefuroxime. When this protein is not modified by heat treatment, it migrates in the same position as the 36 K outer membrane protein in SDS-polyacrylamide gels, so that an alteration to reduced sensitivity to heat modification would not be detected in our system. Nevertheless, the surface structure of the filament form was altered, as observed in the strong tendency of filament cell walls to aggregate, which was not characteristic of the other cell forms of P. mirabilis VI. Studies to resolve this question are presently being carried out.

The outer membrane protein pattern of the spheroplast L-form was similar to that of the bacterial form (14). The cytoplasmic membrane protein pattern of the protoplast L-form showed no resemblance to that of the bacterial cell wall proteins (4).

Response in Mice to LPS Contained in Surface Structures of the Various Cell Forms of P. mirabilis VI

Table 3 presents the data for the secondary IgM and IgG subclass responses to LPS contained in cell walls of the bacterial form, the filament form and the spheroplast L-form, and in cytoplasmic membranes of the protoplast L-form of P. mirabilis VI. Compared with the responses to LPS contained in bacterial cell walls, the IgG responses to LPS contained in cell walls of the filament form were much weaker, although the IgG subclass distribution was very similar. No significant quantitative differences in the IgM responses was observed.

Both the IgM and the IgG subclass responses to LPS contained in cell walls of the spheroplast L-form were somewhat stronger than the responses to LPS in bacterial cell walls, but, once again, the distribution of IgG subclasses of PFC was similar.

The responses to LPS contained in cytoplasmic membranes of the protoplast L-form were also strong, despite the reduced amounts of LPS injected (6 nmol beta-hydroxy myristic acid as compared to 30-40 nmol per injection with bacterial, filament or spheroplast cell walls). However, an alteration

Table 3. Secondary IgM and IgG Subclass Responses in Mice to LPS Contained in Cell Walls of the Bacterial Form, the Filament Form and the Spheroplast L-Form, and in Cytoplasmic Membranes of the Protoplast L-Form of P. mirabilis VI

Immunogen[a]	Antibody Type	PFC/10^6 spleen cells[b] on day 18	% IgG Subclass of total IgG
Bacterial cell walls	IgM	199 ± 62	-
	IgG1	94 ± 17	25
	IgG2	207 ± 23	55
	IgG3	75 ± 12	20
Filament cell walls	IgM	184 ± 35	-
	IgG1	32 ± 6	25
	IgG2	74 ± 29	59
	IgG3	20 ± 3	16
Spheroplast L-form cell walls	IgM	473 ± 87	-
	IgG1	400 ± 178	33
	IgG2	586 ± 172	49
	IgG3	216 ± 34	18
Protoplast L-form membranes	IgM	438 ± 10	-
	IgG1	445 ± 39	52
	IgG2	233 ± 89	27
	IgG3	182 ± 47	21

[a]Dosages per injection were 0.25 mg cell walls of the bacterial form, the filament form and the spheroplast L-form, or 0.25 mg cytoplasmic membranes of the protoplast L-form. Mice received a primary injection on day 0 and a secondary injection on day 14.

[b]Geometric means ± standard errors of PFC. Values are the results of 3 separate experiments. Responses were measured against P. mirabilis VI LPS coupled to SRBC.

in the IgG subclass distribution was observed, as reflected in the predominant induction of IgG2 PFC. This was in contrast to the predominant induction of IgG2 PFC when cell walls of the bacterial, filament or spheroplast forms were used as immunogens. It is very likely that this alteration in IgG subclass distribution is due to the modulating effects of cytoplasmic membrane proteins quite different from the types of proteins present in the cell wall of P. mirabilis VI (4). According to the results summarized in Table 1, different proteins in complex with LPS can effect the induction of IgG responses that have different subclass distributions. Phospholipids can also effect the selective induction of IgG1 PFC in this system. However, it is unlikely that the two-fold increase in the amount of phospholipids in protoplast membranes (see Table 2) is entirely responsible for the predominant IgG1 responses, as this same increase in phospholipids in spheroplast cell walls had little effect on the subclass distribution.

Perhaps the most notable result was the lack of enhancement of IgG-producing cells in the case of the responses to LPS contained in filament cell walls (Table 3). The only alteration in the composition of components detected in cell walls of the filament form was the apparent decrease in the 39 K outer membrane protein (Figure 1). If this apparent decrease is real, then one factor determining the lack of enhancement of IgG PFC might be the ratio of 39 K protein to 36 K protein. The 39 K protein is relatively soluble in aqueous buffers, and complexes of this protein with LPS lead to strong enhancement of IgG responses (Table 1). The 36 K protein aggregates more readily (as do filament form cell walls), and solubilized complexes of the protein with LPS give no enhancement of IgG responses to LPS (Karch, Mark and Nixdorff, unpublished results).

It could be that lack of IgG enhancement is due to aggregation of filament cell walls, which might lead to reduced stimulation. However, the normal IgM responses to LPS contained in filament cell walls would speak against this interpretation. Alternatively, either the mixture of LPS with the 36 K protein does not stimulate T cells that are necessary for IgG responses, or the mixture of LPS with the 36 K protein induces a suppression of the IgG responses.

We feel that a suppression of the IgG responses to LPS contained in filament cell walls is indicated. Otherwise, one would expect that various modulators of the IgG responses to LPS present in the filament cell walls (including the reduced amounts of the 39 K protein) would be able to enhance the IgG responses. Thus, the ratio of the amounts of the 36 K protein to the amounts of enhancing components may be critical in this system. Regarding suppression of LPS responses, it has been reported that T cells induced by complexes of myelin basic protein with LPS suppressed mitogenic responses of lymph node cells to both myelin basic protein and LPS (15). Studies designed to determine if a suppression of the IgG responses to LPS is actually induced by complexes of LPS with the 36 K protein of P. mirabilis are now underway.

ACKNOWLEDGEMENT

This work was supported by the Deutsche Forschungsgemeinschaft.

REFERENCES

1. J. Gmeiner and H. H. Martin, Phospholipid and lipopolysaccharide in Proteus mirabilis and its stable protoplast L-form. Difference in content and fatty acid composition, Eur. J. Biochem. 67:487 (1976).
2. N. K. Jerne and A. A. Nordin, Plaque formation in agar by single antibody-producing cells, Science 140:405 (1963).
3. H. Karch, J. Gmeiner and K. Nixdorff, Alteration of the immunoglobulin G subclass responses in mice to lipopolysaccharide: Effects of nonbacterial proteins and bacterial membrane phospholipids or outer membrane proteins of Proteus mirabilis, Infect. Immun. 40:157 (1983).
4. H. Karch and K. Nixdorff, Comparison of quantitative and qualitative antibody-producing cell responses to lipopolysaccharide in cell walls of the bacterial form and in membranes of the protoplast L-form of Proteus mirabilis, Infect. Immun. 30:349 (1980).
5. H. Karch and K. Nixdorff, Antibody-producing cell responses to an isolated outer membrane protein and to complexes of this antigen with lipopolysaccharide or with vesicles of phospholipids from Proteus mirabilis, Infect. Immun. 31:862 (1981).
6. H. Karch and K. Nixdorff, Modulation of the IgG subclass responses to lipopolysaccharide by bacterial membrane components: Differential adjuvant effects produced by primary and secondary stimulation, J. Immunol. 131:6 (1983).

7. H. -P. Kroll, J. Gmeiner and H. H. Martin, Membranes of the protoplast L-form of Proteus mirabilis, Arch. Microbiol. 127:223 (1980).
8. B. Lugtenberg, J. Meijers, R. Peters, P. van der Hoek and L. van Alphen, Electrophoretic resolution of the "major outer membrane protein" of Escherichia coli K12 into four bands, FEBS Lett. 58:254 (1975).
9. M. A. K. Markwell, S. M. Haar, L. L. Bieber and E. Tolbert, A modification of the Lowry procedure to simplify protein determination in membrane and lipoprotein samples, Anal. Biochem. 37:206 (1978).
10. H. H. Martin, Composition of the mucopolymer in cell walls of the unstable and stable L-form of Proteus mirabilis, J. Gen. Microbiol. 36:441 (1964).
11. H. H. Martin, D. Staboulis and W. Schilf, Penicillinbindeproteine als spezifische Wirkorte der beta-Lactam-Antibiotika und als Faktoren der Antibiotika-Resistenz, Immun. Infekt. 3:99 (1981).
12. R. I. Mishell and D. W. Dutton, Immunization of dissociated spleen cell cultures from normal mice, J. Exp. Med. 126:423 (1967).
13. K. Nixdorff, H. Fitzer, J. Gmeiner and H. H. Martin, Reconstitution of model membranes from phospholipid and outer membrane proteins of Proteus mirabilis. Role of proteins in the formation of hydrophilic pores and protection of membranes against detergents, Eur. J. Biochem. 81:63 (1977).
14. K. Nixdorff, H. H. Martin and N. Siegmund-Schultze, Changes in outer membrane composition after treatment of Proteus mirabilis with antibiotics, in: "The Influence of Antibiotics on the Host-Parasite Relationship II," D. Adam, H. Hahn and W. Opferkuch, eds., Springer-Verlag, Berlin, Heidelberg, New York, in press (1985).
15. S. Raziuddin, R. F. Kibler and D. C. Morrison, Immunosuppression of experimental allergic encephalomyelitis. III. In vitro evidence for induction of suppressor T lymphocytes in draining lymph node cells of animals immunized with myelin basic protein complexed to lipopolysaccharides, J. Immunol. 128:2073 (1982).
16. E. Ruttkowski and K. Nixdorff, Qualitative and quantitative changes in the antibody-producing cell responses to lipopolysaccharide induced after incorporation of the antigen into bacterial membrane phospholipid vesicles, J. Immunol. 124:2548 (1980).
17. S. Schlecht and O. Westphal, Uber die Herstellung von Antiseren gegen die somatischen (O-) Antigene von Salmonellen. II. Mitteilung: Untersuchungen uber Hamagglutinintiter, Zentralbl. Bakteriol. Parasitenkd. Infektionskr. Hyg. Abt. I. Orig. 205:487 (1967).
18. D. S. Stephens, Effect of antibiotics on surface proteins of Neisseria gonorrhoeae, in: "The Influence of Antibiotics on the Host-Parasite Relationship," D. Adam, H. Hahn and W. Opferkuch, eds., Springer-Verlag, Berlin, Heidelberg, New York, in press (1985).
19. U. Taubeneck, Untersuchungen über die L-form von Proteus mirabilis Hauser. II. Entwicklung und Wesen der L-form, Z. Mikrobiol. 2:132 (1962).

ANTIBIOTIC MODIFICATION OF BACTERIAL SUSCEPTIBILITY TO HOST IMMUNITY

Herman Friedman[1] and George Warren[2]

[1]Departments of Medical Microbiology and Immunology
University of South Florida College of Medicine
Tampa, Florida, and [2]Thomas Jefferson University School of Medicine, Philadelphia, Pennsylvania

It is axiomatic that antibiotics influence microorganisms directly. However, recent evidence from a number of laboratories, including ours, has focused attention on the influence of antibiotics on host immune mechanisms and alteration of susceptibility of the microorganism to the immune response system (1-9,12,15). For example, studies in this laboratory have shown that the semisynthetic penicillins such as cyclacillin or ampicillin may modify susceptible bacteria, such as Escherichia coli, to increased vulnerability to antibody mediated complement dependent bacterial lysis as well as increased susceptibility to phagocytosis by macrophages. Pretreatment of E. coli with subinhibitory concentrations of such semisynthetic penicillins but not Penicillin G itself markedly increased the susceptibility of the bacteria to host immune factors, even after repeated washing of the bacteria in vitro (2-8). The pretreated bacteria showed markedly increased susceptibility to bacteriolysis by antibody and complement. They were also phagocytized much more rapidly by blood or spleen monocytes, as well as peritoneal macrophages or adherent splenocytes. In addition, macrophages from adjuvant stimulated animals, including those given either Bacillus Calmette Guerin (BCG) or muramyl dipeptide (MDP), the small molecular adjuvant of mycobacteria and other bacteria, showed even greater activity against antibiotic treated E. coli (7). Macrophages which had ingested these E. coli also showed higher levels of immunogenic cell surface components of the bacteria as compared to phagocytes which had ingested untreated bacteria. The macrophages from mice which phagocytized antibiotic-pretreated and washed bacteria contained increased immunogenic moities of the bacteria as shown by subsequent injection of cell free extracts of the cells into recipient animals (4).

General Experimental Methods and Procedures

For these studies a penicillin resistant strain of E. coli was used exactly as described previously (3,5-8). The bacteria were cultured in vitro on brain heart infusion agar and after 18 hours at 37°C were harvested, washed with sterile saline and resuspended to a concentration of 10^8 viable bacteria per ml as determined by standard agar plate count. Cyclacillin and ampicillin, as well as Penicillin G, were obtained from Wyeth Laboratories, Radnor, PA and dissolved in sterile physiological saline before use as described (3,5-8). For antibody studies, rabbits were immunized with 10^8 heat killed E. coli and one to two weeks after final immunization serum was pooled from individual animals. The rabbits were given four to five injections of bacteria at weekly intervals over a period of four to six months prior to obtaining the first blood specimens and about ten days after the last injection serum was obtained. The titer of the pooled serum was generally 1:1280 or higher by microagglutination tests in which serial 0.25 ml dilutions of serum were incubated in 96 well microtiter plates to which were added equal volumes of a 10^8 suspension of heat killed E. coli. After 1 to 2 hours incubation at 37°C and 18 hours at 4°C the titer was determined as the reciprocal of the highest dilution of serum resulting in complete agglutination of the bacteria in each well. Addition of 0.1 ml of a 1:10 dilution of sterile guinea pig serum to individual wells, plus 10^7 viable E. coli, was used for bacteriolytic tests. After two hours incubation at 37°C the number of viable E. coli present in individual wells was determined by quantitative plate assays to calculate bacteriolytic titers (10).

Phagocytic tests were performed with normal cells from Balb/c mice weighing 16 to 18 grams each. The mice were injected intraperitoneally with 5 ml saline 15 minutes earlier. The peritoneal cells were pooled from individual mice sedimented by centrifugation at 1000 x g at 4°C and resuspended in medium 199 containing 10% fetal calf serum. The cells were then washed twice with medium and allowed to adhere to plastic plates for one hour at 37°C. The non-adherent cells were decanted and adherent cells harvested by scrapping with a sterile rubber policeman. The resulting cells were resuspended to a concentration of 10^6 nucleated cells per ml. Microscopic examination indicated over 90% were morphologically similar to macrophages and that these cells readily phagocytized latex particles within fifteen minutes. In some cases, adherent cells were similarly prepared from the spleen of mice and resuspended to a concentration of 10^6 cells per ml. Over 90% of these cells also phagocytized latex particles. For phagocytic assays suspensions of 10^6 nucleated cells were added to individual wells of 24 well Limbro plates. To each well was then added 1 ml of a suspension of 10^7 E. coli either untreated or previously treated with an antibiotic as indicated. The cultures were incubated in an atmosphere of 95% air and 5% CO_2 for varying periods of time, generally up to four hours. Samples of each culture were placed on microscopic slides, which were then stained with Giemsa and examined microscopically. At least 300 cells were examined per sample per slide. The numbers of E. coli present in the macrophages were scored and the percent of macrophages containing two or more phagocytized bacteria was determined (2,5). For killing experiments, the macrophage E. coli suspensions were pelleted by centrifugation at 2000 x G for ten minutes. The bacteria in the supernatant were counted by plate assay, using serial dilutions. The sedimented macrophages were resuspended in medium, disrupted by freezing and thawing three times and the number of viable bacteria determined by plate counting. In some experiments, macrophages were obtained from mice injected intraperitoneally with 1 mg BCG as the non-specific immunologic stimulator (8,15). In other experiments, mice were injected two to three days earlier with 20 μg MDP obtained from the Pasteur Institute (8,10).

EXPERIMENTAL RESULTS

The E. coli used in these experiments were equally susceptible to cyclacillin and ampicillin but not to Penicillin G. As shown in Table 1, the bacteria grew well in the liver, lung, and spleen of control animals which had not been given an antibiotic. When the mice were injected with Penicillin G (1 million units or more) immediately prior to injection of E. coli or one to 24 hours previously, there was essentially no effect on the growth of the E. coli in these organs of the mice. However, animals given ampicillin or cyclacillin at the same time as challenge with E. coli or 24 hours earlier showed a marked decrease in the number of E. coli in the liver, lung and spleen. At 48 to 96 hours the animals were essentially

Table 1. Comparative Effects of Semisynthetic Penicillins and Penicillin G on Survival of E. coli in Mice

In Vivo Treatment with Antibiotic[a]	E. coli in tissue[b]		
	Liver	Lung	Spleen
None (control)	$> 10^6$	$> 10^6$	$> 10^6$
Ampicillin	2.3×10^2	1.4×10^2	3.9×10^3
Cyclacillin	2.9×10^3	1.8×10^2	1.2×10^4
Penicillin G	$> 10^6$	$> 10^6$	$> 10^6$

[a]Mice infected i.p. with 10^5 E. coli and 1.0 mg of ampicillin or cyclacillin or 10^6 units Penicillin G on day 0.
[b]Average number of E. coli per gm indicated tissue 24-48 hours after injection with E. coli and indicated antibiotic.

sterile as far as E. coli was concerned in these organs. The normal control animals and those given penicillin generally succumbed to 10^8 E. coli unless they were treated with other antibiotics (data not shown).

Subinhibitory concentrations of cyclacillin or ampicillin had marked effects on the susceptibility of the E. coli to lysis by antibody and complement. Pretreatment of the bacteria with these antibiotics, but not Penicillin G, made these bacteria much more susceptible to lysis (Table 2). For example, pretreatment of the bacteria with either cyclacillin or

Table 2. Effect of Pretreatment of E. coli with Graded Doses of Antibiotics on In Vitro Bacteriolytic Titers with Antisera and Complement

Antibiotic addition to E. coli in vitro (μg/10^7 bacteria)[a]		Bacteriolytic titer[b]	
		with complement	no complement (control)
None (control)		1:160	< 1:10
Cyclacillin	10.0	1:320	1:20
	5.0	1:1280	1:20
	2.5	1:960	1:40
	1.0	1:320	< 1:10
Ampicillin	10.0	1:640	< 1:10
	5.0	1:1220	1:20
	2.5	1:960	1:10
	1.0	1:960	< 1:10
Penicillin G	100 U	1:240	< 1:10
	50	1:160	< 1:10
	10	1:160	< 1:10

[a]Washed 18 hour cultures of E. coli (10^8 bacteria/ml) incubated at 4° with graded concentrations of indicated antibiotic before washing and incubation at 37° with serial two fold dilutions of anti-E. coli rabbit serum, with or without 1:10 dilution of sterile guinea pig complement.
[b]Average bacteriolytic titer for 3-4 duplicate titrations.

Table 3. Effect of Time of Pretreatment of E. coli In Vitro with Antibiotic on Susceptibility to Bacteriolysis by Serum and Complement

Antibiotic treatment of E. coli[a]	Time of incubation (hrs)	Serum dilution 1:80	1:160	1:320	1:640	1:1280	1:2560
None (control)	4	0[b]	1+	2+	4+	4+	4+
Ampicillin	1	0	0	2+	4+	4+	4+
	2	0	0	1+	2+	4+	4+
	4	0	0	0	±	2+	4+
Cyclacillin	1	0	0	2+	4+	4+	4+
	2	0	0	0	±	2+	4+
	4	0	0	0	±	1+	4+
Penicillin G	4	0	±	2+	3+	4+	4+

[a]Suspensions of 10^8 E. coli per ml medium containing 2.0 μg ampicillin or cyclacillin or 100V Penicillin G; bacteria incubated for indicated time in hours at 4°C before washing and testing for susceptibility to bacteriolysis by indicating dilution of rabbit anti-E. coli serum and 1:10 dilution of guinea pig complement.
[b]Growth of E. coli after 18 hour culture at 37°C in presence of indicated dilution of serum and complement; 0 = no growth, 4 = complete growth.

ampicillin increased the apparent titer of the serum antibody several fold compared to treatment of the same bacteria with Penicillin G or no treatment. There was greater killing by the antibody and complement using cyclacillin or ampicillin pretreated E. coli by two hours as compared to controls. However, even one hour pretreatment resulted in some increase in susceptibility of the pretreated bacteria (Table 3). No killing occurred in the absence of specific antibody or complement.

Pretreatment of E. coli with similar amounts of cyclacillin or ampicillin also increased the uptake of the bacteria and their destruction in the liver and spleen of normal animals. As seen in Table 4, E. coli after

Table 4. Uptake of Antibiotic Pretreated E. coli in Normal Mice

Antibiotic Treatment of E. coli		E. coli in tissue[b] Blood (30 min.)	Liver (24 hr.)	Spleen (24 hr.)
None (control)		2.1×10^2	8.3×10^3	3.9×10^5
Ampicillin	5.0 μg	0.9×10^2	3.1×10^3	1.8×10^3
	1.0	1.0×10^2	2.1×10^3	7.3×10^2
Cyclacillin	5.0	1.0×10^2	1.1×10^3	6.9×10^4
	1.0	1.2×10^2	8.6×10^2	6.5×10^3
Penicillin G	20.0	3.8×10^2	5.1×10^4	2.1×10^5

[a]Suspensions of 10^8 E. coli pretreated for 2 hours at 4°C with indicated doses of antibiotic prior to washing and injection into Balb/c mice.
[b]Average number of E. coli cfu per ml blood or gram tissue determined by bacterial plate count at indicated time after injection into normal mice.

Table 5. Effect of Antibiotic Treatment on Subsequent Phagocytosis of E. coli by Normal Mouse Peritoneal Cells

Antibiotic treatment of E. coli in vitro[a]		E. coli presence: Macrophage culture — Whole cell extract	Macrophage culture — Cell free extract[b] ($\times 10^2$)	Cell free medium ($\times 10^3$)[c]
None (control)		7.5 ± 1.3	14.8 ± 21.0	36.5 ± 2.3
Ampicillin	5.0 μg	26.5 ± 2.5	2.1 ± 0.4	12.5 ± 1.2
	1.0	21.3 ± 2.7	1.3 ± 0.5	18.6 ± 2.5
Cyclacillin	5.0	28.2 ± 3.4	3.2 ± 0.7	14.2 ± 2.1
	1.0	22.1 ± 2.5	2.0 ± 0.5	15.5 ± 3.1
Penicillin G	20 U	9.3 ± 1.2	10.3 ± 0.9	32.5 ± 3.0

[a]Suspensions of 10^6 washed E. coli pretreated for 2 hours with indicated antibiotic before exposure to 10^6 adherent peritoneal cells from normal mice.

[b]Percent macrophages, ± S.D., with 2 or more E. coli after 60 minutes incubation with untreated or antibiotic pretreated E. coli.

[c]Presence of viable E. coli (number ± S.D.) for 0.5 ml cell-free macrophage extracts or culture supernatant.

treatment with subinhibitory concentrations of these antibiotics, followed by washing, were much more rapidly removed from the blood of injected mice within 30 minutes and fewer viable organisms were present. At 24 hours there was little difference in survival of untreated E. coli or E. coli pretreated with Penicillin G.

Similar results occurred in terms of in vitro phagocytosis, i.e. pretreatment of E. coli with cyclacillin or ampicillin at subinhibitory concentrations increased their phagocytosis by the mouse peritoneal cells (Table 5). More macrophages contained two or more bacteria after incubation with antibiotic pretreated bacteria as compared to macrophages incubated with nontreated bacteria or those which had been pretreated with Penicillin G as a control. Furthermore, assessment of the number of viable bacteria per cell-free lysate of these macrophages showed fewer viable E. coli present when antibiotic pretreatment occurred prior to washing of the bacteria and exposure to the phagocytes. In addition, determination of the number of extracellular bacteria in the medium after exposure of the pretreated bacteria to the phagocytes showed that more bacteria were taken up by macrophages incubated with cyclacillin or ampicillin pretreated E. coli as compared to those which had been incubated previously with Penicillin G.

Even more enhanced phagocytosis occurred when cyclacillin or ampicillin pretreated bacteria were exposed to macrophages from mice which had been injected with BCG or MDP as adjuvants to activate macrophages (Table 6). Although more phagocytosis occurred with macrophages from these animals after incubation *in vitro* with nonantibiotic treated E. coli as compared uptake of E. coli pretreated with Penicillin G or not treated at all, there was a two to three-fold greater increase in the percentage of macrophages which ingested ampicillin or cyclacillin pretreated E. coli when the macrophage donors were injected with BCG or MDP (Table 6).

Antibiotic pretreatment appeared to make the E. coli much more susceptible to antibody mediated bacteriolysis or phagocytosis. Thus, experiments

Table 6. Effect of Antibiotic Pretreatment of E. coli on Subsequent Phagocytosis by Peritoneal Macrophages from Normal or Adjuvant-Treated Mice

Antibiotic pretreatment of E. coli[a]		Mouse macrophage tested[b]		
		Normal	BCG treated[c]	MDP treated[c]
None (control)		6.5 ± 2.1	13.2 ± 4.1	11.3 ± 2.3
Ampicillin	5.0 µg	21.4 ± 3.4	36.1 ± 4.5	30.1 ± 2.8
	1.0	19.3 ± 2.1	30.3 ± 2.6	27.3 ± 3.1
Cyclacillin	5.0	21.5 ± 4.2	39.3 ± 4.0	36.5 ± 3.8
	1.0	18.4 ± 3.1	36.2 ± 2.8	30.3 ± 4.0
Penicillin G	20 U	6.9 ± 1.9	10.6 ± 2.8	11.9 ± 2.4

[a]Indicated antibiotic used to pretreat 10^8 E. coli for 2 hours before assay for phagocytosis.
[b]Average percentage of PE cells, ± S.D., phagocytizing 2 or more E. coli after incubation for 2 hours at 37°C.
[c]Donor mice injected 7 days earlier with 1.0 mg BCG or 2-3 days earlier with 50 µg MDP.

were performed to determine whether antibiotic pretreatment of the E. coli before exposure to macrophages resulted in more immunogenic bacterial material in the cells as compared to macrophages containing E. coli which had not been pretreated with an antibiotic. As shown in Table 7, cyclacillin or ampicillin pretreated E. coli, but not the control E. coli or those which had been pretreated with Penicillin G, resulted in much more immunogenic components present in the macrophage extracts upon injection into normal indicator mice, inducing a higher level of antibody to E. coli. In addition, these macrophage extracts, when injected into normal mice, resulted

Table 7. Effect of Antibiotic Pretreatment of E. coli on the Ability of Phagocytized Bacteria to Induce Anti-E. coli Antibody Forming Cells in Recipient Mice

Antibiotic Pretreatment of E. coli		Antibody response[b]	
		Agglutinin titer	Anti-E. coli PFC
None (control)		1:480	383 ± 72
Ampicillin	5.0 µg	1:1280	650 ± 48
	1.0	1:1280	495 ± 32
Cyclacillin	5.0	1:1280	586 ± 47
	1.0	1:960	542 ± 30
Penicillin G	20.0 U	1:480	310 ± 60

[a]Indicated antibiotic used to pretreated 10^8 E. coli for 2 hours prior to phagocytosis by 10^6 normal mouse peritoneal cells.
[b]Average antibody response for 3-4 normal mice per group injected 8-10 days earlier with 1.0 ml of cell-free extract of PE cells which phagocytized E. coli; control mice given extract of 10^6 normal peritoneal cells had anti-E. coli titer of 1:20 and fewer than 100 PFC per spleen.

Table 8. Effect of Antibiotic on Immunogenicity of E. coli Shown by Ability of Treated Bacteria to Induce Bacteriolytic PFC

Antibiotic pretreatment of E. coli[a]		Anti-E. coli PFC on day[b]			
		+3	+6	+10	+15
None (control)		121 ± 15	865 ± 32	652 ± 42	210 ± 16
Ampicillin	5.0 μg	265 ± 40	1830 ± 240	1445 ± 62	325 ± 40
	1.0	210 ± 32	1750 ± 138	1230 ± 130	428 ± 60
Cyclacillin	5.0	242 ± 19	1563 ± 120	1230 ± 41	652 ± 30
	1.0	152 ± 20	1410 ± 193	1140 ± 160	570 ± 48

[a]Indicated antibiotic used to pretreat 10^8 E. coli for 2 hours before washing and injection into recipient mice.
[b]Average number of anti-E. coli PFC, ± S.D., on indicated day for spleen cells from 3-4 mice per group.

in increased numbers of anti-E. coli antibody plaque forming cells. In addition, greater responses were apparent when these macrophage extracts were injected into mice which had been primed four to five weeks earlier with E. coli vaccine (data not shown). Thus, the cyclacillin or ampicillin pretreated E. coli incubated with macrophages from normal mice not only were taken up in greater numbers but also were much more immunogenic and components of the bacteria appeared in the macrophages as shown by the ability of extracts of these cells to increase antibody responses to E. coli in recipient animals, either normal or antigen primed. Control experiments showed that these macrophage extracts did not induce increased antibody responses to other bacteria such as Salmonella or Legionella, so that the immunogenic component appeared to be a specific antigen(s) of the E. coli.

In order to study in more detail whether antibiotic pretreated E. coli, as compared to controls consisting of Penicillin G treated bacteria, were indeed more immunogenic, the bacteria were injected directly into mice and specific anti-E. coli PFCs determined at various times thereafter (Tables 7 and 8). The untreated E. coli, as a control, induced a large number of PFCs upon injection directly into normal recipient mice. Injection of similar numbers of E. coli which had been pretreated with cyclacillin or ampicillin for 1 to 2 hours resulted in even greater numbers of PFCs to E. coli, indicating that these bacteria, although not inhibited in their growth capacity by these antibiotics, nevertheless appeared to develop more potent immunogenic capacity as shown by their ability to induce larger numbers of specific antibody forming cells.

DISCUSSION AND CONCLUSIONS

There is now much evidence that antibiotic pretreated bacteria become more susceptible to a host's defense system, either cellular or humoral, as compared to untreated bacteria. This probably occurs because the bacteria may be altered after exposure to an antibiotic even at a subinhibitory concentration. Filamentous forms of a bacteria often develop after exposing the organism to even subinhibitory concentrations of an effective antibiotic (9,13,15). Such doses of the antibiotic do not appear to interfere with the viability of the bacteria in vitro. Similar numbers of colony-forming units are usually observed for such antibiotic pretreated bacteria as compared to untreated ones. Moreover, a number of previous studies from many laboratories, including this one, have shown that antibiotic pretreatment of some bacteria with subinhibitory doses of antimicrobial agents results in increased susceptibility of the bacteria to phagocytosis by macrophages, both in vivo and in vitro. As shown in the present study, as well as in previous ones, peritoneal cells from normal mice or even mice treated with conventional adjuvants such as BCG or MDP show an increased ability to phagocytize and kill E. coli pretreated with subinhibitory doses of the semisynthetic penicillins, cyclacillin and ampicillin, but not with an antibiotic to which they are resistant such as Penicillin G. This effect appeared due to a direct influence of the antibiotic on the bacteria since the organisms were washed extensively before injection into the animals or addition to macrophages from normal or adjuvant pretreated animals.

Macrophages appeared to be able to degrade E. coli into more potent immunogens when the bacteria were pretreated with the subinhibitory doses of the semisynthetic antibiotic as compared to bacteria which had not been so pretreated. In addition, incubation of peritoneal cells from normal mice or mice which had been pretreated with BCG or MDP showed increased immunogenicity in terms of the ability of cell-free extracts to result in increased numbers of specific anti-E. coli antibody forming cells upon subsequent injection into normal recipient mice. There is some question, however, as to whether or not the increased immunogenicity of the macrophage extracts could be due to increased amounts of antigen or because larger numbers of bacteria were present in each macrophage. Since the macrophages exposed to cyclacillin or ampicillin pretreated bacteria contained more bacteria, it is possible that this could account for the apparent increased immunogenicity. It is also possible, however, that the bacteria which were more readily phagocytized could have been digested readily into larger amounts of immunogenic fragments after being first pretreated with the antibiotic.

Further studies quantitating the amount of immunogen in macrophages should be performed, including experiments in which different amounts of an extract of macrophages which had been exposed to different numbers of E. coli treated for different time periods with antibiotics are used in similar experiments. The role of pretreatment of the bacteria in resistance to further infection should also be determined. Exposure of a host to larger amounts of immunogenic components of a bacteria may be important in secondary resistance to infection. The ability of antibiotic pretreatment to make a bacterium such as E. coli more susceptible to antibody, as well as phagocytosis, may be important in the early events following infection and thus antibiotic treatment even with subinhibitory doses may be of value. More studies are warranted to investigate these possibilities in depth.

REFERENCES

1. H. Friedman and G. H. Warren, Antibacterial activity of cyclacillin in vivo and in vitro: Effects on Gram negative organisms, Prog. Chemother. 2:119 (1984).
2. H. Friedman and G. H. Warren, Enhanced susceptibility of penicillin-resistant staphylococci to phagocytosis after in vitro incubation with low doses of nafcillin, Proc. Soc. Exp. Biol. Med. 146:207 (1974).
3. H. Friedman and G. H. Warren, Antibody-mediated bacteriolysis: Enhanced killing of Cyclacillin treated bacteria, Proc. Soc. Exp. Biol. Med. 153:301 (1976).
4. H. Friedman and G. H. Warren, Cyclacillin-induced potentiation of Escherichia coli immunogenicity in vivo and in vitro, Chemotherapy 23:324 (1977).

5. H. Friedman and G. H. Warren, Increased phagocytosis of Escherichia coli pretreated with subinhibitory concentrations of cyclacillin or ampicillin, Proc. Soc. Exp. Biol. Med. 169:301 (1982).
6. H. Friedman and G. H. Warren, Increased susceptibility of bacteria treated with subinhibitory concentrations of antibiotics to phagocytosis and killing, Interscience Conf. Antibiotic Chemotherapy 23:178 (1983).
7. H. Friedman and G. H. Warren, Muramyl dipeptide-induced enhancement of phagocytosis of antibiotic pretreated Escherichia coli by macrophages, Proc. Soc. Exp. Biol. Med. 176:765 (1984).
8. H. Friedman, Synergism between the Host Defense Mechanism and Antibiotic Treatment of Bacteria, Zbl. Bakt. Suppl. 13:104 (1985).
9. G. Gillissen, Antibiotics and immune response, concomitant effect of chemotherapy, Immunitat und Infektion 8:79 (1980).
10. E. Lederer, Immunomodulation by muramylpeptides: Recent developments, Clin. Immunol. Newsletter 3:83 (1982).
11. P. J. McDonald, B. L. Wetherall and H. Druel, Post-antibiotic leukocyte enhancement. Increased susceptibility of bacteria pretreated with antibiotics to activity of leukocytes, Rev. Infect. Dis. 3:38 (1981).
12. A. M. Munster, C. B. Loodholdt, A. G. Leary and M. A. Barnes, Effect of antibiotics on cell-mediated immunity, Surgery 81:692 (1977).
13. R. K. Root, R. Istunz, A. Molavi, J. A. Metcalf and H. L. Malech, Interaction between antibiotics and human neutrophile in the killing of staphylococci. Studies with normal and cytochalasin B treated cells, J. Clin. Invest. 67:247 (1981).
14. P. W. Taylor, H. Gaunt and F. M. Unger, Effect of subinhibitory concentrations of mecillinam on the serum susceptibility of E. coli strains, Antimicrob. Agents Chemother. 19:786 (1981).
15. K. Vosbeck, H. Handschin, A. -B. Menge and G. Zak, Effects of subinhibitory concentrations of antibiotics on adhesiveness of Escherichia coli in vitro, Rev. Infect. Dis. 1:845 (1979).
16. Y. Yamamura and I. Azuma, Immunostimulation in cancer patients by biological response modifiers, Adv. Exp. Med. Biol. 166:1 (1982).

SECTION III
INFLUENCE OF ANTIBIOTICS ON HOST DEFENSES IN VIVO

ANTIBIOTICS AND HOST DEFENSE IN IMMUNOCOMPROMISED PATIENTS

Paul G. Quie

American Legion Heart Research
University of Minnesota Medical School
Minneapolis, Minnesota

INTRODUCTION

The clinical success of antibiotics permits patients with primary and acquired immune deficiency to survive infections. As a consequence, it is possible for investigators to compare functional aspects of the immune system in these patients with normal persons. These studies have contributed greatly to our knowledge of human host defense systems. The topic of this chapter will be host defenses in patients with identifiable defects in their immune system. We are grateful to these patients for what they have taught us about human physiology.

FACTORS OF THE IMMUNE SYSTEM INVOLVED IN HOST DEFENSE

The immune system is a highly complex integration of cellular and humoral factors with striking interdependence and exquisite control mechanisms. Normal host resistance to infection requires functional integrity of all aspects of the immune system but it is necessary to divide the system in separate parts for clarity of presentation.

Phagocytic System

The phagocytic system consists of circulating and fixed phagocytes. The primary circulating phagocytic cells are the granulocytes and the primary fixed phagocytic cells are macrophages which reside in juxtaposition to blood and lymph in all organ systems of the body. Several examples of congenital and acquired deficiency of the circulating granulocytes have been described but macrophage disorders are less common. The clinical syndrome, chronic granulomatous disease, clearly demonstrates the importance of normal granulocyte function for normal host defense (8). Dysfunction of macrophages occur in patients that have had a splenectomy or who suffer acute hemolytic disorders.

Complement System

The complement system consists of nine essential serum proteins which are designated C1 through C9 and several other proteins which have either co-factor or inhibitory activity. There may be primary dysfunction of the complement system on the basis of congenital absence of one of the sequential proteins or secondary to inappropriate complement activation. Low serum complement levels are found in patients with severe septic shock.

Activated components of the complement system function in host defense against invading microbes as factors involved in chemotaxis, opsonization and actual killing of microbes. A recognition unit of complement either combines with the Fc fragment of antibody molecules attached to antigens or is activated by the alternative pathway and this specific combination of complement proteins has enzymatic activity for activating C3 into biologically active opsonins. Complement opsonins attach to bacteria or other particles and are ligands for phagocytic cells which have appropriate receptors. Other complement proteins become chemotactic factors which attract phagocytic cells to inflammatory sites.

Complement may also be involved in direct killing of susceptible bacteria. _Neisseria meningitidis_ and _Neisseria gonorrhoeal_ septicemia occur in patients with absent C6, 7, 8 or 9, since this combination of serum proteins is the complement "attack unit" (6).

Immunoglobulin System

The lymphocyte directed immunoglobulin production system gives specificity to the immune response for specific antigens. Receptors on the surfaces of lymphocytes bind to antigens, replicate and secrete lymphokines. Lymphokines stimulate plasma cells to produce specific antibodies which neutralize toxins and act as ligands between microbes and phagocytic cells. Subclasses of lymphocytes may provide helper/inducer activity or suppressor/cytotoxic activity for the host defense system. Systemic infections in patients with a defective immunoglobulin system are typically "pyogenic" including _Streptococcus pyogenes_, _Hemophilus influenzae_, _E. coli_ and _Staphylococcus aureus_.

Cell-Mediated Immune System

Cell-mediated immunity involves a complex series of interactions between lymphocytes and macrophages. Lymphokines secreted by lymphocytes in response to specific microbial antigens modulate function of macrophages. Macrophages are ordinarily long-lived and relatively inactive but when influenced by lymphokines acquire a primary role in host defense against obligate intracellular parasites, viruses and fungi. Typical infecting organisms in patients with defective cell-mediated immunity include herpes viruses, candida, mycobacteria and pneumocystis.

Patients with a Defective Phagocytic System

Patients with a defective phagocytic system suffer recurrent abscess-type infections with _Staphylococcus aureus_, gram-negative aerobic enteric bacilli and the fungal species, aspergillus and candida. Patients may have insufficient numbers of phagocytic cells or circulating phagocytes which are defective. Patients with deficient numbers of phagocytes include those with cyclic neutropenia, aplastic anemia, leukemia or cytotoxic therapy.

Patients also may have normal numbers but defective function of phagocytes. Examples of phagocyte dysfunction include Chronic Granulomatous Disease, Hyperimmunoglobulinemia E - Recurrent Infection Syndrome and the MAC-1 (glycoprotein-150) deficiency syndrome.

Granulocytopenia

Patients with chronic neutropenia as their sole host defense abnormality have relatively infrequent episodes of infection. In contrast, when neutropenia develops in patients with hematological malignancy, an extremely high incidence of serious bacterial and fungal infections is seen. In this clinical context neutropenia, especially when the granulocyte count falls

Table 1. Defective Phagocyte Function

Granulocytopenia
Chronic granulomatous disease
Glucose-6-phosphate dehydrogenase deficiency
Chediak-Higashi syndrome
Myeloperoxidase deficiency
Glutathione-system defect
Malignancy
Down's syndrome
Thermal injury
Protein-calorie malnutrition
Ichthyosis
Glycoprotein (150) MAC-1 defect
Hyperimmunoglobulinemia E - Recurrent Infections (Job's Syndrome)
Schwachman syndrome
Kartagener syndrome
Acrodermatitis enteropathica
Mannosidosis

below 500/mm, not only predisposes to the development of infections but also has a significant effect on the outcome of antibiotic therapy.

Because of poor prognosis of systemic gram-negative bacterial infections in patients with severe profound granulocytopenia, initiation of empirical treatment with antibiotics (beta lactams together with aminoglycosides) at the onset of fever has become routine practice (3). When treating patients with persistent, severe granulocytopenia and systemic bacterial infections, rapid identification of biological agents and antibiotic susceptibility data is necessary. Maximum therapeutic doses of antibiotics should be given and combinations of synergistic bactericidal antibiotics which easily diffuse into sites of infection should be selected. Until the granulocyte count has risen above 500/mm, empirical antibiotic therapy should be continued in patients who have become afebrile (7).

Deep-seated fungal infections, caused by either *Candida* or *Aspergillus* species, pose a major threat to granulocytopenic patients, and previous antibacterial therapy may play a role in predisposing these patients to infections with fungi. Fungal infections are particularly troublesome because of the difficulty in establishing a diagnosis before necropsy. The prognosis of aspergillus infection in granulocytopenic patients is poor; nevertheless, amphotericin B, in combination with 5-flucytosine, should be used since early aggressive therapy does increase survival of granulocytopenic patients with deep-seated fungal disease (5). Another important approach to the management of infectious-disease complications of granulocytopenic cancer patients is prophylactic oral antibiotics to eliminate pathogenic enteric organisms. Several non-absorbable, oral antibiotic regimens have been demonstrated to decrease the incidence of serious infections.

Granulocyte Dysfunction

Patients with defective phagocytic-cell locomotion may have increased susceptibility to infection. Cutaneous and pulmonary infections caused by *S. aureus* are major problems and fungal species, especially *Candida* and *Cryptococcus*, may be associated with chronic lesions. The recalcitrant and recurrent nature of abscesses in patients with chemotactic dysfunction dictates need for antibiotic therapy, initiated early and continued for relatively long periods. Recurrent serious infections are a continual threat in patients with defects in granulocyte microbicidal function. Neutrophils of patients with chronic granulomatous disease, one of the most common and important of these disorders, have an abnormality in the plasma-membrane-associated oxidase system responsible for conversion of oxygen to microbicidal oxygen species (4). Consequently, these patients suffer from recurrent pyogenic infections of the skin, lymph nodes, lungs, intraabdominal organs and bones. *S. aureus*, several species of gram-negative bacilli, and aspergillus are the pathogens most frequently isolated in these patients. Typically, patients respond slowly to antibiotic therapy, and agents with appropriate antibacterial activity, which will penetrate neutrophils such as clindamycin, are useful clinically.

Clinical examples of the importance of normal function of the phagocytic defense system are patients who have undergone splenectomy or who are functionally asplenic. These patients have an increased incidence of serious and often fatal pneumococcal and *Haemophilus influenzae* infections. Although the role of the spleen in host defense is multifaceted, including the production of immunoglobulins (primarily IgM), certain complement components and a population of T helper cells, it acts as a critical filtering mechanism for bacteria in the bloodstream. Antibiotic therapy in splenectomized patients with fulminating pneumococcal sepsis may be ineffective, again demonstrating the need for the contribution of host factors for recovery. Pneumococcal vaccine is given to these high risk patients; however, concern that it may not prove effective usually prompts chronic prophylactic antibiotics as well.

Patients with Complement Defects. Unusually severe infections are frequent in patients with congenital absence of the C3 component of the complement system. Patients with deficiencies of other complement components have problems with *S. pneumoniae*, *S. aureus*, group A streptococci, aerobic gram-negative bacilli, *H. influenzae*, and *N. meningitidis*. The unusual severity of infections in patients with C3 deficiency is related to the central role of the third component of complement, C3b, in bacterial opsonization.

Neisseria meningitidis and *gonorrhoeae* are killed and lysed by the complement system in the absence of phagocytic cells. Therefore, patients with deficiencies of the terminal components of the complement system, C5, C6, C7, C8 or C9, have problems with serious neisserial infections (6). Patients with recurrent or unusually severe gonococcal or meningococcal infections should be evaluated for the possibility of a deficiency of one of these complement components, and in such patients initial antibiotic therapy should include activity against *Neisseria*.

Patients with Immunoglobulin Deficiency. Major infectious disease problems in patients with primary or secondary disorders of specific adaptive immune (antibody) responses include recurrent serious respiratory infections or septicemia with encapsulated bacteria such as *Streptococcus pneumoniae* or pyogenes, *Hemophilus influenzae*, and *Neisseria meningitidis* (1). Therefore, initial selection of antibiotics should generally be directed toward *S. pneumoniae* and *H. influenzae*. In addition to antibiotics, regular administration of gammaglobulin is an important part of the management of patients with defective capacity to produce specific antibodies.

Patients with Defective Cell-mediated Immunity. Serious problems with obligate intracellular microorganisms are associated with primary or secondary defects in cell-mediated immunity (CMI) (2). Prominent bacterial species include staphylococci, mycobacteria, listeria and nocardia; protozoan species include *Pneumocystis carinii* and *Toxoplasma gondii* and the herpes group predominate among the viruses.

Patients with primary defects in CMI, such as thymic hypoplasia (DiGeorge syndrome), ataxia telangectasia, combined immunodeficiency (Swiss type) and the Wiskott-Aldrich syndrome, frequently die of recurrent severe infections before reaching adulthood. The most common and important group of adult patients with compromised CMI are those with T-cell abnormalities secondary to immunosuppressive or cytotoxic chemotherapy. Allograft recipients, lymphoma patients and patients with collagen vascular diseases on high-dose steroid therapy fall into this category. Herpes virus infections are extremely common in renal transplant recipients and in bone marrow transplant patients.

The course of many of the infections occurring in patients with severe defects in CMI is similar to that observed in patients with other host-defense abnormalities: the infections are more severe, caused by unusual organisms, rapidly progressive, and less responsive to antimicrobial therapy.

SUMMARY

Therapeutic decisions involving antimicrobial agents are critically important when infections occur in patients with major defects in host defense. Empirical decisions are necessary and antibiotics with broad spectrum must be given in high dosage by the intravenous route. Clinical signs are unpredictable since the inflammatory response is abnormal. Knowledge of components of immune system most seriously compromised in individual patients does not allow informed empiricism for making therapeutic decisions. For example, patients with complement and antibody deficiency are susceptible to septicemia and meningitis from streptococcal species or Hemophilus. Patients with phagocyte disorders suffer recurrent abscess disease from staphylococci and enteric gram-negative bacteria. Patients with defective cell-mediated immunity have prolonged infections with fungi or viruses. These patients are also susceptible to chronic bacterial infections.

Microbial identification and antibiotic sensitivity testing are critically important when caring for patients with defective host defenses. The need for precise identification is necessary since relatively toxic antibiotics may be necessary and recurrence of infection is a frequent clinical problem. Prolonged hospitalization of these patients favors colonization with multiple resistant hospital strains of microbes and continued development of new antimicrobial agents effective against unusual or resistant microbes is necessary.

Surgical procedures for removal of functionless tissue, or abscesses which are heavily colonized with resistant microbes may be life-saving. As more is learned about the immune system through study of patients with primary specific immunodeficiency, more specific therapies will be developed. Progress in developing effective immunostimulants is a source of optimism.

REFERENCES

1. P. E. Hermans and W. R. Wilson, Immunoglobulin deficiency pathogenesis and types of infections, in: "Infections in the Immunocompromised Host - Pathogenesis, Prevention, and Therapy," J. Verhoef, P. K. Peterson and P. G. Quie, eds., Elsevier/North-Holland Biomedical Press, Amsterdam (1980).
2. J. Klastersky, Therapy of bacterial infections in cancer patients, in: "Infections in the Immunocompromised Host-Pathogenesis, Prevention, and Therapy," J. Verhoef, P. K. Peterson and P. G. Quie, eds., Elsevier/North-Holland Biomedical Press, Amsterdam (1980).

3. L. J. Love, S. C. Schimpff, C. A. Schiffer and P. H. Wiernik, Improved prognosis for granulocytopenic patients with gram-negative bacteremia, Am. J. Med. 68:643 (1980).
4. E. L. Mills and P. G. Quie, Congenital disorders of the functions of polymorphonuclear neutrophils, Rev. Infec. Dis. 2:505 (1980).
5. J. E. Pennington, Successful treatment of Aspergillus pneumonia in hematologic neoplasia, N. Engl. J. Med. 295:426 (1976).
6. B. H. Peterson, T. J. Lee, R. Snyderman and G. F. Brooks, Neisseria gonorrhoeae bacteremia associated with C6, C7 or C8 deficiency, Ann. Intern. Med. 90:917 (1979).
7. P. A. Pizzo, K. J. Robichaud, I. A. Gill, F. G. Witebsky, A. S. Levine, A. B. Deisseroth, D. L. Glanbiger, J. D. Maclowry, I. T. Magrath, D. G. Poplack and R. M. Simon, Duration of empiric antibiotic therapy in granulocytopenic patients with cancer, Am. J. Med. 67:194 (1979).
8. P. G. Quie, Pathology of bactericidal power of neutrophils, Semin. Hematol. 12:143 (1975).

AMPHOTERICIN-B INDUCED IMMUNOMODULATION OF RESISTANCE AGAINST CANDIDA ALBICANS INFECTION

F. Bistoni[1], A. Vecchiarelli[1], P. Marconi[1], G. Verducci[1], P. Puccetti[2] and E. Garaci[3]

[1]Institute of Medical Microbiology, University of Perugia Perugia, Italy
[2]Institute of Pharmacology, University of Perugia, Perugia Italy
[3]Institute of Microbiology, Department of Experimental Medicine, II University of Rome, Rome, Italy

INTRODUCTION

Amphotericin B (AmB) is a polyene antifungal antibiotic used principally in the treatment of systemic infections. The drug has been shown to possess immunoactive properties (7) which include stimulation of humoral (3) and cell-mediated (9) immunity in mice. Not suprisingly, therefore, AmB can also exert protective effects in experimental infection models (2,8,10).

In the present study, we evaluated the hypothesis that the immunoactive effects of AmB may contribute significantly to its overall antifungal activity in vivo. For this purpose, we investigated the impact of AmB treatment on mouse resistance to systemic *Candida albicans* infection; moreover, experiments were also performed in vitro to ascertain whether exposure of candidacidal effectors to AmB may affect their cytotoxic potential.

We found that a single dose of AmB to mice was followed by a dramatic increase in the in vivo resistance of the animals to *Candida* infections, an event which was mirrored by remarkable modifications in *in vitro* functions of cells with anti-*Candida* reactivity.

MATERIALS AND METHODS

Mice

Hybrid (Balb/c Cr x DBA/2 Cr) F_1 (CD2F1:H-2^d/H-2^d) mice were obtained from Charles River, Calco, Milan. In the in vivo experiments, groups consisted of ten mice. For the in vitro assays effector cells from five to ten animals were pooled.

Chemicals

Amphotericin B (Fungizione), kindly supplied by E. R. Squibb & Sons, Princeton, N.J., was provided in vials containing 50 mg of AmB and 41 mg of sodium deoxycholate with 25.2 mg of sodium phosphate as a buffer. The drug was dissolved in sterile, non-pyrogenic 5% glucose in water and injected intraperitoneally in the amount of 0.1 ml/10 g of body weight.

Cyclophosphamide (CY, Endoxan Asta, Asta Werke, West Germany) was dissolved in 0.85% NaCl sterile solution immediately before use and injected intraperitoneally in an amount of 0.1 ml/10 g of body weight.

Microorganisms

The C. albicans strain used throughout this study was isolated from a clinical specimen and identified according to the taxonomic criteria of Lodder (5,6). The yeast was grown at 28°C under slight agitation in low-glucose Winge medium composed of 0.2% (wt/vol) glucose and 0.3% (wt/vol) yeast extract (BBL, Microbiology Systems, Cockeysville MD, U.S.A.) until a stationary phase of growth was reached (about 24 hr.). Under these conditions, the culture gave a yield of approximately 2.8×10^8 cells per ml, and the organism grew as an essentially pure yeast-phase population. After the 24 hour culture, cells were harvested by low-speed centrifugation, washed twice in saline, and diluted to the desired concentration.

Preparation of Effector Cells

Spleen cell suspensions were obtained by standard methods. Peritoneal polymorphonuclear neutrophils (PMN) were induced by intraperitoneal injection of 1 ml of 10% thioglycollate broth (Bacto Brewer thioglycollate medium, Difco Labs., Detroit MI, U.S.A.), 18 hours before testing. The elicited cells were harvested by peritoneal washing and approximately 95% were found to be PMN by morphological examination. Resident peritoneal exudate cells (PEC) were harvested by washing the peritoneal cavity of normal non-induced mice with cold RPMI medium. Effector cells were washed twice, resuspended in complete RPMI and adjusted to the desired concentration.

^{51}Cr-Release Assay Against C. albicans (CRA)

Candidacidal activity of various effector cell populations was assessed by means of a previously described method (1). Briefly, 2×10^8 C. albicans cells were incubated for 2 hours at 37°C under 5% CO_2 with 300 µCi of $Na_2{}^{51}CrO_4$ (Amersham International Ltd., Amersham, U.K.), washed three times in saline, counted and resuspended in medium to a concentration of 5×10^5 ml^{-1}.

Under standard labelling conditions 5×10^4 C. albicans gave 2,000 ± 500 ct. min^{-1}. Various numbers of effector cells in 0.1 ml were mixed in U-shaped 96-well microtiter plates with 5×10^4 radiolabelled C. albicans in 0.1 ml. After 4 hours incubation at 37°C under 5% CO_2, the plates were centrifuged at 800 g for 10 minutes and radioactivity in 0.1 ml of the supernatant was measured on a γ-scintillation counter. The baseline ^{51}Cr release was that of C. albicans incubated alone in complete RPMI 1640 medium and in no case did it exceed 20% of total cpm incorporated by target cells.

Experimental results have been expressed as the percentage lysis in the experimental group (quadruplicate samples) above the baseline control according to the following formula:

$$\text{specific } {}^{51}\text{Cr release} = \frac{\text{ct. min}^{-1}\ (\text{experimental group}) - \text{ct. min}^{-1}\ (\text{spontaneous release})}{0.5 \times \text{total ct. min}^{-1}} \times 100$$

where total ct. min^{-1} is the radioactivity incorporated by 5×10^4 C. albicans cells.

Statistical Analysis

Differences in survival times were analyzed by the Mann-Whitney U test. Differences in specific radiolabel release in the in vitro microtoxicity assays were determined by the Student's "t" test. Each experiment was repeated five times.

RESULTS

Effect of Cyclophosphamide Administration on Survival of Mice Treated with AmB After Challenge with C. albicans

In a preliminary series of experiments we investigated the role of the immune system on the resistance of mice challenged with *C. albicans* and then given AmB as a chemotherapeutic agent. Male CD2F1 mice were treated with the immunosuppressive drug cyclophosphamide (Cy, 150 mg/Kg, i.p.) three days before challenge with different inocula of *C. albicans*. Groups of mice also received AmB (10 mg/Kg, i.p.) at various times after challenge. Table 1 summarizes the results. It is apparent that the outcome of the challenge was largely conditioned by the host immune status at the time of *Candida* injection. Moreover, the efficacy of AmB chemotherapy was also affected by the Cyinduced immunodepression.

Effect of Cy Administration on Survival of Mice Pretreated with AmB and Challenged with C. albicans

We have already shown (2) that AmB, if administered 2-14 days before *C. albicans* challenge, can exert considerable protection against the infection. In the present study we extended such previous observations and investigated any possible antagonistic effect of Cy on the increased resistance induced by AmB. CD2F1 mice were given AmB, 10 mg/Kg, two, four, six or

Table 1. Effect of Cy Administration on Survival of CD2F1 Mice Treated with AmB After Systemic Challenge with *C. albicans* Cells

In vivo treatments: Cy[a]	AmB[b] time (hrs)	Challenge i.v. with *C. albicans* cells	MST[c]	D/T[d]
-	-	5×10^5	4	10/10
-	+ 3h	5×10^5	>60	0/10
-	+ 12h	5×10^5	>60	0/10
-	+ 48h	5×10^5	>60	2/10
-	-	1×10^5	9	10/10
+	-	1×10^5	2	10/10
+	+ 3h	1×10^5	>60	1/10
+	+ 12h	1×10^5	2	10/10
+	+ 24h	1×10^5	2	10/10

[a] Cy (150 mg/Kg) was given as a single i.p. injection 3 days before *C. albicans* challenge (day 0).
[b] AmB (10 mg/Kg) was given as a single i.p. injection at various times after *C. albicans* challenge.
[c] MST, median survival time (days).
[d] D/T, dead mice at 60 days over total animals tested.

Table 2. Effect of Cy Administration on Survival of CD2F1 Mice Pretreated with AmB and Challenged In Vivo with C. albicans Cells

In vivo treatment		Mice challenged with 1 x 10^5 C. albicans cells	
AmB[a] time (days)	Cy[b]	MST[c]	D/T[d]
-	-	9	10/10
- 2	-	>60	0/10
- 4	-	>60	0/10
- 6	-	>60	0/10
- 8	-	>60	0/10
-	+	3	10/10
- 2	+	>60	2/10
- 4	+	12	7/10
- 6	+	4	9/10
- 8	+	4	10/10

[a]AmB (10 mg/Kg) was given as a single injection a number of days before C. albicans challenge (day 0).
[b]Cy (150 mg/Kg) was given as a single i.p. injection 3 days before C. albicans challenge.
[c]MST, median survival time (days).
[d]D/T, dead mice at 60 days over total animals tested.

eight days before i.v. challenge with 1 x 10^5 C. albicans cells. Groups of mice also received Cy, 150 mg/Kg, three days before the infection (Table 2).

The results showed that the beneficial activity exerted by AmB treatment was largely abrogated by subsequent exposure of mice to Cy. Only when treatment with AmB was performed on day -2, i.e., one day after Cy exposure, did the efficacy of AmB appear to be unaffected. Under these conditions, it is possible that the chemotherapeutic activity of the drug may play a major role by means of a direct interaction between AmB and Candida (2).

Effect of Different Doses of AmB on Survival of Mice Challenged with C. albicans and Cytotoxic Properties of Spleen Cells In Vitro

In a subsequent series of experiments we investigated how different dosages of AmB would affect both the in vivo resistance of mice and the in vitro expression of anti-Candida acitivity by splenic or peritoneal effectors. For this purpose, mice treated with a range (1.2 -40 mg/Kg) of AmB doses were either infected in vivo with Candida or used as a source of effector cells to be reacted in vitro against ^{51}Cr-labelled Candida cells. Table 3 shows that doses above the 10 mg/Kg threshold value resulted in in vivo protection and activation of the candidacidal effectors. However, no clear dose-response effect could be demonstrated in this experiment.

Effect of Time of AmB Administration on Both Survival of Mice Challenged with Candida and In Vitro Reactivity of Spleen Cells

To assess the kinetics of development of the increased resistance induced by AmB, the animals were treated at different times with 2.5, 10 and 40 mg/Kg and then challenged with 1 x 10^6 Candida cells. The in vitro reactivity of spleen cells was also assayed (Table 4). It is apparent that,

Table 3. Effect of Different Doses of AmB on Both Survival of CD2F1 Mice Systemically Challenged with *C. albicans* Cells and Candidacidal Activity of Spleen Cells

	Mice challenged with 1×10^6 *C. albicans*			% ^{51}Cr specific release					
				Spleen cells			Peritoneal exudate cells		
AmB (mg/Kg)[a]	MST[b]	D/T[c]	P[d]	10:1[e]	5:1	2.5:1	10:1	5:1	2.5:1
-	3	10/10	-	15.4	9.4	6.4	2.6	2.4	1.6
1.2	4	10/10	NS	14.0	10.8	5.8	2.0	1.6	1.0
2.5	3.4	10/10	NS	12.3	11.2	8.0	1.8	1.0	0.7
5.0	4	10/10	NS	NT	NT	NT	NT	NT	NT
10	>60	0/10	<0.01	28.4*	18.3*	11.4*	7.2*	6.8*	6.1*
20	>60	0/10	<0.01	32.6*	20.3*	10.9*	6.4*	5.6*	5.0*
40	>60	0/10	<0.01	36.2*	25.7*	13.2*	9.6*	7.0*	5.4*

[a] AmB was given as a single i.p. injection 8 days before *C. albicans* challenge or the in vitro assay (day 0).
[b] MST, median survival time (days).
[c] D/T, dead mice at 60 days over total animals tested.
[d] P, AmB-treated versus untreated controls; NS, not statistically significant.
[e] Effector to target cell ratios.
*P < 0.01 (AmB-treated versus untreated controls).
NT, not tested.

Table 4. Effect of Time and Dose of AmB Administration on Both Survival of CD2F1 Mice Systemically Infected with *C. albicans* and Candidacidal Activity of Spleen Cells

AmB administration[a] (days)	AmB (2.5 mg/Kg)			AmB (10 mg/Kg)			AmB (40 mg/Kg)		
	Survival[b]		% ^{51}Cr specific release[c]	Survival		% ^{51}Cr specific release[c]	Survival		% ^{51}Cr specific release[c]
	MST[d]	D/T	10:1[e]	MST	D/T	10:1	MST	D/T	10:1
2	>60*	2/10	13.2	>60*	1/10	18.3*	>60*	0/10	NT
4	7	10/10	11.3	>60*	2/10	21.1*	>60*	0/10	12.2
6	4	10/10	10.9	>60*	2/10	31.3*	>60*	0/10	15.4
8	4	10/10	12.6	>60*	3/10	24.1*	>60*	2/10	28.1*
15	4	10/10	11.8	5	10/10	11.5	6	10/10	NT

[a]AmB was given as a single i.p. injection a number of days before *C. albicans* challenge or in vitro assay (day 0).
[b]Mice were infected by i.v. route with 1 x 10^6 *C. albicans* cells.
[c]Candidacidal activity of spleen cells was evaluated in a 4 hr. ^{51}Cr release assay against radiolabelled *C. albicans* cells.
[d]MST = median survival time (days).
[e]Effector to target cell ratio.
*$P < 0.01$ (AmB-treated versus untreated controls). The MST of untreated mice was 4 days (D/T:10/10) and the in vitro activity of spleen cells from such donors was 11.4 (A/T ratio 10:1).
NT = not tested.

Table 5. Effect of Cy Administration on Candidacidal Activity of Spleen and Peritoneal Exudate Cells from AmB-Treated CD2F1 Mice

In vivo treatment		% ^{51}Cr specific release					
		Spleen cells			Peritoneal exudate cells		
AmB(mg/Kg)[a]	Cy(mg/Kg)[b]	10:1[c]	5:1	2.5:1	10:1	5:1	2.5:1
-	-	16.8	13.8	8.8	1.0	0.2	0.1
-	150	9.6*	6.0*	5.6*	0.5	0.1	0
10	-	32.0	23.4	17.3	9.6	6.4	3.7
10	150	12.7*	9.3*	6.0*	1.0*	0.3*	0.1*

[a]AmB was given as a single i.p. injection 8 days before the in vitro assay (day 0).
[b]Cy was given as a single i.p. injection 3 days before the in vitro assay.
[c]Effector to target cell ratios.
*, P <0.01 (Cy-treated versus untreated mice).

using AmB in the optimal range of 10-40 mg/Kg, considerable activation was detectable up to eight days after drug exposure. Parallelism was found between the pattern of in vivo resistance and the expression of cytotoxic activity in vitro.

Effect of Cy Administration on Candidacidal Activity of Spleen and Peritoneal Cells from AmB-Treated Mice

The possible antagonistic effect of Cy treatment on the in vitro expression of candidacidal activity of splenic and peritoneal effectors was studied in an experiment in which animals treated with AmB (10 mg/Kg, i.p., day -8) plus Cy (150 mg/Kg, i.p., day -3) were used as donors of cells to be reacted against the labelled yeast in a ^{51}Cr release assay. Table 5 shows the results. It is apparent that Cy treatment greatly antagonized the boosting activity of AmB.

Candidacidal Activity of Different Effector Cells Activated In Vitro by AmB

The possibility was also explored that activation of candidacidal effectors by AmB might occur in vitro following exposure of the cells to the drug. Spleen cells, resident peritoneal macrophages and thioglycolate-induced peritoneal cells (a population consisting of 95% polymorphonuclear neutrophils) were cultured in vitro for two hours in the presence of AmB (10 γ/ml). At the end of the incubation period, the cells were harvested, washed and reacted against labelled Candida. Table 6 shows the results: of the tested populations, spleen cells and peritoneal resident cells appeared to be susceptible to in vitro activation by AmB, while PMN showed a decreased candidacidal activity.

DISCUSSION

AmB is currently used as a primary agent for the treatment of many systemic mycoses. It is known that the drug can considerably enhance host immune response (1,3,9) while inducing macrophage activation (4). In experimental infection models, AmB administration can protect mice against bac-

Table 6. Candidacidal Activity of Various Effector Cells After In Vitro Exposure to AmB

Effector cells[a]	Treatment with AmB	% ^{51}Cr specific release 10:1[b]	5:1	2.5:1
Spleen cells	-	11.4	5.7	4.6
Spleen cells	+	19.8*	12.6*	7.5*
Peritoneal resident cells	-	0.5	0.3	0.1
Peritoneal resident cells	+	7.8*	6.2*	4.5*
Polymorphonuclear cells	-	40.4	31.6	20.4
Polymorphonuclear cells	+	20.6*	18.6*	12.6*

[a]Spleen cells, peritoneal resident cells or thioglycolate induced peritoneal resident cells were cultured on plastic Petri dishes for 2 hours with 10 γ/ml of AmB. After that the cells were used as effector cells against radiolabelled C. albicans cells in a 4 hour ^{51}Cr release assay.

[b]Effector to target cell ratios.

*P <0.01 (AmB-treated versus controls).

terial (10) and helmintic challenge (8). We have recently reported that the drug is also capable of inducing increased resistance to Candida infection (2).

The present study follows and extends those previous observations. It is shown that in vivo or in vitro application of AmB activates cells in the host with fungicidal properties and that this event may be related to the increase in resistance to challenge with C. albicans. In a preliminary series of experiments (Table 1) we obtained evidence that the host immune status plays a considerable role in the therapeutic activity of AmB even when the drug is expected to exert a primary chemotherapeutic effect. We went on to investigate the possible involvement of the immune system in the adjuvant activity of AmB (Table 2). It was shown that the protection afforded by exposure of mice to AmB, up to eight days before Candida challenge, was reversed by subsequent treatment of the animals with Cy. Thus it appeared that the cells of the host immune system might be activated by AmB treatment to become candidacidal. As a matter of fact, spleen and peritoneal exudate cells from AmB-treated donors exerted a strong anti-Candida activity (Table 3), which was maximal when the donor mice had been treated six days earlier with AmB 10 mg/Kg (Table 4). Similar to that observed in vivo, also the in vitro expression of anti-Candida reactivity displayed by AmB-activated cells was impaired by exposure of the donors to Cy. Finally, two of the major candidacidal populations, i.e., spleen cells and peritoneal macrophages, could be activated in vitro to become cytotoxic.

In conclusion, the present study, which follows a previous report on the subject by our group (2) provides additional support to the concept that the immuno-adjuvant effect of AmB may contribute significantly to its therapeutic activity. Studies are under way to determine the effects of repeated AmB administrations, similar to the dosages given to patients with systemic mycoses who experience long-term treatments.

ACKNOWLEDGMENTS

This work was supported by Contract n. 83.00628.52 and Contract n. 83.00654.52 within the Progetto Finalizzato per il Controllo delle Malattie da Infezione from the Consiglio Nazionale delle Ricerche, Italy. We are grateful to Eileen Zannetti for her assistance in the preparation of the manuscript.

REFERENCES

1. F. Bistoni, M. Baccarini, E. Blasi, P. Puccetti and P. Marconi, A radiolabel release microassay for phagocytic killing of _Candida albicans_, _J. Immunol. Meth._ 52:369 (1982).
2. F. Bistoni, A. Vecchiarelli, R. Mazzola, P. Puccetti, P. Marconi and E. Garaci, Immunoadjuvant activity of Amphotericin B as displayed in mice with _Candida albicans_, _Antimicrob. Agents Chemother._ 22:625 (1985).
3. T. J. Blanke, J. R. Little, S. F. Shirley and R. G. Lynch, Augmentation of murine immune responses by Amphotericin B, _Cell. Immunol._ 33:180 (1977).
4. H. Lin, G. Medoff and G. S. Kobayashi, Effects of Amphotericin B on macrophages and their precursor cells, _Antimicrob. Agents Chemother._ 11:154 (1977).
5. I. Lodder, "The Yeasts: A Taxonomic Study," North Holland Publishing Company, Amsterdam (1970).
6. P. Marconi, F. Bistoni, L. Boncio, A. Bersiani, P. Bravi and M. Pitzurra, Utilizzazione di una soluzione salina ipertonica di cloruro di potassio (3M KCl) per l'estrazione di antigeni solubili da _Candida albicans_, _Ann. Sclavo_ 18:61 (1976).
7. G. Medoff, F. Valeriote, J. Ryan and S. Tolen, Response of transplanted AKR leukemia to combination therapy with Amphotericin B and 1,3-Bis (2-chloroethyl)-1-nitrosourea-dose and schedule dependency, _J. Natl. Cancer Inst._ 58:949 (1977).
8. G. R. Olds, S. J. Stewart and J. J. Ellner, Amphotericin B-induced resistance to _Schistosoma mansoni_, _J. Immunol._ 126:1667 (1981).
9. S. F. Shirley and J. R. Little, Immunopotentiating effects of Amphotericin B. I. Enhanced contact sensitivity in mice, _J. Immunol._ 123:2878 (1979).
10. M. Z. Thomas, G. Medoff and G. S. Kobayashi, Changes in murine resistance to _Lysteria monocytogenes_ infection induced by Amphotericin B, _J. Infect. Dis._ 127:373 (1973).

THE INFLUENCE OF ANTIBIOTICS ON THE SERUM RESISTANCE OF ENTEROBACTERIACEAE

Christoph Wiemer, Britta Kubens and Wolfgang Opferkuch

Ruhr-Universität Bochum
Medizinische Mikrobiologie und Immunologie
Bochum, F.R.G.

INTRODUCTION

Resistance to the bactericidal activity of serum is an important virulence factor of gram-negative bacteria. This serum resistance is responsible for the ineffectiveness of a main host defense mechanism, the attack and killing by the complement system.

The literature about the influence of β-lactam antibiotics on the serum resistance of bacteria is controversial. A decrease in serum resistance of E. coli was found by Traub (7) using ampicillin, by Friedman and Warren (3) for cyclocillin, Dutcher and associates (4) for ampicillin and Taylor and co-workers (6) for mecillinam. Lorian and Atkinson (4) reported about an increase in serum resistance of Enterobacteriaceae in the presence of ampicillin or mecillinam. Fierer and Finley (2) found no influence of ampicillin or cephalothin on the serum resistance of an E. coli and a Klebsiella pneumoniae strain (Table 1). These variations can probably be explained by differences between the definitions of serum resistance and the methods of determination.

The aim of this investigation was to study whether the newly developed β-lactam antibiotics have any influence on the serum resistance of Enterobacteriaceae. In this study serum resistance is defined on the basis of growth curves, using the agar-plate method. We designated a strain as "serum sensitive" if no further growth takes place after incubation with 5% NHS, and as "serum resistant" if there was growth or no decrease of viable counts even in 20% NHS.

MATERIALS AND METHODS

Bacteria

All strains used were originally isolated from blood cultures, except E. coli WF 52, which is a urine isolate, and were kindly provided by Prof. A. Glynn, London. The strains of E. coli, Enterobacter cloacae, Klebsiella pneumoniae, Proteus mirabilis, and Proteus morganii, grew after incubation in 20% NHS, whereas the strains of Serratia marcescens only tolerated a maximum of 8% NHS. The serogroups of the two E. coli strains were: BK 615: 09a; WF 52: 026:K13:H11.

Table 1. Influence of β-lactam Antibiotics on the Serum Resistance of Enterobacteriaceae

Strain	Antibiotic	Test serum	Serum resistance	Ref.
E. coli	Ampicillin	NHS	↓	7
E. coli	Cyclacillin	HRS	↓	3
E. coli	Ampicillin	NHS	↓	1
Enterobacteriaceae	Ampicillin/ Mecillinam	NHS	↑	4
E. coli Klebs. pneumoniae	Ampicillin/ Cephalothin	NHS	∅	2
E. coli	Mecillinam	NHS	↓	6

NHS = normal human serum
HRS = hyperimmune rabbit serum
∅ = no influence
↑ = increase
↓ = slight decrease

Serum, Antibiotics

Blood was obtained from healthy volunteers, allowed to clot for two hours at 4°C, and centrifuged at 3000 rpm at 4°C; serum was stored in aliquots at -20°C and thawed shortly before use. Inactivation serum was heated at 56°C for 30 minutes. Complement activity was tested by determination of CH50, and ranged between 25 and 36 units.

The antibiotics were obtained from Merck, Sharp & Dohme, Munich, F.R.G. (imipenem, cefoxitin), Hoechst A. G., Frankfurt, F.R.G. (cefotaxime, cefuroxime, cefodizime-HR 221), Leo Pharmaceuticals, Bellerup, Denmark (mecillinam) and Takeda-Grunenthal, Stolberg, F.R.G. (cefsulodin).

Serum Bactericidal Assay

Bacteria were inoculated from a nutrient agar slant into 0.9% sodium chloride up to a concentration of 0.5 McFarland standards, then transferred

Table 2. MIC of Six New β-Lactam Antibiotics for the Strains BK 615, WF 52, and BK 319

Antibiotic	BK 615	MIC (μg/ml) WF 52	BK 319
Cefsulodin	64	64	2048
Cefoxitin	4	2	2048
Cefuroxime	4	4	512
Cefotaxime	0.032	0.016	128
Cefodizime	0.125	0.125	128
Mecillinam	0.25	0.25	256

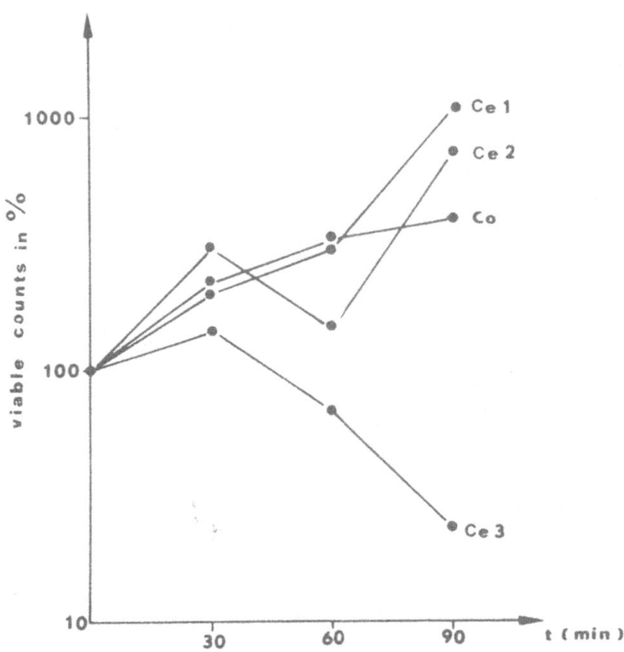

Figure 1. Influence of 1/2 MIC cefuroxime on the serum resistance of BK 319. Ce 1, 20% heat-inactivated serum; Ce 2, 15% active serum; Ce 3, 20% active serum.

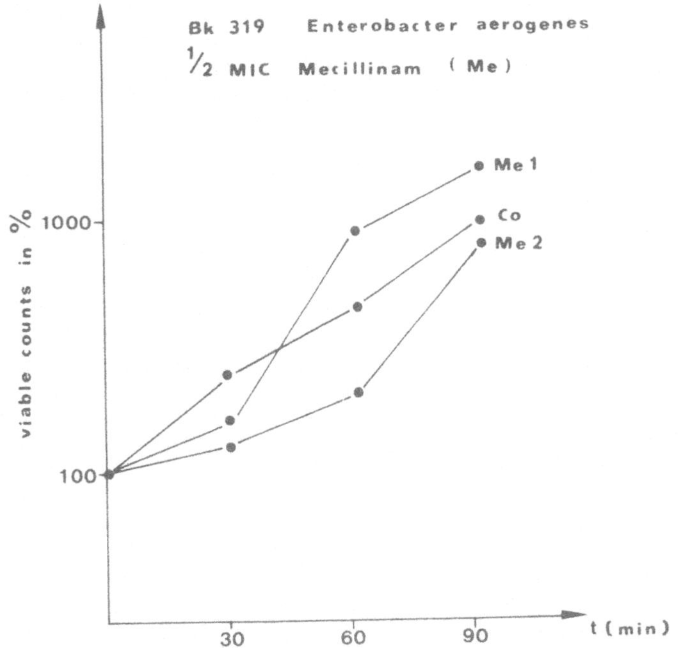

Figure 2. Influence of 1/2 MIC mecillinam on the serum resistance BK 319. Me 1, 20% heat-inactivated serum; Me 2, 20% active serum.

Table 3. MIC Imipenem for Twelve Enterobacteriaceae

	Strains	MIC µg/ml	Before treatment	After treatment
WF 52	Escherichia coli	0.125	20	15
BK 615	Escherichia coli	0.25	20	3
BK 28	Enterobacter aerogenes	0.5	20	15
BK 319	Enterobacter aerogenes	0.5	20	3
BK 383	Enterobacter cloacae	0.25	20	20
BK 967	Enterobacter cloacae	0.5	20	20
BK 177	Klebsiella pneumoniae	0.25	20	20
BK 1171	Klebsiella pneumoniae	0.25	20	20
BK 1435	Proteus mirabilis	4	20	15
BK 74	Proteus morganii	2	20	20
BK 31	Serratia marcescens	1	8	8
BK 1292	Serratia marcescens	0.5	8	8

Serum resistance as the maximal serum concentration in % (v/v) tolerated by the bacteria before and after treatment with 1/4 MIC imipenem.

into a nutrient broth containing 1/4 MIC of the different antibiotics and incubated at 37°C for 18 hours. 100 µl of this overnight culture were added to 900 µl of a medium containing the same concentration of the antibiotic and incubated in a shaking water bath for three hours in order to obtain a log-phase culture. Thereafter, the cultures were standardized to a concentration of 0.5 McFarland standards, and the final test mixture contained 0.8 ml of this bacterial suspension, 0.2 ml freshly thawed serum and 1/4 MIC of the antibiotic. The control mixtures contained either heat inactivated serum with or without antibiotics or active serum without antibiotic. The pH of the test mixtures ranged between 7.3 and 7.5. The bacteria were incubated for another 90 minutes in a shaking water bath, and samples were taken every 30 minutes to estimate the number of viable counts.

RESULTS AND DISCUSSION

The MIC of the used antibiotics for E. coli (BK 615, WF 52) and Enterobacter aerogenes (BK 319) are listed in Table 2. A slight decrease in serum resistance from 20% to 15% NHS (serum resistance is given as the maximal serum concentration in % (v/v), tolerated before and after treatment with the antibiotic) could be observed if 1/2 MIC of cefoxitin, cefodizime (HR 221), cefsulodin or cefuroxime was added. As shown in Figure 1, the killing rate of NHS in the presence of 1/2 MIC cefuroxime is still less than 90%. Comparable results were obtained after treatment with cefoxitin, cefodizime and cefsulodin (data not shown). Serum resistance of the investigated strains was not influenced by addition of 1/2 MIC mecillinam (Figure 2) and 1/2 MIC cefotaxime (data not shown).

All strains used to investigate the influence of imipenem on serum resistance are listed in Table 3. The MIC and the serum resistance with or without 1/4 MIC imipenem are also given. As can be seen from these data, serum resistance of the strains WF 52, BK 615, BK 28, BK 319 and BK 1435 was altered. The decrease in serum resistance was especially impressive for the strains BK 615 and BK 319. The other seven strains did not show any alterations. Treatment of BK 28, BK 1435 and WF 52 with 1/2 MIC imipenem in 20% NHS caused a killing rate of about 90%, while the untreated cells grew at their normal rate. Under the same conditions more than 99.9% of the inoculum of BK 615 and BK 319 was killed. Even a serum concentration of only 5% NHS led to a reduction of viable counts by more than 90% of the inoculum, whereas heat inactivated serum showed no influence (Figure 3). This phenomenon of "induced serum sensitivity" (from 20% to 3% NHS) proved to be dose-dependent as shown in Figure 4. The decrease of viable counts is two logs of growth smaller if a concentration of 1/8 MIC instead of 1/4 MIC imipenem is added. After transfer into antibiotic-free medium, the bacteria recovered their original resistance which indicates that the induced sensitivity is reversible.

A comparison of the serum resistance after treatment with imipenem and mecillinam is shown in Table 4. While imipenem caused a decrease in serum

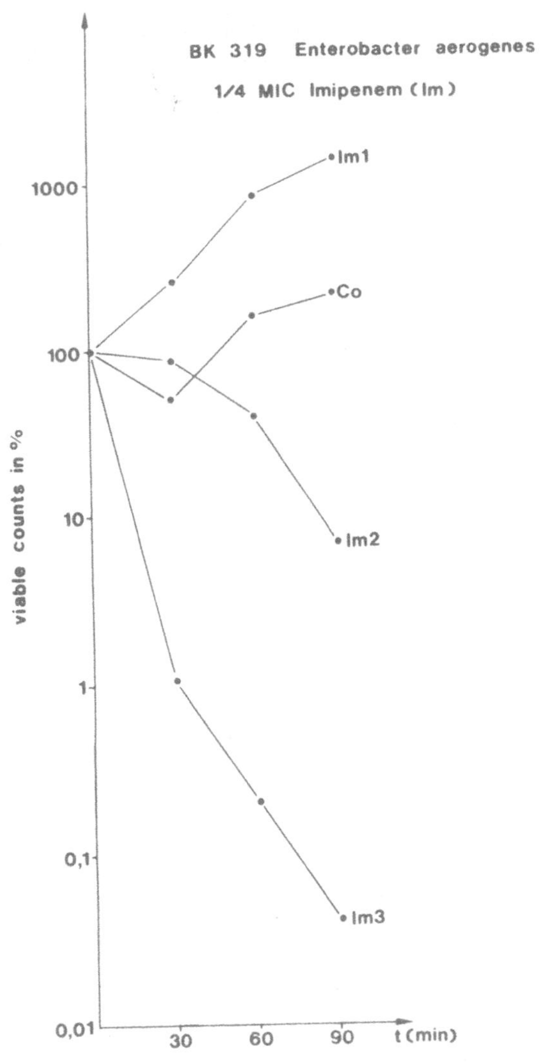

Figure 3. Influence of different serum concentrations on the imipenem-treated serum-resistant bacteria of BK 319. Im 1, 20% heat-inactivated serum; Im 2, 5% active serum, Im 3, 20% active serum.

Table 4. Comparison of Serum Resistance in % (v/v) After Treatment with Mecillinam and Imipenem

Antibiotic	BK 615	Serum resistance in % WF 52	BK 319
Control	20	20	20
Mecillinam	20	20	20
Imipenem	3	15	3

resistance, mecillinam had no influence at all. Taylor and associates (6) found a decrease in serum resistance in E. coli after treatment with 1/2 MIC or lower concentrations of mecillinam, whereas the strains used for this study were not killed under similar conditions. As both mecillinam and imipenem are round cell-forming β-lactam antibiotics and their main biochemical target is the penicillin-binding protein (PBP) 2, these results

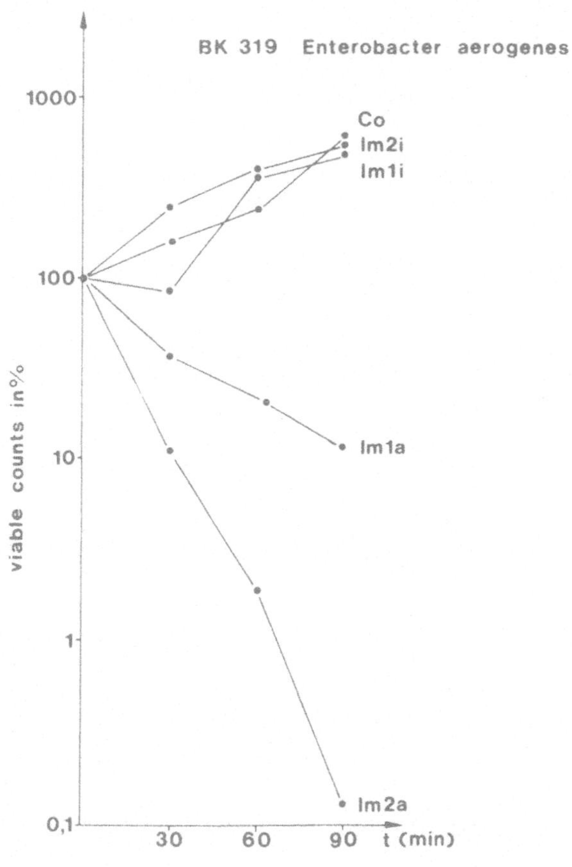

Figure 4. Influence of different concentrations of imipenem on the serum resistance of BK 319. Im 1i, 1/8 MIC + heat-inactivated serum; Im 1a, 1/8 MIC + active serum; Im 2i, 1/4 MIC + heat-inactivated serum; Im 2a, 1/4 MIC + active serum. Serum concentration: 20%.

are of special interest. From our data it can be concluded that PBP 2 cannot be responsible for the observed phenomenon.

To be sure that there was a real change in serum resistance and not an additional effect of the antibiotic itself, it is very important to reduce the serum concentration. When the experiments were carried out under the same conditions using filament-forming antibiotics, no killing could be observed if the serum concentration was reduced. Imipenem was the only antibiotic which influenced serum resistance of the strains BK 615 and BK 319 to such an extent that even 3% NHS (instead of more than 20%) was able to kill the bacteria.

To answer the question of how complement kills the imipenem-treated cells, by the classical or by the alternative pathway, experiments were carried out with serum preincubated with bacteria to absorb antibodies or Mg^{++} EGTA containing serum: no killing effect could be observed in the cases of absorbed serum or EGTA-containing serum (Figure 5). It was assumed that the killing works via the antibody dependent classical pathway. In order to find a serum protein responsible for the described effect of induced serum sensitivity, serum proteins were fractionated by ammonium sulfate precipitation and gel chromatography. But up to now it has not been possible to restore the killing potency of the serum by adding frac-

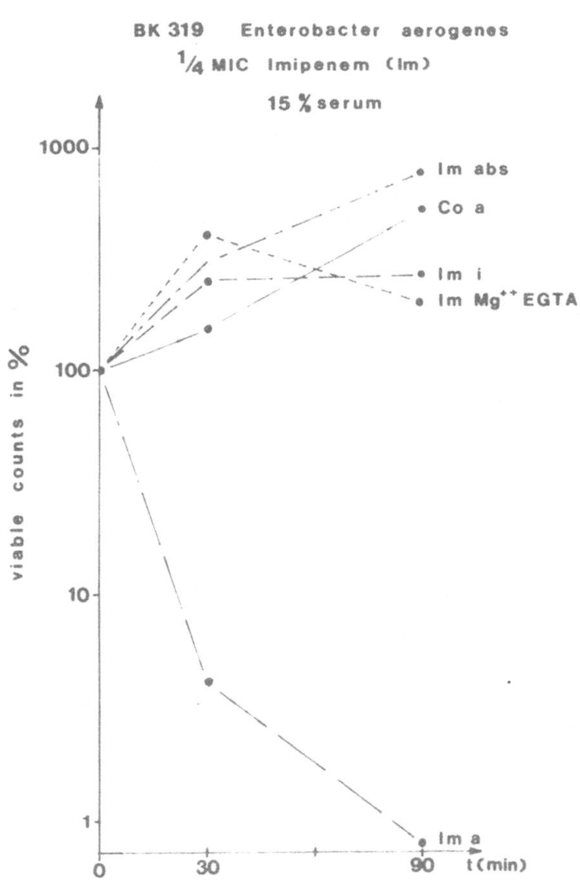

Figure 5. Growth curves of imipenem-treated bacteria of BK 319 in absorbed or Mg^{++} EGTA-containing serum. Abs, absorbed serum; a, active serum; i, heat-inactivated serum.

Table 5. CH50 of the Classical and the Alternative Pathway in Normal and Absorbed Serum (in U/ml)

CH50 in U/ml	serum	absorbed serum
classical pathway	37.9	35.3
alternative pathway	30.7	30.7

tions to absorbed serum. Neither the CH50 of the classical nor of the alternative pathway was altered by the absorption, as can be seen in Table 5.

To examine whether the bactericidal activity was impaired, the serum sensitive E. coli strain WF 96 was incubated in normal and in absorbed serum. There was no growth in 3% normal serum, whereas there was growth up to 15% absorbed serum. Addition of an antiserum to the absorbed serum had no effect on the growth of the bacteria. A non-specific factor necessary for the killing process has to be postulated. The nature of this factor is still unknown. Further studies are necessary to clarify the identity of the responsible factor.

REFERENCES

1. B. S. Dutcher, A. M. Reynard, M. E. Beck and R. K. Cunningham, Potentiation of antibiotic bactericidal activity by normal human serum, Antimicrob. Agents Chemother. 13:820 (1978).
2. J. Fierer and F. Finley, Lethal effect of complement and lysozyme on polymyxin-treated, serum-resistant gram-negative bacilli, J. Infect. Dis. 140:581 (1979).
3. H. Friedman and G. H. Warren, Antibody-mediated bacteriolysis: Enhanced killing of cyclacillin-treated bacteria, Proc. Soc. Exp. Biol. Med. 153:301 (1976).
4. V. Lorian and B. A. Atkinson, Effect of serum and blood on Enterobacteriaceae grown in the presence of subminimal inhibitory concentrations of ampicillin and mecillinam, Rev. Infect. Dis. 1:797 (1979).
5. M. M. Mayer, Complement and complement fixation, in: "Experimental Immunochemistry," E. A. Kabat and M. M. Mayer, eds., 2nd edition, C. C. Thomas, Springfield (1964).
6. P. W. Taylor, H. Gaunt and F. M. Unger, Effect of subinhibitory concentrations of mecillinam on the serum susceptibility of Escherichia coli strains, Antimicrob. Agents Chemother. 19:786 (1981).
7. W. H. Traub and J. C. Sherris, Studies on the interaction between serum bactericidal activity and antibiotics in vitro, Chemotherapy 15:70 (1970).

UPTAKE AND ANTIBACTERIAL EFFECTS OF ANTIBIOTICS WITHIN CELLS

Charles S. F. Easmon

Department of Medical Microbiology
Wright-Fleming Institute
St. Mary's Hospital Medical School
London, England

INTRODUCTION

In order to be effective, antimicrobial agents must reach the site of infection. Even where infection presents as septicaemia, the primary source is usually extravascular. Good tissue penetration may not be sufficient as a wide range of microorganisms can survive within host cells (Table 1).

There are three main methods of studying the cellular uptake of antimicrobial agents in vitro. First by observing the killing of intracellular target organisms. Second by measuring the bactericidal capacity of cell sonicates following exposure to the agent being studied. Third by using radiolabelled antimicrobial agents and measuring the cellular accumulation of the label by autoradiography or direct counting disintegrations per minute. Although these methods are simple in theory, there are a number of technical problems that must be overcome.

KILLING OF INTRACELLULAR ORGANISMS

Cells are mixed with opsonized organisms so that ingestion can occur. Then the cells, with ingested organisms, are incubated in the presence of antimicrobial agents and the subsequent reduction in viable counts measured by removing aliquots of cells at regular intervals, disrupting them and counting surviving organisms.

Table 1. Genera with Potential for Intracellular Survival

Mycobacterium	Staphylococcus
Listeria	Streptococcus
Salmonella	Pseudomonas
Brucella	Neisseria
Mycoplasma	Haemophilus
Chlamydia	

There are several problems that have to be overcome. Non-professional phagocytes (e.g. epithelial cells) do not take up ingested organisms readily. The work of Ginsburg and his colleagues has shown that opsonization with some cationic polypeptides will improve bacterial and fungal uptake by epithelial cells in culture (7).

Cell adherent organisms present another potential problem. If cell adherent organisms remain when antimicrobial agents are added to the system, they introduce two sources of error. First, these organisms can be killed readily without any cellular uptake of the drug. Secondly, phagocytosis of adherent organisms will continue and the antimicrobial agent may be taken up by "piggy-back phagocytosis".

The phagocytic system must either be checked to see that few adherent uningested organisms remain, or alternatively they must be removed. An ideal agent for removing adherent organisms should have a broad spectrum of activity, be neither cytotoxic nor taken up by cells and lyse organisms rapidly. No such agent exists. Lysostaphin, an enzyme complex that lyses Staphylococcus aureus, has been used most widely but is limited to this organism (6). It should be used in the lowest concentration for the shortest period possible, particularly when working with macrophages.

Using this technique rifamycins, quinolones, macrolides, chloramphenicol and aminoglycosides have been shown to act against intracellular bacteria (1,2,4,5,11). However, as shown in Table 2, the failure of an antimicrobial agent to kill intracellular bacteria does not necessarily mean that it has not been taken up. Antimicrobials that are bacteriostatic or only slowly bactericidal can present difficulties (3). Where intracellular killing is seen, resistant strains of the organisms should be used to check that killing is due to the direct action of the drug and is not secondary to the stimulation of intracellular killing mechanisms (2).

There are limits to this method of studying cellular uptake that cannot be overcome. Many of these can be solved by other techniques which also offer a better degree of quantitation.

BACTERICIDAL ACTIVITY OF CELL SONICATES AND USE OF RADIOLABELLED ANTIBIOTIC

With both methods the main problem is the separation of cells from antibiotic without allowing elution of drug from the cells. Normal washing in antibiotic-free medium allows this to occur. The alternative is to centrifuge cells rapidly through a water excluding gradient, thus avoiding the need for washing (8).

When measuring the bactericidal activity of cell sonicates following antibiotic exposure, the limiting factor is the sensitivity of the assay for the very small volumes of cell pellet involved. If the available assays are relatively insensitive and uptake poor it may be necessary to

Table 2. Reasons for Failure to Kill Intracellular Organisms

1. Agent not taken up
2. Intracellular bacteria not susceptible to antibiotics
3. Intracellular antibiotic not biologically active
4. Intracellular antibiotic active but not in phagolysosome
5. Antibiotic bacteriostatic or slowly bactericidal

increase the concentration of extracellular antibiotic above the physiological range. Any possible cytotoxic effects of such high concentrations should be assessed.

The use of radiolabelled antimicrobial agents depends on availability. While a few antibiotics such as benzylpenicillin and gentamicin can be bought easily, the only source of many compounds will be the relevant pharmaceutical company. Labels used will usually be tritium or Carbon-14, both beta emitters. The sensitivity of the method will depend upon the specific activity of the labelled antimicrobial agent.

To measure uptake by either bioassay or radiolabelled drug, the intracellular volume of the cell pellet must be calculated. This is normally done by subtracting from the total pellet volume (found by using tritiated water) the extracellular volume (found by using labelled insulin or polyethylene glycol) (8,10).

CONCLUSIONS

No one method is satisfactory for measuring the cellular uptake of antibiotics. Properly controlled functional assays of intracellular killing using appropriate target organisms must form the basis of the work. However, they should be combined with more quantitative assays of uptake that do not rely on intracellular targets. Experiments with radiolabelled agents alone will not show whether intracellular antibiotic is biologically active. Finally, the precise intracellular location of antibiotics can be determined by cellular disruption with differential centrifugation using marker enzymes to identify intracellular organelles (9).

REFERENCES

1. K. N. Brown and A. Percival, Penetration of antimicrobials into tissue culture cells and leucocytes, Scand. J. Infect. Dis. Suppl. 14:251 (1978).
2. C. S. F. Easmon, Effect of antibiotics on the intracellular survival of Staphylococcus aureus in vitro, Br. J. Exp. Pathol. 60:24 (1979).
3. C. S. F. Easmon and J. P. Crane, Cellular uptake of clindamycin and lincomycin, Br. J. Exp. Pathol. 65:725 (1984).
4. C. S. F. Easmon and J. P. Crane, Comparative uptake of rifampicin and rifapentine (DL 473) by human neutrophils, J. Antimicrob. Chemother. 13:585 (1984).
5. C. S. F. Easmon and J. P. Crane, Uptake of ciprofloxacin by macrophages, J. Clin. Pathol. 38:442 (1985).
6. C. S. F. Easmon, H. Lanyon and P. J. Cole, Use of lysostaphin to remove cell adherent staphylococci during in vitro assays of phagocytic function, Br. J. Exp. Pathol. 59:381 (1978).
7. I. Ginsburg, M. N. Sela, A. Morag, Z. Ravid, Z. Duchan, M. Ferne, S. Rabinowitz-Bergner, P. P. Thomas, P. Davies, J. Niccols, J. Humes and R. Bonney, Role of leukocyte factors and cationic polyelectrolytes in phagocytosis of group A streptococci and Candida albicans by neutrophils, macrophages, fibroblasts and epithelial cells, Inflammation 5:289 (1981).
8. J. D. Johnson, W. L. Hand, J. B. Francis, N. King Thompson and R. W. Corwin, Antibiotic uptake by alveolar macrophages, J. Lab. Clin. Med. 95:429 (1980).
9. D. B. Lowrie, T. J. Peters and A. Scoging, Benzylpenicillin transport and subcellular distribution in mouse peritoneal macrophage monolayers, Biochem. Pharmacol. 31:423 (1982).

10. G. L. Mandell, Interaction of intraleukocytic bacteria with antibiotics, J. Clin. Invest. 52:1673 (1972).
11. G. L. Mandell and T. K. Vest, Killing of intraleukocytic Staphylococcus aureus by Rifampin. In vitro and in vivo studies, J. Infect. Dis. 125:486 (1972).

EFFECTS OF SURAMIN ON THE MOUSE IMMUNE SYSTEM

Maud Brandely, Iris Motta, Bruno Hurtrel,
Paolo Truffa-Bachi and Philippe H. Lagrange

Institut Pasteur
Paris, France

INTRODUCTION

Virtually all virus infections lead to some degree of immune depression. This is especially significant in cases of viruses infecting lymphocytes or lymphocyte subpopulations (C.M.V., EBV, Measles and Rubella virus). The most dramatic one has been described recently; non-oncogenic retroviruses isolated from humans associated with the Acquired Immunodeficiency Syndrome (AIDS). The retroviruses are unique RNA viruses that contain an RNA-dependent DNA polymerase: the reverse transcriptase (RT), which enables them to replicate by reverse transcription of the RNA genome into a double stranded DNA. Three compounds, shown to be selective inhibitors of the RT, are candidates for the antiviral treatment of AIDS patients: Ribavirin (11), a mineral condensed ion; HPA 23, (ammonium-5-tungsto-2-antimoniate) (6); and a very old drug already licensed for clinical use, the Suramin (Germanin R, Bayer) (7), which has been used for the therapy of African Trypanosomiasis (17). Concerning the latter, apart from its inhibitory action on phagosome-lysosome fusion in macrophage (1,9), no attempt has been made to assess its own potential immunomodulating effects. The ratio of minimal antiviral concentration to the minimal immunosuppressive concentration must be formally evaluated indirectly to assess the best dosage of such a drug that is used to restore indirectly the host immune response, but may, by its own immunomodulating activities delay the quality and the speed of the recovery process.

Knowledge of mechanisms underlying such effects will be important to dictate the choice of associative reconstitutive immunotherapy (8). It is the purpose of this short review to describe the recent results obtained in murine models with Suramin in our laboratory.

IN VIVO EFFECTS OF SURAMIN ON INFECTIONS EVOKED BY INTRACELLULAR MULTIPLYING BACTERIA

Overall results presented recently (3) did confirm previous observations, namely that in vivo treatment of mice with Suramin (100 to 400 mg/kg) interferes with macrophage functions and increases the susceptibility to *Listeria monocytogenes* (14), and to *Mycobacterium tuberculosis* (15). Suramin meets the blocking properties of ployanions on both resident and sessile blood-born macrophages since a significant decrease of resistance to *L. monocytogenes* was observed in the early macrophage-monocyte mediated phase of resistance detected three to six hours after challenge. The depressive effect of Suramin at its maximum 48 hours after one single intraperitoneal injection, was followed ten days later by an increased resistance, corresponding to the observed splenomegaly. However, such rebound was not observed in Suramin-treated mice infected with an attenuated M. bovis, strain B.C.G. Suramin was shown to inhibit a non-specific defense mechanism to low dose (1×10^4/mouse) of BCG, common to naturally susceptible (C57BL/6) and resistant (C3H) mice. Similar treatment also entailed a depression of the 48 hour but not of the 24 hour delayed-type hypersensitivity (DTH) reaction to tuberculin in mice infected subcutaneously (SC) with living BCG. This alteration was also associated with a greater multiplication of BCG locally and in the draining lymph node after SC inoculation. These observations suggest that Suramin might interfere with cell mediated immunity (CMI) not only at the macrophage but also at the T lymphocyte level and has led us to assess the influence of Suramin and its mode of action on CMI and humoral immune responses, using a non-replicating antigen, namely sheep red blood cells (SRBC), in order to avoid any additive suppressive effect of antigen overloading resulting from the unrestricted intracellular bacterial replication. Moreover, in mice, DTH and antibody to SRBC tend to be mutually exclusive and modulation of the immune response can produce striking changes in the balance between humoral and CMI (10).

The dosage of Suramin which has been used in mice in order to obtain the in vivo and in vitro immunodepression was 6 to 8 µg/mouse (300-400 mg/kg) given through one single intraperitoneal injection. This dosage of Suramin used was selected from published data on in vivo immunomodulation in experimental animals (2). That dosage is far in excess from the Suramin dosage usually given to AIDS patients (15 mg/kg body weight, every five days for 35 days (5,14).

IN VIVO EFFECTS OF SURAMIN ON IMMUNE RESPONSES GENERATED TO SRBC

Administration of Suramin by IP route at various times, before, during or after antigenic sensitization (either IV or SC), resulted in a profound inhibition of DTH responses but did not seem to have any adverse effect on antibody production as detected by plaque forming cells (PFC) of circulating hemmagglutinin levels (4). Suramin was particularly effective when given during the effector phase of DTH. However, this DTH suppression was only transient. Evidence was obtained showing that this short term (no more than 48 hours) Suramin-induced suppressive effect on the expression of DTH, was related to a defective recruitment by sensitized T lymphocytes of accessory cells at the site of antigen injection, as it occurred after sublethal irradiation. Transfer of 10^7 peritoneal exsudate cells from normal syngeneic mice to Suramin-treated or sublethally irradiated recipients restored to normal or subnormal levels of the DTH reaction induced with a local adoptive transfer of T sensitized lymphocytes. In addition to the short term suppressive effect, Suramin administration given eight days before SRBC sensitization blocked the subsequent expression of the DTH effector cells, which was correlated with the abnormal enlargement of different organs: splenomegaly being particularly marked. Hence this DTH anergy appeared to result from a more extensive antigenic degradation since it was reversed by a 100-fold higher sensitizing antigen dose. However, this mechanism cannot account for the depression of DTH when mice were treated one hour prior to the IV or SC immunization with SRBC. This suppression was also short-lived, since positive DTH reactions recovered within eight days; and was observed independently of the dose of sensitizing antigen. Analysis of the sensitized lymphocyte population in these mice indicates that Suramin does neither prevent the induction of DTH mediating cells, nor the induction of helper T-cells, but suggests that the expression of the former might be inhibited by the presence of suppressive cells which are generated as a result of drug treatment. Evidence that Suramin causes the generation of a suppressive T-cell subpopulation was studied further with the in vitro analysis of immunocompetence of T-cell, B-cell and adherent cell population harvested in Suramin-treated mice.

EFFECTS OF SURAMIN ON IN VITRO ANTIBODY PRODUCTION TO SRBC

Action of Suramin on a thymus-dependent immune response was investigated in mice immunized with SRBC and treated with Suramin on the subsequent in vitro humoral anti-SRBC response (13). Evidence was obtained that in vivo treatment of Suramin during priming to SRBC led to a modification of some T-cell functions resulting in the suppression of the in vitro secondary immune response. Non-specific quantitative alteration in the relative proportion of T and B lymphocyte populations was ruled out by fluorescence activated cell sorter analysis. However, a large increase in the esterase positive cells was found. Nevertheless, the immune unresponsive state of SRBC Suramin-treated spleen cells cannot be ascribed to the adherent cells since these later can replace normal accessory cells in the normal anti-SRBC response and, on the other hand, did not exert any suppressive activity on normal cells. Using the same method of depletion reconstruction it was shown that the inability of Suramin-treated SRBC sensitized spleen cells to respond in vitro was not due to a dysfunction of the B-cells since upon addition to normal T lymphocytes, these cells are secreting antibodies. The addition of low concentrations of enriched nylon wool filtrated T-cells from SRBC + Suramin-treated spleen cells to normal T depleted population allowed the recovery of an immune response to SRBC, indicating that a defect of T helper cells was not by itself responsible for the lack of the in vitro response. However, as observed for DTH local transfer, addition to larger quantities of the same T-cells from SRBC Suramin-treated spleen cells, resulted in a lower degree of reconstitution, suggesting the presence of a suppressive compartment in this population. The suppressive population was demonstrated after an enrichment using the Wheat Germ Agglutinin (WGA). The WGA+ contained a population of cells able to suppress the in vitro response, and was abolished by irradiation and anti-Thy 1 plus complement treatment. This suppressive population was absent in non-treated SRBC primed mice. It should be noted also that the in vitro demonstrated Suramin-induced immunosuppression was not observed in situ, in SRBC + Suramin-treated mice, as reported, a secondary in vivo challenge given to these mice leads to an enhanced anti-SRBC response, which was related to a non-specific increase in the number of spleen cells. An explanation for the opposite effects of Suramin on the in vivo antibody production and CMI/DTH is that the Suramin-induced suppressor T-cells leave the spleen compartment as a result of in situ challenge and exert their activity on circulating DTH mediating T-cells.

EFFECTS OF SURAMIN ON THE IN VITRO LYMPHOCYTE PROLIFERATION

In vitro proliferation responses of spleen cells from Suramin-treated mice were shown to be suppressed, when both T-cell and B-cell mitogens were used. This effect was still observed in mice treated four and eight days before the test (Figure 1), and did occur for the optimal and suboptimal doses of the mitogens used. The observed excess of esterase (+v¢) cells was not responsible for this depressive effect of Suramin, since adherent cell depletion did not abrogate the suppression. Moreover, the treatment of spleen cells from Suramin-treated mice with anti-Thy 1 antibody plus complement was not able to alter the suppressed LPS proliferative response, but was able to completely abrogate the Con A response. Possible alterations of in vitro mediators production were tested next, with spleen cells from mice being treated four days previously. Adherent spleen cells from normal and from Suramin-treated mice, being stimulated with LPS, produced the same level of interleukine 1 (IL1) measured by the levels of PHA (5 g/ml) stimulation on thymocytes from C3H/HeJ mice. However, using a CTLL assay, it was observed that spleen cells from Suramin-treated mice (primed or not by SRBC) stimulated by Con A were markedly less able to produce IL2 (Figure 2) when compared to normal spleen cells. Also supernatants from Con A stimulated spleen cells from Suramin-treated mice, were not able to restore the in vitro antibody response of T-cell depleted population (results not shown), indicating a frank inhibition of the T replacing factor (TRF).

CONCLUSIONS

The capacity of Suramin to inhibit the RT of animal retroviruses was reported in 1979 (7) and also was recently confirmed effective on human nononcogenic retroviruses associated with AIDS (12). Preliminary results did show also some immunological improvements in four AIDS patients (16). However, a part of a number of recognized toxicities of Suramin in human beings, such as renal damage, shock, coma and our reported recent results in mice, are in favor of multiple effects on the immune responses which might impede the normal recovery after the in vivo inhibition of retrovirus replication. The first effect of Suramin involved its activity on the accessory cells of the mononuclear phagocyte system. It alters a killing mechanism, being independent of the H_2O_2 killing mechanism, associated with

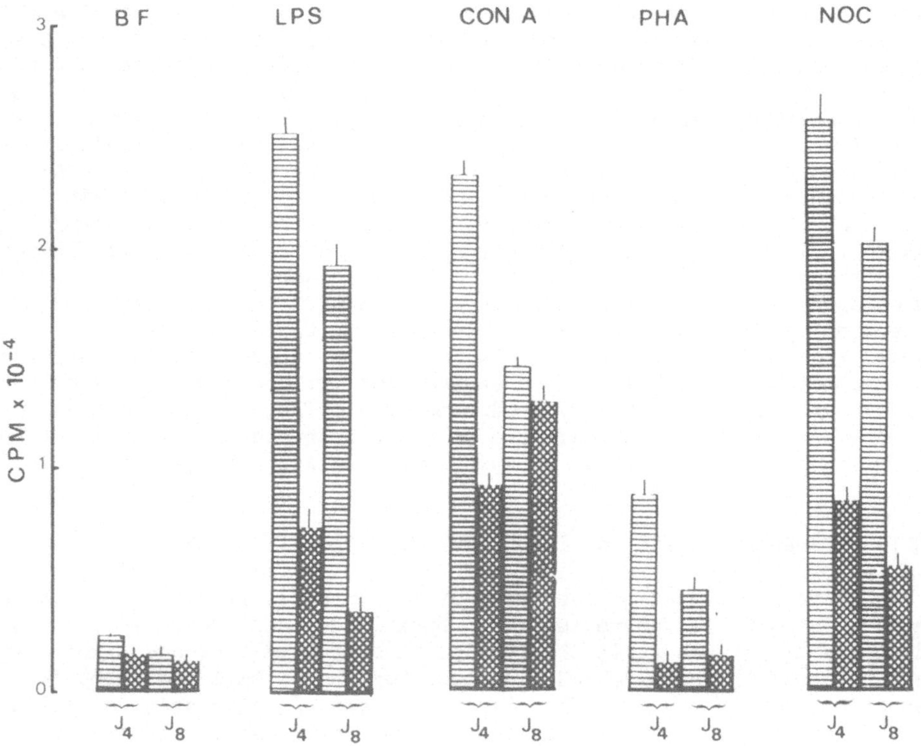

Figure 1. Proliferative responses to B (LPS: 200 µl/ml, Nocardia: 50 µl/ml) or T cell (Con A: 4 µl/ml, PHA: 10 µg/ml) mitogens of 1×10^6 cells/ml harvested from normal mice (hatched bar) and from mice treated 4 or 8 days previously with suramin (400 mg/kg) (dark bars). BF represent the background stimulation without mitogen in the culture medium. Culture in triplicate ± SEM.

the inhibition of the phagosome lysosome fusion. It impedes the recruitment of the accessory cells at the site of the specific antigen deposition during the DTH reaction. However, in contrast to the hypothesis concerning its action on the antigen presentation through induced membrane alterations, such effect was observed neither for the expression of DTH after an in vitro local transfer of primed T-cells, nor for the in vitro antibody production. Moreover, equivalent numbers of LPS stimulated macrophages from Suramin-treated mice produced the same quantity of IL1 as macrophages from normal mice.

The second effect of Suramin involved its ability to stimulate the production of suppressor T-cells, suspected in vivo for the DTH reaction to tuberculin after BCG vaccination, or after SRBC sensitization, and evidence in vitro for the secondary antibody response. This helper T-cell anergy is related in part to the suppressive T-cell activity demonstrated in the SRBC + Suramin-treated spleen cell populations, and the associated reduced ability of such cells to produce IL2 and TRF. An explanation for the opposite

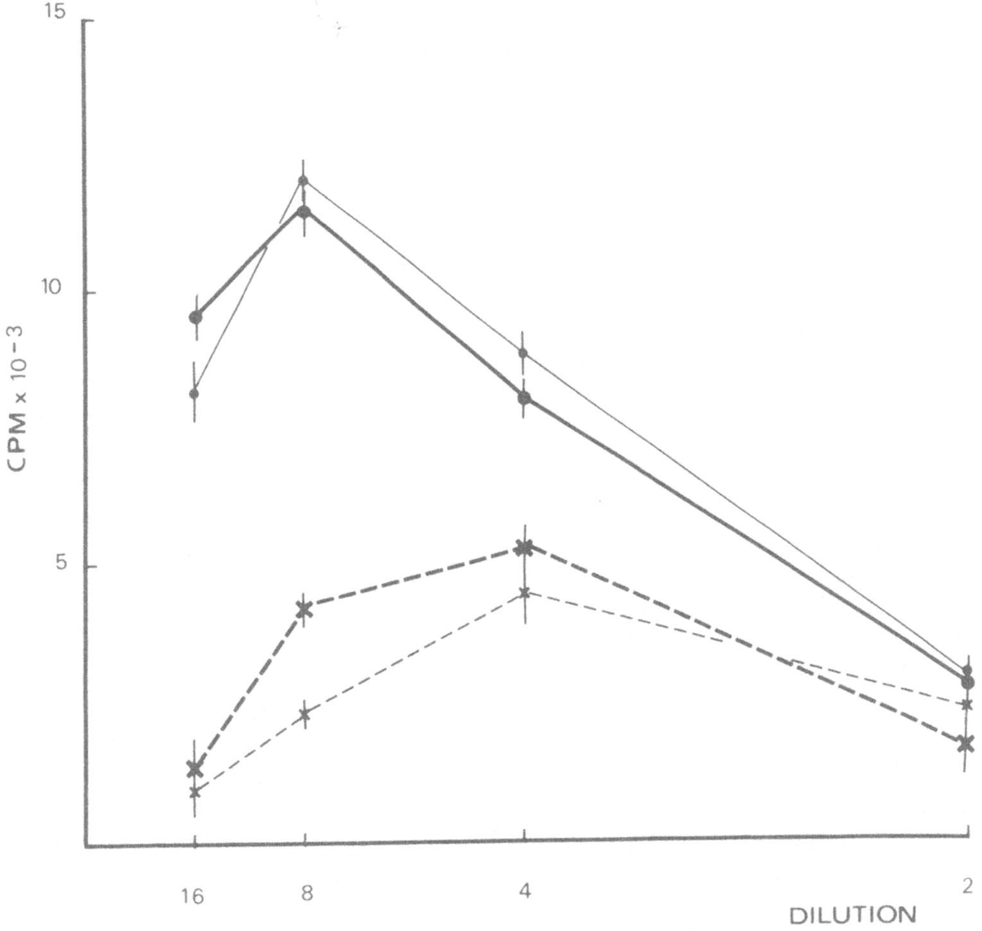

Figure 2. Proliferative responses of CTLL, IL2 dependent cultivated in presence of varying dilutions of supernatants from Con A stimulated spleen cells harvested from normal (heavy line), SRBC primed (light line) and from Suramin-treated mice (heavy dotted line and light dotted lines correspond to non-primed mice). Mean of four cultures per group ± SEM.

effects of Suramin on in vivo antibody production and cell- mediated DTH (or in vitro antibody response) is that these Suramin-induced T suppressive cells leave the spleen compartment as a result of in situ antigenic challenge and exert their activity on circulating DTH mediating T-cells.

These results suggest that Suramin treatment will not substantially benefit patients with late stage AIDS by downgrading the potential remains of the immune system. Therefore, there may be rationale for using this drug early in the disease associated with pro-host immunotherapy in order to restore both the retroviruses induced immune defects and the immune alterations associated with the Suramin treatment.

REFERENCES

1. J. A. Armstrong and P. D. A. Hart, Response of cultured macrophages to Mycobacterium tuberculosis, with observation of fusion of lysosomes with phagosomes, J. Exp. Med. 134:713 (1971).
2. N. Bloksma, M. J. DeReuver, and J.M.N. Willers, Influence on macrophage functions as a possible basis of immunomodification by polyanions, Ann. Immunol. Inst. Pasteur 131D:255 (1980).
3. M. Brandely, P. H. LaGrange and B. Hurtrel, Effects of Suramin on the in vivo antimicrobial resistance against Listeria monocytogenes and Mycobacterium bovis (BCG) in mice, submitted for publication (1985).
4. M. Brandely, P. H. LaGrange, B. Hurtrel, I. Motta and P. Truffa-Bachi, Effects of Suramin on the immune responses to sheep red blood cells in mice, I. In vivo studies., Cell. Immunol. 93:in press (1985).
5. S. Broder, AIDS Meeting Antiviral Agents Workshop, National Institutes of Health, Bethesda, Maryland (1985).
6. J. C. Chermann, F. Sinoussi and C. Jasmin, Inhibition of RNA-dependent DNA polymerase of murine oncornaviruses by ammonium 5 tungsto-2-antimoniate, Bio. Chem. Biophys. Res. Comm. 65:1229 (1975).
7. E. DeClercq, Suramin: a potent inhibitor of the reverse transcriptase of RNA tumor viruses, Cancer Lett. 8:9 (1979).
8. J. W. Hadden, Immunostimulation therapy in the treatment of infectious diseases: the pro-host approach, EOS, Rev. Immunol. Immunofarm. 5:51 (1985).
9. P. D. A. Hart and M. R. Young, Interference with normal phagosome-lysosome fusion in macrophages, using ingested yeast cells and Suramin, Nature (London) 256:47 (1975).
10. P. H. LaGrange, G. B. Mackaness and T. E. Miller, Influence of dose and route of antigen injection on the immunological induction of T cells, J. Exp. Med. 139:528 (1974).
11. J. B. McCormick, J. P. Getchell, S. W. Mitchell and D. R. Hicks, Ribavirin suppresses replication of lymphadenopathy-associated virus in cultures of humans adult T lymphocytes, Lancet 2:1367 (1984).
12. H. Mitsuya, M. Popovic, R. Yarchoan, S. Matsushita, R. C. Gallo and S. Broder, Suramin protection of T cells in vitro against infectivity and cytopathic effect of HTVL-III, Sciences 226:172 (1984).
13. I. Motta, M. Brandely, P. Truffa Bachi, B. Hurtrel and P. H. LaGrange, Effects of Suramin on the immune responses to sheep red blood cells in mice, II. In vitro studies, Cell. Immunol. 93: in press (1985).
14. E. L. Pesanti, Suramin effects on macrophage phagosome lysosome fusion formation and antimicrobial activity, Infec. Immun. 20:503 (1978).
15. J. R. W. Rees and P. D. A. Hart, Enhancement of experimental tuberculosis in the mouse by Suramin, Tubercle 37:327 (1956).
16. D. Rouvroy, J. Bogaerts, J. B. Habyarimana, D. Nzaramba and P. Van de Perre, Short term results with Suramin for AIDS related conditions, Lancet 1:878 (1985).

17. J. Williamson, Review of chemotherapeutic and chemoprophylactic agents, in: "The African Trypanosomiasis," M. W. Mulligan, ed., Wiley, New York (1970).

IMMUNOMODULATION BY ANTIVIRAL AGENTS

Mario R. Escobar

Medical College of Virginia
Virginia Commonwealth University
Richmond, Virginia

ABSTRACT

Most commonly clinical or subclinical viral infections are self-limited by the effective immune response of the host leading to recovery. Occasionally, the infectious process may continue uncontrolled contributing to the demise of the patient or resulting in a number of sequelae, if the patient survives. This unfavorable outcome in a number of viral infections (e.g., those associated with herpes virus) usually reflects immunoincompetence (e.g., in transplant, cancer and AIDS patients). Conversely, dysregulation of immune functions (e.g., in autoimmunity) may triggered during the aftermath of certain viral infections. Recently, accumulated knowledge about the molecular biology of viruses has opened the way to more rational approaches to the development of more potent and more selective antiviral agents. In fact, some of these compounds have already been licensed for clinical use. Nonetheless, some of these antivirals which effectively affect viral replication may also possess significant immunosuppressive activity. Only in a few instances have antiviral agents been investigated for this interaction with the immune system and no attempts have been made to assess their potential immunosuppressive effects in the wide variety of assay systems for measuring the level of immunoreactivity. A correlation between the minimal antiviral concentration of the chemotherapeutic agent required to inhibit virus replication in cell culture and its minimal immunosuppressive concentration measured by lymphocyte responsiveness to mitogens or specific viral antigens has revealed different levels of efficacy (i.e., highest antiviral effect and lowest immunosuppressive activity): highest level as in the case of acyclovir (ACV) and bromovinyldeoxiuridine (BVDU) for HSV-1; moderate level as in the case of trifluridine (TFT). There are other chemotherapeutic agents whose efficacy is presently being evaluated regarding their interaction with the immune system. Other aspects of the management of the patient with viral disease include the clinical evaluation of biologic antivirals (e.g., interferon) and immunoenhancing substances designed to act through immunopotentiation of normal host responses. These studies should take into account: 1) the effect of these antiviral agents on each immune parameter of the host, particularly that which plays a major role in the resistance against the virus concerned; and, 2) the ratio of minimal antiviral concentration to the minimal immunosuppressive concentration to identify those agents or dosages that may impair the host's immune response and, therefore, delay rather than speed the recovery process.

ANTIVIRAL AGENTS IN THE TREATMENT OF HERPES VIRUS INFECTIONS IN IMMUNOSUPPRESSED PATIENTS

Erik De Clercq

Rega Institute for Medical Research
Katholieke Universiteit Leuven
Leuven, Belgium

INTRODUCTION

Immunosuppressed patients, particularly patients with hematologic malignancies, are much more vulnerable to virus infections, i.e. herpes virus infections, than are healthy persons in the population at large. This is illustrated not only by such fatal diseases as AIDS (acquired immunodeficiency syndrome), CMV (cytomegalovirus) pneumonia and EBV (Epstein-Barr virus)-associated lymphoproliferative disorders, but also by those virus infections, i.e. HSV (herpes simplex virus) and VZV (varicella-zoster virus), that are usually mild and benign in healthy individuals but often serious and occasionally fatal in the immunosuppressed host.

Along with the marked success obtained in recent years in the treatment of some cancers, there has been a parallel increase in the relative importance of infectious diseases which represent serious and often life-threatening complications in these patients. In many instances, it is a virus infection that undermines the potentially effective antitumor therapy and causes death of the patient (43). Thus, an effective antiviral drug may be of critical importance for an immunosuppressed patient with a severe viral infection, as it could make the difference between life and death.

Since the herpes viruses HSV, VZV, CMV and EBV are of great importance as the etiologic agents of severe viral infections in immunocompromised patients, the present report will be focused on the new antiviral drugs and therapeutic modalities that have recently been developed to treat these viral infections. It should be recognized that those patients that are most prone to herpes virus infections and hence likely to benefit most from an effective antiviral chemotherapy, are the severely immunocompromised. These patients are the least able to sustain further immuno- or myelosuppression. It is obvious, therefore, that any antiviral agent, if it were to be used successfully in the chemotherapy of virus infections in immunocompromised patients, should not further impair the host's immune responsiveness, and thus, be free of immuno- or myelotoxicity at therapeutically useful doses (15,16).

ANTIVIRAL COMPOUNDS

Cytarabine

Cytarabine (Ara-C) (Figure 1) has been abandoned for clinical use as an antiviral agent essentially because it was found to prolong, rather than shorten the dissemination of herpes zoster in immunocompromised patients (52). This deleterious action could be attributed to a suppressive effect of Ara-C on the hematopoietic and immune defense systems.

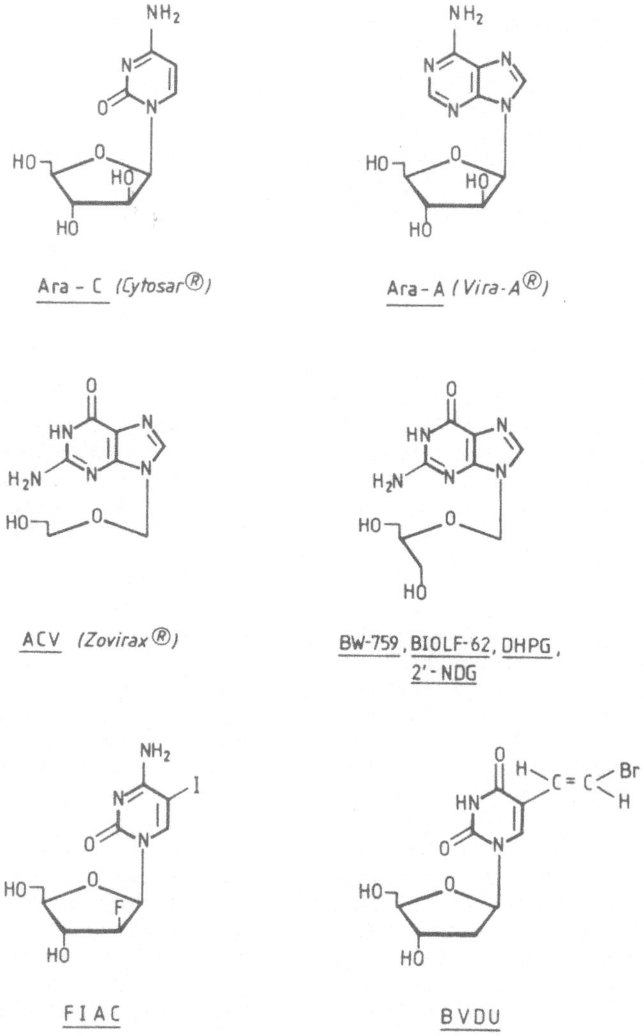

Ara - C *(Cytosar®)*

Ara - A *(Vira-A®)*

ACV *(Zovirax®)*

BW-759, BIOLF-62, DHPG, 2'-NDG

FIAC

BVDU

Figure 1. Structural formulae of selected antiviral compounds: Ara-C (Cytosar®); 1-β-D-arabinofuranosylcytosine, cytosine arabinoside. Ara-A (Vira-A®): 9-β-D-arabinofuranosyladenine, adenine arabinoside. ACV (Zovirax®): 9-[(2-hydroxyethoxy)methyl]guanine, acycloguadenosine, acyclovir. BW-759, BIOLF-62, DHPG, 2'-NDG: 9-[(2-hydroxy-1-(hycroxymethyl)-ethoxy)methyl]guanine, 9-[(1,3-dihydroxy-2-propoxy)-methyl]guanine, 2'-nor-2'-deoxyguanosine. BVDU: (E)-5-(2-bromovinyl)-2'-deoxyuridine, bromovinyldeoxyuridine. FIAC: 1-(2'-fluoro-2'-deoxy-β-D-arabinofuranosyl)-5-iodocytosine, fluoroiodoaracytosine.

Vidarabine

Vidarabine (Ara-A) (Figure 1) is of some benefit in the treatment of HSV and VZV infections in immunocompromised patients. It accelerates cessation of new vesicle formation by 1-2 days (60-62). This is accompanied by a more rapid resolution of existing lesions, and these results are achieved with minimal evidence of laboratory or clinical drug toxicity. However, the drug has to be given at the intravenous route, and its poor solubility in aqueous medium (∿ 0.45 mg/ml) necessitates the administration of large volumes of water. Furthermore, vidarabine treatment has to be instituted within 72 hours of the onset of the disease to favorably affect the cutaneous healing process (VZV or HSV lesions).

Acyclovir

Therapy of HSV and VZV infections by ACV. Several placebo-controlled trials have been carried out with acyclovir (ACV) (Figure 1), which indicate that it is highly efficacious in the treatment of HSV infections: it significantly shortens the period of new lesion formation, pain, crusting and healing, and, in particular, the time of virus shedding (36,38,57). Shortening of the period of virus shedding is much less demonstrable following vidarabine administration over a similar time frame.

Acyclovir is also considered efficacious for the treatment of VZV infection in immunocompromised patients (37). Yet, the study conducted by Balfour et al. (1983) indicated that, although ACV, when administered intravenously at 1500 mg/m^2/day for 7 days, prevented progression, i.e. dissemination of zoster in immunocompromised patients, it did not exert a significant effect on the duration of virus shedding, new lesion formation, healing or pain. Nor did it prevent post-therapeutic neuralgia.

In immunocompromised children with varicella, acyclovir prevents visceral complications, i.e. pneumonitis, but does not accelerate the resolution of existing lesions (39). Boguslawska and associates (6) claimed that acyclovir, in comparison with Ara-C, shortens the period of formation of new VZV lesions, but, since Ara-C has by itself a deleterious effect on the course of VZV infections (52), the beneficial effect noted for acyclovir by Boguslawska et al. should be interpreted cautiously. If any beneficial effect were to be expected from acyclovir therapy for VZV infections in immunocompromised patients, treatment should be started within 72 hours of the onset of rash (2).

Prophylaxis of HSV infections by ACV. Acyclovir has been the subject of several double-blind placebo-controlled trials to assess its efficacy in the prophylaxis of HSV infections in high-risk immunosuppressed patients, i.e. bone-marrow transplant recipients or patients receiving remission induction chemotherapy for acute leukemia (26,41). Acyclovir proved clearly effective in preventing the recurrence of HSV infection during the treatment period. Once acyclovir was discontinued, however, herpes infections developed at the same rate as in the placebo group, indicating no effect of ACV on latent virus. Indications for prophylactic acyclovir in the immunosuppressed host are few: i.e. patients with frequently recurrent and severe herpes simplex who are undergoing a short but intense period of immunosuppression. ACV may be of great utility in such patients, especially if, as reported by Gluckman et al. (25), it could be given by the oral route (800 mg/day) for the prevention of HSV infections in high-risk patients.

Dihydroxypropoxymethylguanine

Dihydroxypropoxymethylguanine (DHPG) (Figure 1) is structurally related to acyclovir and has been referred to as BW-759, BIOLF-62 and 2'NDG (24,46,48). As compared to acyclovir, DHPG is at least ten-fold more potent in inhibiting CMV and EBV replication in vitro (10,24); and the potent and selective activity of DHPG against CMV in vitro (31,53,55) has prompted clinical investigations with the drug in the therapy and prophylaxis of CMV infections in immunosuppressed patients (data forthcoming). An addition of DHPG is that it is about 50-fold more efficacious than ACV in vivo, i.e. when administered orally or parenterally to mice infected with HSV-1 or HSV-2 (1,24,46).

Fluoroiodoaracytosine

Fluoroiodoaracytosine (FIAC) (Figure 1) is a candidate antiviral drug with potent in vitro activity against a number of herpes viruses, including HSV, VZV, CMV and EBV (11,28,30,32,58). FIAC has been shown to stabilize cutaneous VZV lesions in immunosuppressed patients within 48 to 72 hours after starting treatment (64). However, the therapeutic index of FIAC is far from impressive, since it causes myelosuppression, nausea and vomiting at a dosage of 400 and 600 mg/m^2/day, that is three- to five-fold higher than the effective dose (120mg/m^2/day).

Bromovinyldeoxyuridine

Activity spectrum of BVDU. Bromovinyldeoxyuridine (BVDU) (Figure 1) is the most potent and most selective of all anti-HSV-1 and anti-VZV agents that are currently being pursued for their therapeutic potentials in the clinic (19,20,21,44). It is active against HSV-1, VZV and several other herpes viruses, i.e. suid herpes virus type 1 (pseudorabies virus), bovid herpes virus type 1 (infectious bovine rhinotracheitis virus), simian varicella virus (SVV) and herpes virus platyrrhinae at a concentration of 0.01 µg/ml or lower (13). A remarkable characteristic of BVDU is that it is much less inhibitory for HSV-2 than for HSV-1 (21), and, consequently,

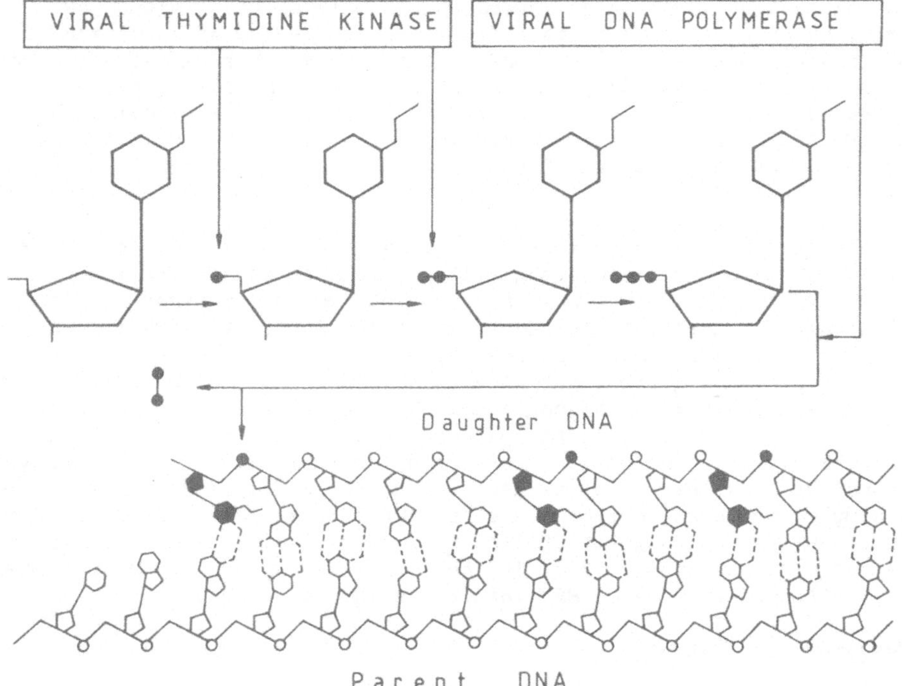

Figure 2. Mechanism of antiviral action of BVDU (14).

BVDU can be used as an accurate marker for the identification of type 1 and type 2 HSV strains in clinical isolates.

<u>Mechanisms of antiviral action of BVDU.</u> The mechanism of action of BVDU (14) is based upon a specific interaction with two virus-encoded enzymes: 1) viral thymidine kinase which converts the compound successively to its 5'-monophosphate (BVDUMP) and 5'-diphosphate (BVDUDP) (which is then further converted to BVDU 5'-triphosphate (BVDUTP) by an as yet unidentified cellular kinase); and 2) viral DNA polymerase which may either be inhibited by BVDUTP, in competition with the natural substrate dTTP, or, alternatively, recognize BVDUTP as substrate and incorporate it into DNA (Figure 2). The selectivity of BVDU as an anti-herpes agent would primarily depend on its phosphorylation by the herpesvirus-specified thymidine kinase. This specific phosphorylation restricts the further antimetabolic action of BVDU to the virus-infected cell.

Other anti-herpes agents, i.e. ACV, FIAC and DHPG, achieve their selective antiviral activity by a mechanism that is similar to that of BVDU (14). A major difference in the mechanism of action of ACV and BVDU is that BVDU is incorporated into DNA via an internucleotide linkage, whereas ACV has to be incorporated at the 3'-terminal of DNA, since it lacks the necessary 3'-hydroxylgroup for further chain elongation.

<u>Efficacy of BVDU in animal models.</u> Beneficial effects have been noted with BVDU in a wide variety of experimental HSV-1 and VZV model infections, reminiscent of the major HSV and VZV manifestations in humans, i.e. mucocutaneous herpes, herpetic keratitis, genital herpes, herpetic encephalitis, disseminated herpes simplex or zoster, and varicella [as reviewed in (22)]. Illustrated in Figure 3 is the reduction in the mortality rate of athymic nude mice infected with HSV-1, upon systemic (intraperitoneal or peroral) treatment with BVDU (23). This model can be considered as representative of generalized HSV infection in immunosuppressed patients.

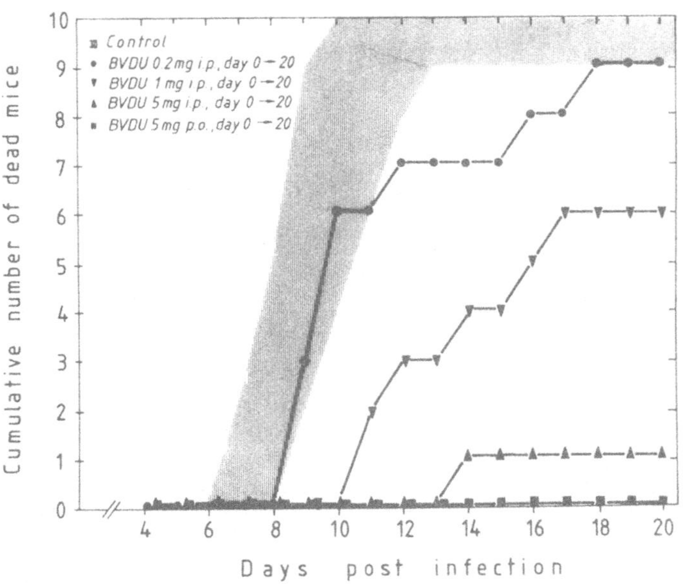

Figure 3. Mortality rate of athymic-nude mice inoculated intracutaneously with HSV-1 (strain KOS) and treated intraperitoneally (i.p.) or perorally (p.o.) with BVDU [as based on the data of (23)].

Efficacy of BVDU in humans. Initial clinical studies have been conducted with BVDU in five groups of patients: 1) BVDU 0.1% eyedrops in the topical treatment of patients with herpetic keratitis (35,33); 2) oral BVDU at 7.5 mg/kg/day for 5 days, together with BVDU 0.1% eyedrops, in the treatment of ophthalmic zoster in elderly patients (34,33); 3) oral BVDU at 7.5 mg/kg/day for 5 days in the treatment of localized or disseminated herpes zoster in cancer patients (63); 4) oral BVDU at 15 mg/kg/day for 5 days in the treatment of varicella or zoster in children with cancer (4,17) and 5) oral BVDU at 7.5 mg/kg/day for 5 days in the treatment of mucocutaneous herpes simplex or herpes zoster in severely immunosuppressed patients (including bone-marrow transplant recipients) (54). From these studies BVDU appeared as a safe and highly efficacious drug for both topical treatment of herpetic keratitis and oral treatment of HSV-1 and VZV infections in immunosuppressed patients. In the majority of the patients, BVDU arrested progression of the HSV-1 or VZV infection within 1 day of treatment (Figure 4). This was more remarkable as several patients had been suffering from progressive HSV or VZV for one week or longer (54).

BVDU as compared to Ara-A and ACV. At present, Ara-A and ACV are the only antiviral drugs licensed for clinical use in the systemic treatment of herpes virus infections. The following considerations make BVDU a potentially more attractive candidate than Ara-A and ACV for the systemic treatment of HSV-1 and, in particular, VZV infections in immunocompromised patients.

a. In vitro, BVDU is about five-fold more potent than ACV and 1000-fold more potent than Ara-A in inhibiting the replication of HSV-1 (21), and about 500- to 1000-fold more potent than ACV and Ara-A in inhibiting the replication of VZV (5,44). The relative potencies of BVDU and ACV as inhibitors of HSV-1, HSV-2, VZV, CMV and EBV are compared in Figure 5. From this diagram it is clear that all herpesviruses, with one remarkable exception (HSV-2), are more sensitive to BVDU than ACV.

b. BVDU is highly effective against simian varicella virus infection in monkeys (an animal model that is reminiscent of generalized VZV infections in humans) (51); at dosage levels (5, 10 and 15 mg/kg/day) which are

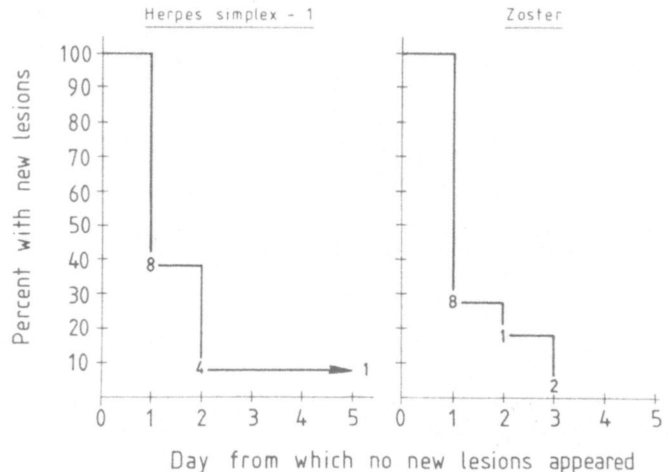

Figure 4. Formation of new herpes simplex-1 or zoster lesions in severely immunosuppressed patients (including bone marrow transplant recipients) upon initiation of oral BVDU treatment (7.5 mg/kg/day). Number of patients enrolled in this study: 13 (herpes simplex-1) and 11 (zoster) [as based on data of (54)].

readily applicable in man. At the same dosage regimens, ara-A and ACV are either ineffective or only marginally effective (49,50).

c. BVDU is very well absorbed orally (up to 90%), whereas oral ACV is absorbed poorly (only about 20% of an oral dose of 200 mg) (42); Ara-A has never been given by the oral route to patients.

d. Although neither BVDU nor ACV are immuno- or myelotoxic at the concentrations required to inhibit the replication of HSV-1 or VZV, BVDU is undoubtedly the least immuno- or myelotoxic of the two; i.e., taken several immuno- and myelotoxicity tests together (15,16), the immuno- or myelotoxic doses are 100 μg/ml (on average) for BVDU and 20-40 μg/ml for ACV; Ara-A starts to be myelo- and immunotoxic from a concentration of 1-2 μg/ml.

e. From the studies of Tricot et al. (54) and Wildiers and De Clercq (63), it appears that BVDU is still effective when treatment is initiated after a prolonged (several weeks) duration of the VZV infection (even if unresponsive to ACV). In contrast, ACV must be given within three days of the onset of the disease to be clinically effective (2,3).

LIMITATIONS OF ANTI-HERPES COMPOUNDS

There are some limitations in the clinical usefulness of the anti-herpes agents, which should caution against their indiscriminate use. The in vitro activity spectrum of the compounds should be carefully examined before embarking upon clinical trials: i.e. based on their in vitro potency against CMV (Figure 5), neither BVDU nor ACV may be expected to offer much benefit in the therapy or prophylaxis of CMV infections. Following the same reasoning it would not seem justified to pursue BVDU for its clinical potentials in the treatment of HSV-2 infections. Vice versa, the minimum concentration of BVDU required to inhibit the replication of EBV (0.02 μg/ml; 27), appears to be sufficiently low to envisage clinical trials with BVDU in the treatment of patients with EBV-associated diseases, especially during the phase of active virus replication. In fact, of a series of antiviral agents which were evaluated for their inhibitory effects on EBV replication, BVDU emerged as the most selective inhibitor (therapeutic index: 6500; 27).

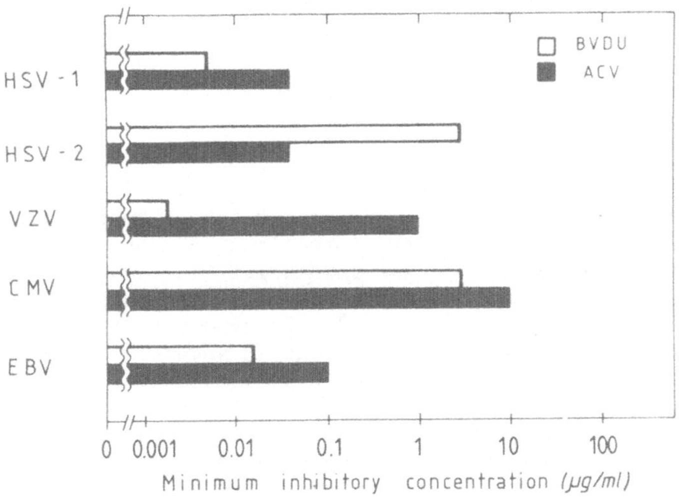

Figure 5. Comparative antiviral potencies of BVDU and ACV in vitro (as based on the data of (5,13,14,21,27,29,44,47).

A limitation in the use of ACV is its low oral absorption (as already been mentioned above). The plasma drug levels achieved with the recommended oral dosage of acyclovir (5 x 200 mg/day) may be sufficient to control HSV infections but inadequate to affect VZV infections. Recently, an analogue of acyclovir has been developed, designated BW A515U (6-deoxyacyclovir), which generates plasma concentrations of ACV that are comparable to those obtained with intravenous ACV (42,59). The plasma ACV concentrations achieved with the analogue may be high enough for it to be effective against VZV infections. Whether 6-deoxyacyclovir is an effective and safe drug for oral treatment of VZV infections, remains to be determined.

An inevitable problem linked to all anti-herpes agents is their inability to cope with virus latency and to eradicate latent virus from the sensory ganglia. Although BVDU, ACV and their congeners may prevent the establishment of virus latency as well as recolonization of the ganglia following each new recurrence, latent virus infections once established are not amenable to antiviral chemotherapy.

Resistance of herpesviruses to antiviral drugs, i.e. ACV, is not a clinical problem at the moment, but it can be induced in vitro and detected in vivo. ACV-resistant HSV mutants have been isolated from immunosuppressed patients treated with acyclovir (7,12,45,56). The mutants isolated by Burns et al. (7), Sibrack et al. (45) and Wade et al. (56) were specifically defective in phosphorylating ACV, whereas the mutant isolated by Crumpacker et al. (12) possessed diminished thymidine kinase activity. Mutants based on an altered DNA polymerase have so far not been isolated from patients, or at least not been reported in the literature.

No toxic side effects have been observed with BVDU at the doses used (4,33,54,63). Also, acyclovir is essentially non-toxic at the recommended dosage regimens, although care must be exercised in patients with poor renal function or patients who are inadequately hydrated. The possible long-term side effects of the antiviral drugs, especially after prolonged prophylactic use, remain to be assessed. It is noteworthy that in the sister-chromatid exchange induction test (8,9), which can be considered as a sensitive parameter of chromosomal damage and mutagenic potential, BVDU turned out to be harmless up to a concentration of 75 μg/ml, which is 7500-fold higher than its minimum antiviral concentration. BVDU thus achieved a specificity index of 7500. When evaluated under the same conditions, ACV, FIAC and DHPG achieved a specificity index of 2857, 225 and 64, respectively (18); which means that BVDU is at least as safe, if not safer, from a mutagenicity viewpoint than other antiviral drugs.

SUMMARY

Acyclovir (ACV, Zovirax ®) and vidarabine (Vira-A ®) are at present the only antiviral drugs licensed for the treatment of herpes simplex virus (HSV) and varicella-zoster virus (VZV) infections in immunosuppressed patients. The recommended doses are for vidarabine (intravenous) 10 mg/kg/day for ten days, and for acyclovir (intravenous) 750 mg/m^2/day for seven days (up to 5000 mg/m^2/day for VZV infections). Intravenous or oral ACV can also be used for prevention of HSV infections in severely immunosuppressed patients, i.e. bone-marrow transplant recipients. However, oral ACV has not been shown to be effective against VZV infections. Bromovinyldeoxyuridine (BVDU) seems to be an attractive candidate for the systemic treatment of HSV-1 and VZV infections in immunosuppressed patients. BVDU is a more potent inhibitor of HSV-1 and VZV replication than ACV or ara-A, and non-toxic for bone-marrow progenitor cells and lymphocytes at doses far in excess of those required to inhibit HSV-1 or VZV replication. Moreover, BVDU is very well absorbed orally, highly effective in experimental model infections in animals, and several open clinical studies suggest that it is a safe and efficacious drug in oral treatment of HSV-1 and VZV infections in man. For the treatment of cytomegalovirus (CMV) and Epstein-Barr virus (EBV) infections no particular drug can at present be recommended. Several nucleoside analogues, i.e. fluoroiodoaracytosine (FIAC) and dihydroxypropoxymethylguanine (DHPG), show rather potent in vitro activity against CMV, and clinical studies have been undertaken with DHPG in immunosuppressed patients with CMV infections. Since ACV, FIAC, DHPG and BVDU are rather selective inhibitors of EBV replication, it would be worth pursuing their role in the chemotherapy of EBV-associated diseases in immunosuppressed patients.

REFERENCES

1. W. T. Ashton, J. D. Karkas, A. K. Field and R. L. Tolman, Activation by thymidine kinase and potent antiherpetic activity of 2'-nor-2'-deoxyguanosine (2'NDG), Biochem. Biophys. Res. Commun. 108:1716 (1982).
2. H. H. Balfour, Jr., Intravenous acyclovir therapy for varicella in immunocompromised children, J. Pediatr. 104:134 (1984).
3. H. H. Balfour, Jr., B. Bean, O. L. Laskin, R. F. Ambinder, J. D. Meyers, J. C. Wade, J. A. Zaia, D. Aeppli, L. E. Kirk, A. C. Segreti, R. E. Keeney and The Burroughs Wellcome Collaborative Acyclovir Study Group, Acyclovir halts progression of herpes zoster in immunocompromised patients, New Engl. J. Med. 308:1448 (1983).
4. Y. Benoit, G. Laureys, M. -J. Delbeke and E. De Clercq, Oral BVDU treatment of varicella and zoster in children with cancer, Eur. J. Pediatr. 143:198 (1985).
5. K. K. Biron and G. B. Elion, Effect of acyclovir combined with other antiherpetic agents on varicella zoster virus in vitro, Am. J. Med. 73(A):54 (1982).
6. J. Boguslawska-Jaworska, E. Koscielniak and B. Rodziewicz, Acyclovir therapy for chickenpox in children with hematological malignancies, Eur. J. Pediatr. 142:130 (1984).
7. W. H. Burns, R. Saral, G. W. Santos, O. L. Laskin, P. S. Lietman, C. McLaren and D. W. Barry, Isolation and characterization of resistant herpes simplex virus after acyclovir therapy, Lancet i:421 (1982).
8. J. J. Cassiman, E. De Clercq, A. S. Jones, R. T. Walker and H. Van den Berghe, Sister chromatid exchange induced by anti-herpes drugs, Brit. Med. J. 283:817 (1981).
9. J. J. Cassiman, E. De Clercq and H. Van den Berghe, Induction of sister-chromatid exchange by 5-substituted 2'-deoxyuridines, Mutation Res. 117:317 (1983).
10. Y. -C. Cheng, E. -S. Huang, J. -C. Lin, E. -C. Mar, J. S. Pagano, G. E. Dutschman and S. P. Grill, Unique spectrum of activity of 9-[(1,3-dihydroxy-2-propoxy)methyl]guanine against herpesviruses in vitro and its mode of action against herpes simplex virus type 1, Proc. Natl. Acad. Sci. USA 80:2767 (1983).
11. J. M. Colacino and C. Lopez, Efficacy and selectivity of some nucleoside analogs as anti-human cytomegalovirus agents, Antimicrob. Agents Chemother. 24:505 (1983).
12. C. S. Crumpacker, L. E. Schnipper, S. I. Marlowe, P. N. Kowalsky, B. J. Hershey and M. J. Levin, Resistance to antiviral drugs of herpes simplex virus isolated from a patient treated with acyclovir, New Engl. J. Med. 306:343 (1982).
13. E. De Clercq, The antiviral spectrum of (E)-5-(2-bromovinyl)-2'-deoxyuridine, J. Antimicrob. Chemother. 14, Suppl. A:85 (1984a).
14. E. De Clercq, Biochemical aspects of the selective antiherpes activity of nucleoside analogues, Biochem. Pharmacol. 33:2159 (1984b).

15. E. De Clercq, Antiherpesvirus agents and the immune system, Zbl. Bakt. Suppl. 13:39 (1985a).
16. E. De Clercq, Antiviral agents and the immune system, in: "Antimicrobial Agents and Immunity," J. Jeljaszewicz and G. Pulverer, eds., Academic Press Inc., London, in press (1985b).
17. E. De Clercq, Y. Benoit, G. Laureys and M. J. Delbeke, Clinical potentials of bromovinyldeoxyuridine (BVDU): in particular for oral treatment of varicella-zoster virus infections in children with cancer, in: "Proceedings of the International Symposium on Pharmacological and Clinical Approaches to Herpes Viruses and Virus Chemotherapy," Oiso, Japan. Excerpta Medica International Congress Series (ICS 667), Elsevier Science Publishers, Amsterdam, in press (1985).
18. E. De Clercq and J. -J. Cassiman, Mutagenic potential of anti-herpes agents, Submitted for publication (1985).
19. E. De Clercq, J. Descamps, P. De Somer, P. J. Barr, A. S. Jones and R. T. Walker, (E)-5-(2-Bromovinyl)-2'-deoxyuridine: a potent and selective anti-herpes agent, Proc. Natl. Acad. Sci. USA 76:2947 (1979).
20. E. De Clercq, J. Descamps, M. Ogata and S. Shigeta, In vitro susceptibility of varicella-zoster virus to E-5-(2-bromovinyl)-2'-deoxyuridine and related compounds, Antimicrob. Agents Chemother. 21:33 (1982).
21. E. De Clercq, J. Descamps, G. Verhelst, R. T. Walker, A. S. Jones, P. F. Torrence and D. Shugar, Comparative efficacy of antiherpes drugs against different strains of herpes simplex virus, J. Infect. Dis. 141:563 (1980).
22. E. De Clercq and R. T. Walker, Synthesis and antiviral properties of 5-vinylpyrimidine nucleoside analogs, Pharmac. Ther. 26:1 (1984).
23. E. De Clercq, Z. -X. Zhang, J. Descamps and K. Huygen, E-5-(2-Bromovinyl)-2'-deoxyuridine vs. interferon in the systemic treatment of infection with herpes simplex virus of athymic nude mice, J. Infect. Dis. 143:846 (1981).
24. A. K. Field, M. E. Davies, C. Dewitt, H. C. Perry, R. Liou, J. Germershausen, J. D. Karkas, W. T. Ashton, D. B. R. Johnston and R. L. Tolman, 9-{[2-Hydroxy-1-(hydroxymethyl)ethoxy]methyl}guanine: a selective inhibitor of herpes group virus replication, Proc. Natl. Acad. Sci. USA 80:4139 (1983).
25. E. Gluckman, J. Lotsberg, A. Devergie, X. M. Zhao, R. Melo, M. Gomez-Morales, T. Nebout, M. C. Mazeron and Y. Perol, Prophylaxis of herpes infections after bone-marrow transplantation by oral acyclovir, Lancet ii:706 (1983).
26. I. M. Hann, H. G. Prentice, H. A. Blacklock, M. G. R. Ross, D. Brigden, A. E. Rosling, C. Burke, D. H. Crawford, W. Brumfitt and A. V. Hoffbrand, Acyclovir prophylaxis against herpes virus infections in severely immunocompromised patients: randomized double blind trial, Brit. Med. J. 287:384 (1983).
27. J. -C. Lin, D. J. Nelson, C. U. Lambe and J. S. Pagano, Effects of nucleoside analogues in inhibition of Epstein-Barr virus, Presented at the International Symposium on Pharmacological and Clinical Approaches to Herpes Viruses and Virus Chemotherapy, Oiso, Japan, 10-13 September 1984 (1984a).
28. J. -C. Lin, M. C. Smith, Y. -C. Cheng and J. S. Pagano, Epstein-Barr virus: inhibition of replication by three new drugs, Science 221:578 (1983).
29. J. -C. Lin, M. C. Smith and J. S. Pagano, Prolonged inhibitory effect of 9-(1,3-dihydroxy-2-propoxymethyl)guanine against replication of Epstein-Barr virus, J. Virol. 50:50 (1984b).
30. C. Lopez. K. A. Watanabe and J. J. Fox, 2'-Fluoro-5-iodo-aracytosine, a potent and selective anti-herpes agent, Antimicrob. Agents Chemother. 17:803 (1980).

31. E. -C. Mar, Y. -C. Cheng and E. -S. Huang, Effect of 9-(1,3-dihydroxy-2-propoxymethyl)guanine on human cytomegalovirus replication in vitro, Antimicrob. Agents Chemother. 24:518 (1983).
32. E. -C. Mar, P. C. Patel, Y. -C. Cheng, J. J. Fox, K. A. Watanabe and E. -S. Huang, Effects of certain nucleoside analogues on human cytomegalovirus replication in vitro, J. Gen. Virol. 65:47 (1984).
33. P. C. Maudgal, E. De Clercq and L. Missotten, Efficacy of bromovinyl-deoxyuridine in the treatment of herpes simplex virus and varicella-zoster virus eye infections, Antiviral Res. 4:281 (1984).
34. P. C. Maudgal, L. Dralands, L. Lamberts, E. De Clercq, J. Descamps and L. Missotten, Preliminary results of oral BVDU treatment of herpes zoster ophthalmicus, Bull. Soc. Belge Ophtalmol. 193:49 (1981a).
35. P. C. Maudgal, L. Missotten, E. De Clercq, J. Descamps and E. De Meuter, Efficacy of (E)-5-(2-bromovinyl)-2'-deoxyuridine in the topical treatment of herpes simplex keratitis, Albrecht von Graefes Arch. Klin. Exp. Ophthalmol. 216:261 (1981b).
36. J. D. Meyers, J. C. Wade, C. D. Mitchell, R. Saral, P. S. Lietman, D. T. Durack, M. J. Levin, A. C. Segreti and H. H. Balfour, Jr., Multicenter collaborative trial of intravenous acyclovir for treatment of mucocutaneous herpes simplex virus infection in the immunocompromised host, Am. J. Med. 73(A):229 (1982).
37. J. D. Meyers, J. C. Wade, D. H. Shepp and B. Newton, Acyclovir treatment of varicella-zoster virus infection in the compromised host, Transplantation 37:571 (1984).
38. C. D. Mitchell, B. Bean, S. R. Gentry, K. E. Groth, J. R. Boen and H. H. Balfour, Jr., Acyclovir therapy for mucocutaneous herpes simplex infections in immunocompromised patients, Lancet i:1389 (1981).
39. C. G. Prober, L. E. Kirk and R. E. Keeney, Acyclovir therapy of chickenpox in immunosuppressed children - A collaborative study, J. Pediatr. 101:622 (1982).
40. R. Saral, R. F. Ambinder, W. H. Burns, C. M. Angelopulos, D. E. Griffin, P. J. Burke and P. S. Lietman, Acyclovir prophylaxis against herpes simplex virus infection in patients with leukemia, Ann. Intern. Med. 99:773 (1983).
41. R. Saral, W. H. Burns, O. L. Laskin, G. W. Santos and P. S. Lietman, Acyclovir prophylaxis of herpes-simplex-virus infections. A randomized, double-blind, controlled trial in bone marrow transplant recipients, New Engl. J. Med. 305:63 (1981).
42. P. Selby, R. L. Powles, S. Blake, K. Stolle, E. K. Mbidde, T. J. McElwain, E. Hickmott, P. D. Whiteman and A. P. Fiddian, Amino-(hydroxyethoxymethyl)purine: a new well-absorbed prodrug of acyclovir, Lancet ii:1428 (1984).
43. W. M. Shannon and F. M. Schabel, Jr., Antiviral agents as adjuncts in cancer chemotherapy, Pharmac. Ther. 11:263 (1980).
44. S. Shigeta, T. Yokota, T. Iwabuchi, M. Baba, K. Konno, M. Ogata and E. De Clercq, Comparative efficacy of antiherpes drugs against various strains of varicella-zoster virus, J. Infect. Dis. 147:576 (1983).
45. C. D. Sibrack, L. T. Gutman, C. M. Wilfert, C. McLaren, M. H. St. Clair, P. M. Keller and D. W. Barry, Pathogenicity of acyclovir-resistant herpes simplex virus type 1 from an immunodeficient child, J. Infect. Dis. 146:673 (1982).
46. D. F. Smee, J. C. Martin, J. P. H. Verheyden and T. R. Matthews, Anti-herpes virus activity of the acyclic nucleoside 9-(1,3-dihydroxy-2-propoxymethyl)guanine, Antimicrob. Agents Chemother. 23:676 (1983).
47. C. A. Smith, B. Wigdahl and F. Rapp, Synergistic antiviral activity of acyclovir and interferon on human cytomegalovirus, Antimicrob. Agents Chemother. 24:325 (1983).
48. K. O. Smith, K. S. Galloway, W. L. Kennell, K. K. Ogilvie and B. K. Radatus, A new nucleoside analog, 9-([2-hydroxy-1-(hydroxymethyl)-ethoxy]methyl)guanine. highly active in vitro against herpes simplex virus types 1 and 2, Antimicrob. Agents Chemother. 22:55 (1982).

49. K. F. Soike, A. D. Felsenfeld and P. J. Gerone, Acyclovir treatment of experimental simian varicella infection of monkeys, Antimicrob. Agents Chemother. 20:291 (1981a).
50. K. F. Soike, A. D. Felsenfeld, S. Gibson and P. J. Gerone, Ineffectiveness of adenine arabinoside and adenine arabinoside 5'-monophosphate in simian varicella infection, Antimicrob. Agents Chemother. 18:142 (1980).
51. K. F. Soike, S. Gibson and P. J. Gerone, Inhibition of simian varicella virus infection of African green monkeys by (E)-5-(2-bromovinyl)-2'-deoxyuridine (BVDU), Antiviral Res. 1:325 (1981b).
52. D. A. Stevens, G. W. Jordan, T. F. Waddell and T. C. Merigan, Adverse effect of cytosine arabinoside on disseminated zoster in a controlled trial, New Engl. J. Med. 289:873 (1973).
53. M. J. Tocci, T. J. Livelli, H. C. Perry, C. S. Crumpacker and A. K. Field, Effects of the nucleoside analog 2'-nor-2'deoxyguanosine on human cytomegalovirus replication, Antimicrob. Agents Chemother. 25:247 (1984).
54. G. Tricot, E. De Clercq, M. A. Boogaerts and R. L. Verwilghen, Oral bromovinyldeoxyuridine therapy for herpes simplex and varicella-zoster virus infections in severely immunosuppressed patients, Submitted for publication (1985).
55. A. S. Tyms, J. M. Davis, D. J. Jeffries and J. D. Meyers, BWB759U, an analogue of acyclovir, inhibits human cytomegalovirus in vitro, Lancet ii:924 (1984).
56. J. C. Wade, C. McLaren and J. D. Meyers, Frequency and significance of acyclovir-resistant herpes simplex virus isolated from marrow transplant patients receiving multiple courses of treatment with acyclovir, J. Infect. Dis. 148:1077 (1983).
57. J. C. Wade, B. Newton, C. McLaren, N. Flournoy, R. E. Keeney and J. D. Meyers, Intravenous acyclovir to treat mucocutaneous herpes simplex virus infection after marrow transplantation, Ann. Intern. Med. 96:265 (1982).
58. K. A. Watanabe, U. Reichman, K. Hirota, C. Lopez and J. J. Fox, Nucleosides. 110. Synthesis and antiherpes virus activity of some 2'-fluoro-2'-deoxyarabinofuranosylpyrimidine nucleosides, J. Med. Chem. 22:21 (1979).
59. P. D. Whiteman, A. Bye, A. S. E. Fowle, S. Jeal, G. Land and J. Posner, Tolerance and pharmacokinetics of A515U, an acyclovir analogue, in healthy volunteers, Eur. J. Clin. Pharmacol. 27:471 (1984).
60. R. J. Whitley, M. Hilty, R. Haynes, Y. Bryson, J. D. Connor, S. -J. Soong, C. A. Alford and the National Institute of Allergy and Infectious Diseases Collaborative Antiviral Study Group, Vidarabine therapy of varicella in immunosuppressed patients, J. Pediatr. 101:125 (1982a).
61. R. J. Whitley, S. -J. Soong, R. Dolin, R. Betts, C. Linnemann, Jr., C. A. Alford, Jr. and The NIAID Collaborative Antiviral Study Group, Early vidarabine therapy to control the complications of herpes zoster in immunosuppressed patients, New Engl. J. Med. 307:971 (1982b).
62. R. J. Whitley, S. Spruance, F. G. Hayden, J. Overall, C. A. Alford, Jr., J. M. Gwaltney, S. -J. Soong and The NIAID Collaborative Antiviral Study Group, Vidarabine therapy for mucocutaneous herpes simplex virus infections in the immunocompromised host, J. Infect. Dis. 149:1 (1984).
63. J. Wildiers and E. De Clercq, Oral (E)-5-(2-bromovinyl)-2'-deoxyuridine treatment of severe herpes zoster in cancer patients, Eur. J. Cancer. Clin. Oncol. 20:471 (1984).
64. C. W. Young, R. Schneider, B. Leyland-Jones, D. Armstrong, C. T. C. Tan, C. Lopez, K. A. Watanabe, J. J. Fox and F. S. Philips, Phase I evaluation of 2'-fluoro-5-iodo-1-β-D-arabinofuranosylcytosine in immunosuppressed patients with herpesvirus infection, Cancer Res. 43:5006 (1983).

THE EFFECT OF SOME ANTIBIOTICS ON INTERFERON PRODUCTION

M. Ghione[1], A. Pugliese[2], A. Valpreda[2], C. Salomone[3], P. Martinetto[4], and P. A. Tovo[3]

[1]Instituto di Microbiologia Medica, Università di Milano, [2]Instituto di Malattie Infettive, Università di Torino, [3]Clinica Pediatrica, Università di Torino, and [4]Instituto di Microbiologia, Università di Torino, Italy

INTRODUCTION

The commonly used antibacterial drugs are selected on the basis of their effect on the structure and function of prokaryotic cells but they are not devoid of action on eukaryotic cells. This can be due to the fact that eukaryotic cells include prokaryotic-like structures (such as mitochondria) and have several functions and metabolic mechanisms very similar to the prokaryotic ones.

On the other hand, antibacterial drugs may display pharmacologic properties not necessarily connected with the mechanism(s) of antibacterial action. The study of the possible activity of antibacterial drugs on cells involved in the immune system reaction is particularly interesting (7).

Indeed time-honored preclinical tests and phase I trials aimed to prevent the introduction into the clinical armamentarium of toxic compounds do not take into implicit consideration the possible drug-induced alteration of the immune system. The case in point is of relevance because the integrity of the immune system is an essential prerequisite for the successful outcome of an antibacterial treatment especially when intensive and protracted schedules of therapy are employed.

Antibiotic-dependent immunosuppressive mechanisms revealed by clinical observations have been extensively studied with particular emphasis on humoral and cell mediated reactions including phagocyte functions [see (4-6) for review]. At the same time, only limited and partly contradictory information is available on the possible influence of chemotherapeutic drugs on interferon (IFN) synthesis (2,11-14). The IFN system, whose various components can be activated by viral, bacterial and antigenic stimuli, plays a critical role in the network of immune reactions against infectious agents due to its antiviral and immunomodulating properties (for review see 9).

In this chapter we discuss studies on the type I IFN production in experimental animals or cells of pediatric patients treated with commonly used chemotherapeutic drugs.

MATERIALS AND METHODS

Experimental Animals

Groups of ten CD1 mice (Charles River, Italy), 20 g body weight, were injected intraperitoneally qid for 5 days with either saline or antibiotic solution. Drugs and doses are listed in Table 1. Two hours after the last injection the mice were given i.p. 0.3 ml of Newcastle disease virus (NDV_F haemagglutinating titer 512, propagated in allantoic fluid of embryonated hens' eggs, harvested after three days of incubation and kept at -20°C). Six hours after virus injection the mice were exsanquinated and the blood from five mice was pooled. The serum was separated and adjusted to pH 2 by 1N HCl, was kept at 4°C for three days; then neutralized by 1N NaOH and tested for IFN activity by cytopathogenic inhibition assay on mouse fibroblast cells infected at a low dose (ca 0.01 viral particle/cell) with vesicular stomatitis virus (VSV). A working standard of murine IFN equivalent to 45 Units was included in each titration. The IFN titer was expressed as the reciprocal of the dilution that reduced to 50% the cytopathogenic effect.

A routine examination was carried out to exclude the possible concomitance of viral lesions chiefly of liver and lung. Particular attention was devoted to the conditions of the peritoneal cavity and the morphology of the peritoneal cells was inspected.

Human Peripheral Blood Lymphocytes (PBL) from Pediatric Patients

After having secured the informed consent of the parents, blood samples were taken, before the start of the treatment and after its completion, from eleven tuberculosis patients treated with Rifampicin, six patients affected by respiratory tract infections treated with Thiamphenicol and five patients with predominant streptococcal disease treated with Erythromycin. Doses and length of treatment are listed in Table 2. PBL from Lymphoprep separation suspended (10^6/ml) in Eagle medium (10% calf serum) were activated with NDV_F according to Tovo, Vitale, Tridico et al. (13). The culture fluids adjusted to pH 2.5 were kept at 4°C for a week, then neutralized and tested for IFN activity by measuring the haemagglutinin yield reduction on cell cultures infected by Sindbis virus, according to Oie, Buckler, Uhlendorf et al. (10). A working standard preparation of human IFN equivalent to 10^3 U/ml was included in each titration.

Assays using the identical procedure were carried out simultaneously to determine the IFN produced by PBL isolated from subjects of the same age group not affected by infectious diseases, bled for diverse diagnostic purposes, and found to be clinically normal.

Table 1. IFN Production in Saline and Antibiotic-Treated Mice

Drug	Doses i.p. mg/kg/d d 1-5	Cumulative dose mg/kg	Range of the type I IFN titers
Saline solution	5000	25000	512 - 778
Ampicillin	750	3750	512 - 1024
Thiamphenicol	150	750	256 - 778
Erythromycin	100	500	384 - 1024
Rifampicin	150	750	256 - 384
Tetracycline	100	500	48 - 96

RESULTS

No overt systemic toxic effects ascribable to the treatment were noticed in experimental animals. The examination revealed mild peritoneal inflammation and limited effusion in animals treated with either saline, Ampicillin, Thiamphenicol, Erythromycin, or Rifampicin. The predominant peritoneal cell population was found to be constituted chiefly of morphologically normal macrophages and mononucleated cells. In Tetracycline-treated animals drug residues and consistent signs of peritoneal irritation with hyperemia and scarce effusion were observed. In these animals the scanty peritoneal cell population was represented predominantly by lumps of mesothelial cells and macrophages loaded with drug particles.

In duplicate assays, no significant difference in IFN production was observed between groups of animals treated either with saline (i.e. control group), Ampicillin, Thiamphenicol, Erythromycin or Rifampicin. The IFN titer depression observed in Rifampicin-treated animals was found to fall within the experimental error limits whereas a significant decrease in the IFN titer below the control limits was detected in Tetracycline-treated animals. The range of the titer is given in Table 1.

The IFN produced by PBL of antibiotic-treated pediatric patients was not significantly different, before or after the treatment, from that or age-matched controls. The IFN titers and standard deviations (in log units) are given in Table 2.

DISCUSSION

The present study shows that in mice repeated i.p. injections of fairly high, but not overtly toxic, doses of Rifampicin, Thiamphenicol, Erythromycin and Ampicillin did not significantly modify the production of type I IFN. Conversely, a significant decrease of IFN titer was found in animals repeatedly treated with Tetracycline.

These findings seemed to be partly at variance with some data of the literature. Indeed Rollag and Degrè (12) by using an experimental model

Table 2. IFN Production by PBL of Healthy or Antibiotic Treated Pediatric Subjects

Subjects per group	Age/ range (y)	Affected by	Treated with	Dose/ range (mg/ kg/d)	Length of treatment	IFN titer (x + SD) log units
10	3-12	-	-	-	-	3.125 ± 0.33
10	3-11	Tuberculosis	Rifampicin	11-20	15-100	3.15 ± 0.27
6	3-6	Respiraatory tract	Thiamphenicol	25-30	6-8	2.87 ± 0.27
5	2-10	Streptococc. infections	Erythro-	45-50	3-6	3.18 ± 0.14

analogous to the present one, did not observe modifications of IFN synthesis by single intraperitoneal injections of various doses of a Tetracycline analog (Oxytetracycline) and Rifampicin as well. Whereas, Ustacelebi and Williams (14) reported on the inhibitory activity of Rifampicin on IFN production by some human adenovirus in chick embryo cells and Cortese, Pugliese and Tovo (2) on the inhibition of IFN synthesis induced by poly I:C in syngeneic mice treated with high doses of a Rifampicin analog (Rifamycin SV).

The discrepancies can be explained on the basis of differences among experimental conditions such as animal species or strain, as well as schedule of treatment and, last but not least, physicochemical and kinetic drug characteristics. In fact, parenterally administered Oxytetracycline and Rifampicin display a higher absorption rate than Tetracycline and Rifampicin SV, respectively. Such differences can be of relevance particularly when high drug concentrations are injected in serosal cavities. The rapid water absorption leaves a drug residue in situ, that, in the case of Tetracycline, is known to induce phlogistic phenomena evolving towards the formation of granulomatous tissue.

The irritating property of Tetracycline is well known and is utilized for obtaining the obliteration of serosal cavities as, e.g., in the treatment of malignant effusions (8). From a certain point of view Tetracycline can be considered to act, in this context, as a biological response modifier. Most probably, an array of mediators (such as cytokines etc.) are sequentially involved in the unfolding of the tissue reactive phenomena elicited by this antibiotic. Diverse cell functions are modified by Tetracycline derivatives (1,3). The present study indicated that the morphologically evident early peritoneal reactions induced by Tetracycline injection may be associated with depletion or suppression of IFN enhancer system(s), or derepression of inhibitors.

In clinical terms the relevance of these considerations is applied only to a few types of treatment of rare occurrence in pediatric practice where the use of Tetracycline and its derivatives is usually limited and other antibiotics are preferred. The present study showed that some of them (Rifampicin, Thiamphenicol, Erythromycin) administered at usual doses also for long-term treatment to pediatric patients did not hamper the capability of PBL to synthesize type I IFN. Our data and that of the literature taken as a whole, allow us to conclude that drugs, selected on the basis of their inhibitory activity on prokaryotic organisms, can modify the function of eukaryotic cells (including IFN synthesis) either directly or via complex reactions. On the other hand, the probability that the clinical application of some among the most commonly used antibiotics tested in the present study may hinder the synthesis of type I IFN appears to be remote and scarcely relevant, so that it shall not be considered as a deterrent from employing these drugs in the treatment of cases (of frequent occurrence in pediatric practice) where viral and bacterial infections concur in determining the clinical syndrome.

REFERENCES

1. L. Athlin, L. Domellof and B. Norberg, Adherence and phagocytosis of yeast cells by blood monocytes, effects in vitro of a therapeutic doxyciclin concentration, _Acta Path. Microbiol. Immunol. Scand._ Sect C 92:227 (1984).
2. D. Cortese, A. Pugliese and P. A. Tovo, Effetto di Rifampicina sulla produzione di interferon, Atti XIX Cong. Naz. Soc. Ital. Microbiol., Catania, 5-8 giugno (1980).

3. J. G. R. Elferink and M. Deierkauf, Inhibition of polymorphonuclear leukocyte functions by chlortetracycline, Biochem. Pharmacol. 33:3667 (1984).
4. M. Ghione, Influenza di farmaci antibatterici su processi inflammatori e immunitari, Giorn. Ital. Chemiot. 26:97 (1979).
5. M. Ghione, Toxicology of antimicrobial agents: effect of antimicrobial agents on the immune system, in: "Clinical Chemotherapy," H. P. Kuemmerle, ed., Thieme Stratton 1:373 (1983).
6. M. Ghione, Antibiotici e difese organiche, Medico e Bambino 6:348 (1984).
7. G. Gillissen, Possible mechanisms of immunological side-effects of antibiotics, Zbl. Bakt. Suppl. 13:91 (1985).
8. Martindale, The extra pharmacopeia, 28 ed., J. E. F. Reynolds, ed., The Pharmaceutical Press, London (1982).
9. T. C. Merigan and H. Friedman, eds., "Interferon," UCLA Symposia Mol. Cell. Biol. (1982).
10. H. K. Oie, C. E. Buckler, C. P. Uhlendorf, D. A. Hill and S. Baron, Improved assay for a variety of interferon, Proc. Soc. Exp. Biol. Med. 140:1178 (1972).
11. A. Pugliese and P. A. Tovo, Effect of Distamycin A on the production of interferon induced in vitro by the NDV virus, Acta Virol. 25:62 (1981).
12. H. Rollag, Jr. and M. Degrè, Effect of antibiotics on interferon production in mice, Acta Path. Microb. Scand. Sect. B 84:369 (1976).
13. P. A. Tovo, M. Vitale, F. Tridico and A. Pugliese, Effetto di trattamenti a lungo termine con Rifampicina Cloramfenicolo e Cortisone sulla produzione di interferon virus-indotto, Giorn. Batt. Virol. Immun. 75:1 (1982).
14. S. Ustacelebi and J. F. Williams, Depression of interferon production in chick embryo cells by Rifampicin, J. Gen. Virol. 15:139 (1972).

SECTION IV
ANTIMICROBIAL EFFECTS ON PHAGOCYTIC FUNCTION OF POLYMORPHONUCLEAR LEUKOCYTES, MONOCYTES, AND MACROPHAGES

INFLUENCE OF DIFFERENT TETRACYCLINES ON GRANULOCYTE FUNCTIONS

Håkan Gnarpe, Judy Belsheim, Charlotte Blomqvist, and Lars Wesslen

Department of Clinical Bacteriology
Gävle Central Hospital
Gävle, Sweden

INTRODUCTION

Tetracyclines are bacteriostatic antibiotics that act as inhibitors of the microbial protein synthesis by chelating cation-containing enzymes at the ribosome level (12,13). They are supposed not to influence the protein synthesis in mammalian cells. In later years it has been demonstrated repeatedly that tetracyclines are taken up by mammalian cells and even that they are concentrated intracellularly. Being chelating agents it is reasonable to expect the tetracyclines to have effects also on mammalian cells, dependent on, for example, Ca and Mg ions for their proper function (21,22). It has been shown in several reports that the tetracyclines do affect a number of cellular functions, i.e., those of the granulocytes (1,3-5,20) and lymphocytes (5). However the data presented have been controversial: some reports have found the tetracyclines stimulating, others have found them more or less depressing, depending on the techniques used and the cellular functional step being investigated (5,20).

In this chapter we discuss the influence of four different tetracycline preparations on different granulocyte functions both under rigid in vitro as well as under experimental in vivo conditions.

MATERIALS AND METHODS

Antibiotics

Four different tetracyclines were obtained from the manufacturer in purified form. Doxycyclinepolymethaphosphate sodium complex (DMSC), Batch no. AB08079-1, doxycycline monohydrate, Batch no. AB060120-1, and doxycycline hyclate, Batch no. AB050165-1, were obtained from Hovione Chemicals, Lisboa. Lymecycline, Batch no. 7D5524 was obtained from Farmitalia Carlo Erba, Milan. These drug preparations were used for in vitro experiments. For experimental in vivo investigations, doxycycline polymethaphosphate sodium complex (DMSC) was obtained in capsules corresponding to 100 mg of doxycycline base from Hovione, Lisboa.

Volunteers

Ten healthy volunteers from the laboratory staff were used as blood donors for the in vitro investigations as well as for the experimental in vivo investigations. None of the volunteers were on any medication; the interval between the experimental in vivo treatments was one week. For experimental in vivo investigations, the dosage given was one capsule of DMSC daily for five days.

Preparation of White Blood Cells

Polymorphonuclear granulocytes (PMNs) were prepared from heparinized peripheral venous blood as described earlier (2).

Bacterial Strain

A strain of Escherichia coli was used, originally isolated from a wound culture. The MIC (Minimal Inhibitory Concentration) of the strain for the four tetracyclines was determined in broth and was for all four drugs 1.0 mcg per ml.

Granulocyte Adherence

The granulocyte adherence was measured as the retention in nylon fiber columns according to McGregor et al. (11) as described earlier (5).

Granulocyte Migration

The granulocyte migration was investigated with the leukocyte migration under agarose technique described earlier (2). In the experiments, granulocytes were incubated with the different tetracyclines at increasing concentrations for 30 min.; the chemotactic agents used were fresh serum or E. coli LPS at a concentration of 20 mg per ml, or cell-free supernatant from an E. coli culture, incubated for 4 or 16 hours with the respective antibiotic preparation in the experiments with subinhibitory concentrations (3).

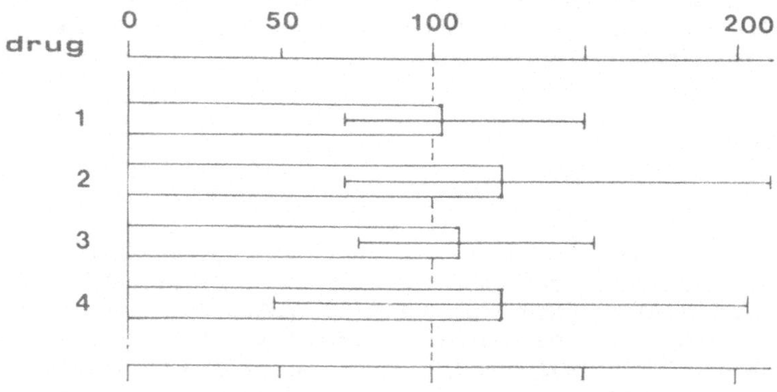

Figure 1. Polymorphonuclear granulocyte adherence measured as retention in nylon fiber columns after incubation with four different tetracyclines at 10 mcg per ml for 30 min. Mean values for ten individuals are given as well as ranges.
drug 1 = doxycycline polymethaphosphate sodium complex (DMSC)
drug 2 = doxycycline monohydrate
drug 3 = doxycycline hyclate
drug 4 = lymecycline

Quantitative Phagocytosis

The quantitative PMN phagocytosis of opsonized yeast cells was investigated with a method described by Hed (7) allowing differentiation of yeast cells attaching to the PMN surface from internalized yeast cells. The PMNs used were incubated for 30 min. with the respective antibiotic. All results were expressed as per cent of number of yeast cells associated with homologous control PMNs at 15 or 20 min.

Granulocyte Chemiluminescence

PMNs were obtained by Dextran 70 sedimentation of venous blood; the RBCs lysed and the remaining PMNs were washed and finally resuspended in PBS buffer containing three per cent Dextran 70 but no Ca^{2+} or Mg^{2+} ions to avoid aggregation and activation of the PMNs. The luminol- (2×10^{-5} M) enhanced chemiluminescence (CL) was measured in a Lumac-Biocounter M2010 and continuously recorded as relative light units per min (RLU) against time. CL was initiated by *Staphylococcus aureus*, strain Wood 46, which had been inactivated by heat and opsonized by pooled human serum.

RESULTS

The granulocyte adherence, measured as retention in nylon fiber columns after incubation with 10 mcg per ml of the respective tetracyclines for 30 min is shown in Figure 1 for ten healthy volunteers. DMSC and doxycycline hyclate gave insignificant deviation from the drug-free PMNs; doxycycline monohydrate and lymecycline showed a tendency towards an increased retention compared to DMSC and doxycycline hyclate. The observed differences were not significant.

The undirected migration of PMNs obtained from ten healthy volunteers preincubated with the four tetracyclines in concentrations from 1 to 50 mcg per ml for 30 min. is shown in Figure 2 expressed as per cent of the

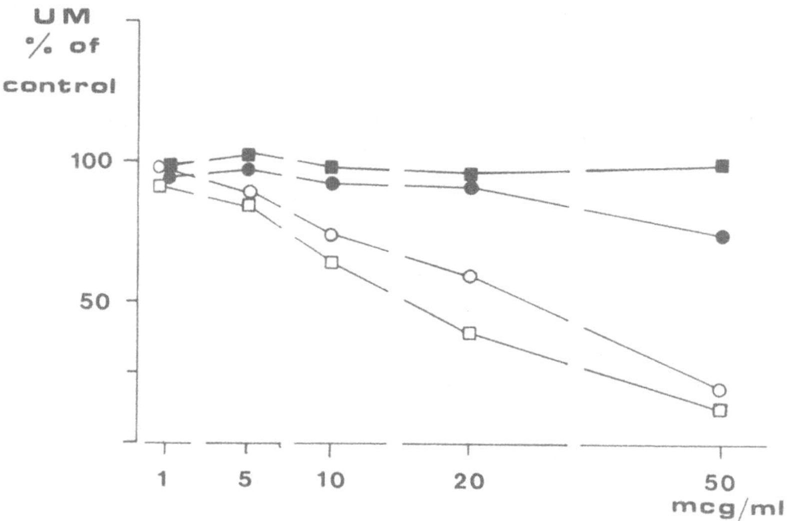

Figure 2. Undirected migration of PMNs from ten individuals incubated for 30 min with increasing concentrations of four diffeent tetracyclines. All values given are mean values expressed as per cent of drug-free PMNs. O = DMSC; ● = doxycycline monohydrate □ = doxycycline hyclate; ■ = lymecycline.

undirected migration of antibiotic-free PMNs. The values given are mean values for all ten volunteers.

All four tetracyclines had no or insignificant influence at low concentrations. At higher concentrations, DMSC and doxycycline hyclate and, at a concentration of 50 mcg per ml, also doxycycline monohydrate depressed the undirected migration.

The directed migration of PMNs obtained from ten volunteers, preincubated with the different tetracyclines for 30 min. is shown in Figure 3 expressed as per cent of directed migration of the antibiotic-free PMNs. All values are mean of ten volunteers. At all concentrations (1 - 50 mcg per ml), doxycycline monohydrate and lymecycline had no significant influence on the directed migration. DMSC and doxycycline hyclate were slightly stimulating at 5 and 10 mcg per ml and very inhibitory at 20 and 50 mcg per ml.

In experiments when E. coli was exposed for 1/20 of MIC of the respective antibiotics and the cell-free supernatant then used as chemotactic factor, no significant influence was found. It was found that both DMSC and doxycycline hyclate induced a prolonged lag phase for the E. coli strain making it necessary for a bacterial exposure time of 16 hours for these drugs as compared to four hours for doxycycline monohydrate and lymecycline.

The in vitro quantitative phagocytosis of opsonized yeast cells by PMNs incubated at various concentrations of the four tetracyclines is shown in Figure 4. All values are expressed as per cent of yeast cells attaching to or engulfed by drug-free PMNs after 15 min (= 100 per cent). At this time 50 per cent of the yeast cells, associated with the PMNs, had been phagocytosed (= internalized). As is shown in the figure, no significant deviations from the drug-free controls were found for doxycycline monohydrate or lymecycline. DMSC had a lower number of cell-associated yeast cells both at 50 and at 10 mcg per ml, and the number of internalized (phagocytosed) yeast cells was low at 50 mcg per ml. Doxycycline hyclate

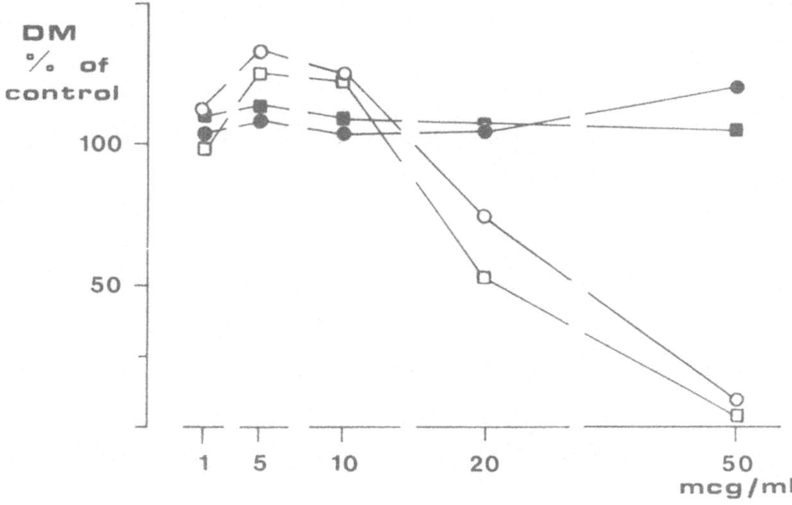

Figure 3. Directed migration of PMNs from ten individuals incubated for 30 min in increasing concentrations of four different tetracyclines. All values are mean values and given as percent of drug-free PMNs. Symbols as in Figure 2.

prevented internalization at 50 mcg per ml. This is further illustrated in Figures 5 and 6, showing the rapid start of phagocytosis in drug-free environment (Figure 5) as compared to the incomplete ingestion of yeast cells after 45 min by doxycycline incubated PMNs (10 mcg per ml) (Figure 6). Otherwise no significant deviations from the control PMNs were observed.

The quantitative phagocytosis of opsonized yeast cells by PMNs exposed to cell-free supernates of an E. coli culture without or with the tetracyclines added in 1/20 MIC is shown in Figure 7. The observed values at 8 and 20 minutes are shown. Yeast to PMN association (attachment and internalization) was rapid: after 8 min 97 per cent had become PMN-associated. Internalization was a slower procedure: 20 per cent at 8 min as compared to 49 per cent after 20 min. All four tetracyclines seemed to induce an increase of the number of PMN-associated yeast cells. Significant increases were found for doxycycline monohydrate and for lymecycline. All four preparations seemed to indirectly stimulate internalization of the yeast cells; however, the increases observed were not significant.

The chemiluminescence of PMNs was affected in a dose-dependent manner at concentrations of 3-18 mcg per ml of DMSC if Ca^{2+} or Mg^{2+} were not present in the reaction mixtures. When the chemiluminescence experiments were per-

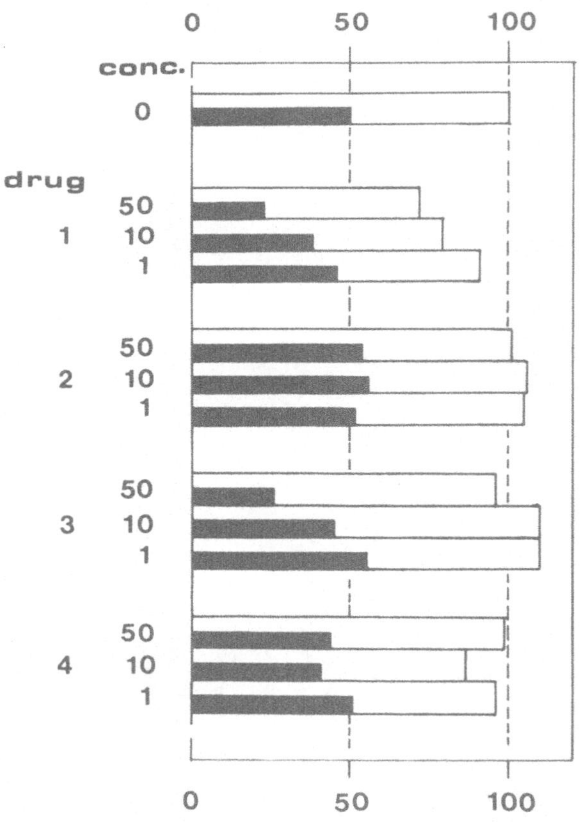

Figure 4. PMN quantitative phagocytosis of opsonized yeast cells after incubation with four tetracyclines at different concentrations. All values are expressed as per cent of PMN-associated yeast cells after 15 min (= 100%). Open bar denotes cell-associated yeast cells; black bar denotes per cent engulfed yeast cells.

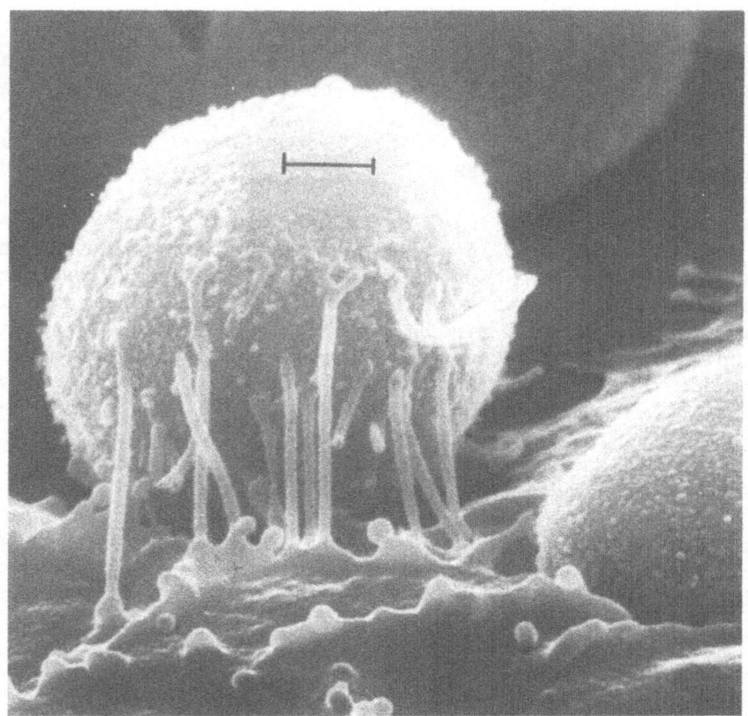

Figure 5. Scanning electron micrograph of early stage of phagocytosis, 8 min after addition of yeast cells to drug-free PMNs on glass. Note number of filopods reaching out for invagination of the yeast cell. Black bar is 1 μm.

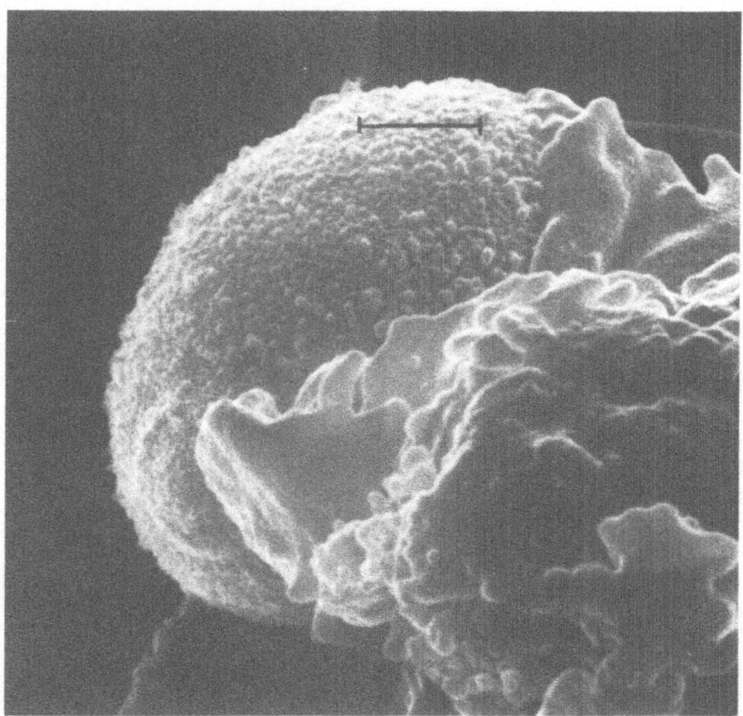

Figure 6. Scanning electron micrograph of late, incomplete phagocytosis of yeast cell after 45 min by doxycycline - incubated PMN on glass (0 mcg/l). More than 2/3 of yeast cell is still outside PMN.

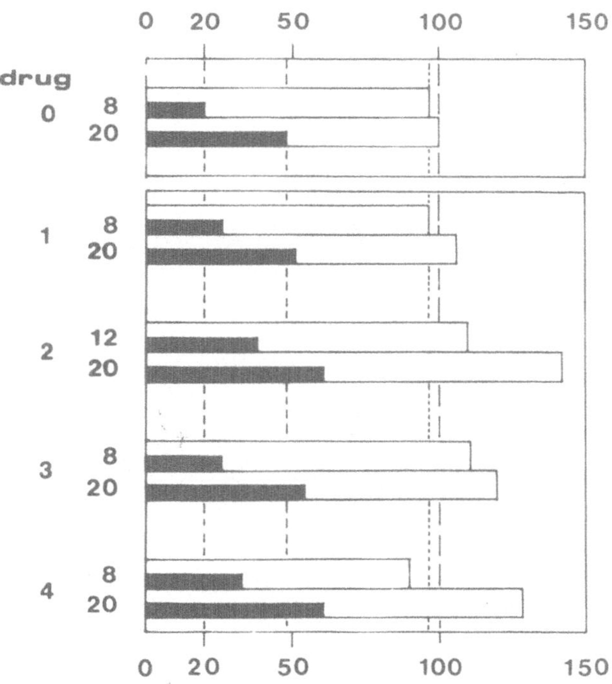

Figure 7. Quantitative PMN phagocytosis of opsonized yeast cells using cell-free supernatants from an E. coli culture incubated with 1/20 of MIC of four tetracyclines for stimulation. Observations are made at 8 and 20 min with one exception, drug 2 (doxycycline monohydrate) where the first observation was made after 12 min. All values are expressed as per cent of PMN-associated yeast cells at 20 min in drug-free supernatant. Drug 1 = DMSC; Drug 2 = doxycycline monohydrate; Drug 3 = doxycycline hyclate; Drug 4 = lymecycline.

formed in buffered systems with Ca^{2+} and Mg^{2+}, or when these ions were added, the results were similar to the controls. This is shown in Figure 8. The influence of DMSC on the chemiluminescence was shown to be temperature dependent as shown in Figure 9.

When volunteers were given DMSC in a dosage of 100 mg daily for five days, no significant differences of the PMN chemiluminescence was found as compared to pre-treatment values.

DISCUSSION

All tetracyclines act as protein synthesis inhibitors (12,13). Additionally, it has been shown that tetracyclines have potential to cause cell membrane defects resulting in leakage of intracellular microbial constituents (13). It has also been shown that the tetracyclines are taken up by microbial cells in a two-step mechanism. The first is a binding of the tetracycline molecule to cations in the outer microbial membrane; the second is an energy-requiring transportation into the effector sites at the ribosomal level (12). Depending on the microbial species exposed, the kind and amount

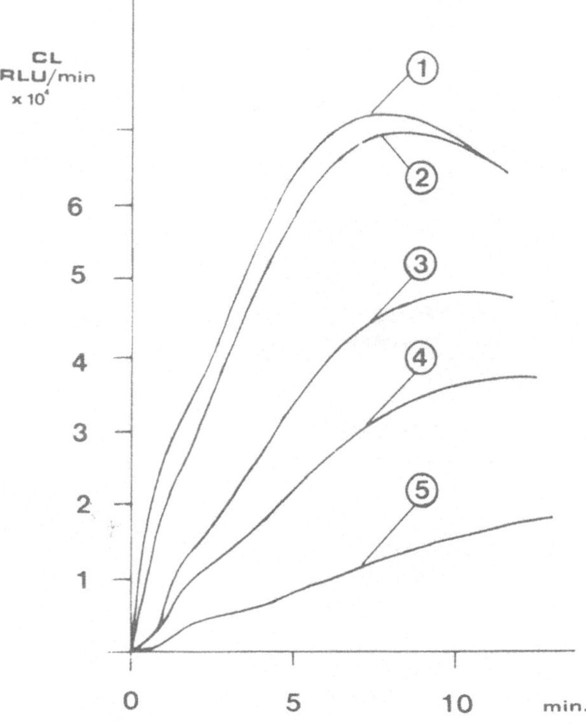

Figure 8. Luminol-stimulated chemiluminescence of PMNs incubated with DMSC at a concentration of 18 mcg/l using Staphylococcus aureus strain Wood 46 for initiation of chemiluminescence. 1 = control cells kept at 25°C for 1 hr before start; 2 = control cells kept at 0° for 1 hr before start; 3 = cells preincubated with 18 mcg/ml DMSC kept at 25°C for 2 hrs after addition of Ca2+ and Mg2+; 4 = same as 3, kept at 25°C for 1 hr after addition of Ca2+ and Mg2+; 5 same as 3, kept at 0°C for 1 hr after addition of Ca2+ and Mg2+.

of intracellular constituents released from the cells vary; Webster et al. (17) found that P. acnes cultures exposed to subinhibitory concentrations of tetracyclines released a diminished amount of chemotactic factors. The results presented here using an E. coli strain as source of chemotactic factor(s) indicate that there are few and small effects. However, there may be differences between the individual drug preparations as doxycycline monohydrate and lymecycline gave an indirect stimulation of the yeast for PMN association at sub-MIC concentrations.

The uptake of tetracyclines over the mammalian cell membrane is related to the lipid solubility of the preparations: doxycycline being more efficiently taken up than tetracycline hydrochloride (4). According to earlier findings (5), doxycycline is even found in higher concentrations intracellularly, i.e., granulocytes, than in serum which might have consequences for the function of the cells as suggested earlier (4,5,18). Our results show that there are pronounced differences between the effects of the different tetracyclines: the highly lipid soluble preparations causing a pronounced depression of both the PMN undirected and directed migration as well as on the rate of internalization of opsonized yeast cells (4). These effects, leading to defective function with possible negative consequences in vivo (14-16), are most likely due to chelate binding of divalent cations, primar-

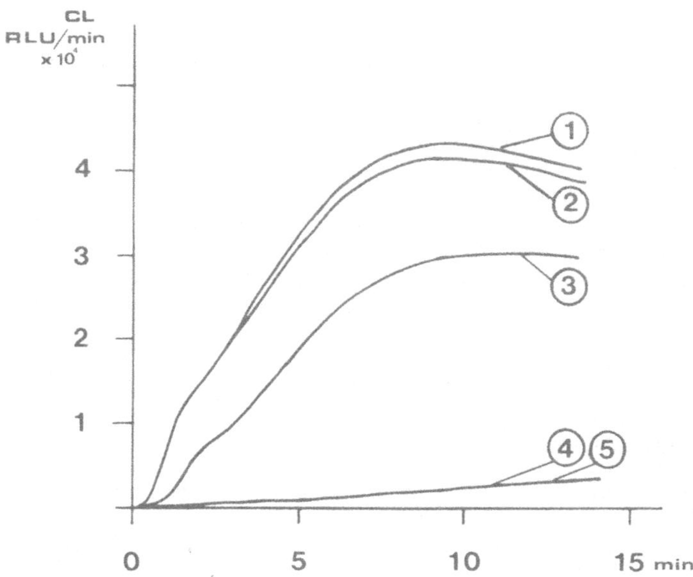

Figure 9. Luminol-stimulated chemiluminescence of PMNs incubated with 18 mcg/ml of DMSC at different temperatures. 1 = Control cells kept at 0°C for 1 hr; 2 = Control cells kept at 25°C for 1 hr; 3 = cells incubated with 18 mcg/ml of DMSC at 0°C for 1 hr; 4 = Cells incubated with 18 mcg/ml of DMSC at 25°C for 1 hr; 5 = as 3 but further incubated at 25°C for 1 hr.

ily Ca^{2+} but also Mg^{2+} being essential for membrane transportation and deformability (6,8,10,21,22). Our results show that the cations are more efficiently bound by the lipophilic substances; however, our results also indicate that the effects are reversible upon addition of Ca^{2+} which is further demonstrated by the in vivo experiments with chemiluminescence on volunteers given DMSC where no deviations were found. This is most likely due to continuous mobilization of Ca^{2+} in vivo. It is also possible that the lack of influence is due to alterations of the PMN functional state during the preparation for chemiluminescence.

We have shown earlier that doxycycline does depress the granulocyte migration more than lymecycline under experimental in vivo conditions (1,5) and that this can be found also in clinical situations (5). If this means that there may be a certain depression of the aggregation of inflammatory cells at the site of infection induced by the tetracyclines, this may be advantageous for the infected patient (9): the tetracyclines exerting antibiotic effects on the invading microbe and, maybe, immunomodulating effects on the nonspecific host defense, reducing the number of granulocytes but not phagocytosis (19).

REFERENCES

1. J. Belsheim, H. Gnarpe and J. Lofberg, Granulocyte function during prophylaxis with doxycycline, Scand. J. Infect. Dis. 11:287 (1979).
2. J. Belsheim, A modified leukocyte migration under agarose technique (LMAT): technical aspects, Acta Path. Microbiol. Scand. Sect. C 89:167 (1981).
3. J. Belsheim and H. Gnarpe, Antibiotics and granulocytes. Direct and indirect effects on granulocyte chemotaxis, Acta Path. Microbiol. Scand. Sect. C 89:217 (1981).

4. J. Glette, S. Sandberg, G. Hopen and C. O. Solberg, Influence of tetracyclines on human polymorphonuclear leukocyte function, Antimicrob. Agents Chemother. 25:354 (1984).
5. H. Gnarpe and J. Belsheim, Interaction of antibiotics with granulocytes and lymphocytes, Zbl. Bakt. 13 (Suppl.):123 (1985).
6. M. B. Hallett and A. K. Campbell, Is intracellular Ca^{2+} the trigger for oxygen radical production by polymorphonuclear leucocytes?, Cell Calcium 5:1 (1984).
7. J. Hed, The extinction of fluorescence by crystal violet and its use to differentiate between attached and ingested organisms in phagocytosis, FEMS Microbiol. Lett. 1:357 (1977).
8. R. L. Hoover, R. Folger, W. A. Haering, B. R. Ware and M. J. Karnovsky, Adhesion of leukocytes to endothelium: roles of divalent cations, surface charge, chemotactic agents and substrate, J. Cell. Sci. 45:73 (1980).
9. A. C. Issekutz, Vascular responses during acute neutrophilic inflammation. Their relationship to in vivo neutrophil emigration, Lab. Invest. 45:435 (1981).
10. P. H. Kazanjian and J. E. Pennington, Influence of drugs that block calcium channels on the microbicidal function of human neutrophils, J. Inf. Dis. 151:15 (1985).
11. R. R. MacGregor, E. J. Macarek and W. A. Kefalides, Comparative adherence of granulocytes to endothelial monolayers and nylon fibers, J. Clin. Invest. 61:697 (1978).
12. L. McMurry and S. B. Levy, Two transport systems for tetracycline in sensitive Escherichia coli: critical role for an initial rapid uptake system insensitive to energy inhibitors, Antimicrob. Agents Chemother. 14:201 (1978).
13. M. L. Pato, Tetracycline inhibits propagation of deoxyribonucleic acid replication and alters membrane properties, Antimicrob. Agents Chemother. 11:318 (1977).
14. P. G. Quie and L. Cates, Clinical conditions associated with defective polymorphonuclear chemotaxis, Amer. J. Pathol. 88:711 (1977).
15. J. E. Repine, C. C. Clawson and F. C. Goetz, Bactericidal function of neutrophils from patients with acute bacterial infections and from diabetics, J. Inf. Dis. 142:869 (1980).
16. J. L. Rubin, R. W. Griffiths and H. R. Hill, Allergen-induced depression of neutrophil chemotaxis in allergic individuals, J. Allergy Clin. Immunol. 62:301 (1978).
17. G. F. Webster, J. J. Leyden, K. J. McGurley and W. P. McArthur, Suppression of polymorphonuclear leukocyte chemotactic factor production in Propionibacterium acnes by subminimal inhibitory concentrations of tetracycline, ampicillin, minocycline and erythromycin, Antimicrob. Agents Chemother. 21:770 (1982).
18. W. D. Welch, D. Davis and L. D. Thrupp, Effect of antimicrobial agents on human polymorphonuclear leukocyte microbicidal function, Antimicrob. Agents Chemother. 20:15 (1981).
19. A. Scheja and A. Forsgren, Functional properties of polymorphonuclear leukocytes accumulated in a skin chamber, Acta Path. Microbiol. Immunol. Scand. Sect. C 93:31 (1985).
20. A. M. Shibl, Effect of antibiotics on adherence of microorganisms to epithelial cell surfaces, Rev. Infect. Dis. 7:51 (1985).
21. J. E. Smolen, H. M. Korchak and G. Weissmann, The roles of extracellular and intracellular calcium in lysosomal enzyme release and superoxide anion generation by human neutrophils, Biochem. Biophys. Acta. 677:512 (1981).
22. J. E. Smolen, P. Noble, R. Freed and G. Weissmann, Metabolic requirements for maintenance of the chlortetracycline-labeled pool of membrane-bound calcium in human neutrophils, J. Cellul. Physiol. 117:415 (1983).

EFFECTS OF ANTIMICROBIAL AGENTS ON SOME PHASES OF NEUTROPHIL CHEMOTAXIS

Giuliana Gialdroni Grassi and Anna Fietta

Chair of Chemotherapy, Institute of Respiratory Diseases
University of Pavia
Pavia Italy

INTRODUCTION

A variety of interactions exists between human phagocytes and antimicrobial agents. On one hand phagocytes may provide a protected environment for microorganisms by either inactivating or preventing entrance of antibiotics (8). On the other hand, chemotherapeutic agents may modify bacterial surface structures or metabolism thus affecting pathogen-phagocyte interaction. They may also act directly on phagocytes by enhancing or suppressing their metabolism and/or functions such as adherence, locomotion, phagocytosis and microbicidal activities.

The knowledge of these possible interactions is of great interest mainly in connection with the problem of treating patients with primary or induced immunodeficiencies. In this class of patients, in fact, phagocytes represent a critical component of the host defense system against invasion by pathogenic bacteria and fungi (15).

The first step in acute response to the invasion of the body by microorganisms is the release of chemoattractants which activate phagocytes causing them to orient and migrate through the vascular endothelium and the interstitial spaces to the area of infection. This process of directed migration is termed chemotaxis.

A number of commonly employed antimicrobial agents inhibit in vitro neutrophil chemotaxis. However, conflicting results have often been obtained in different laboratories and few clinical studies have evaluated the effect of antibiotic administration on neutrophil functions (4-6). Moreover, little experimental work has been devoted to better understand the mechanisms involved in these interactions (7).

The aim of this chapter is to review our data concerning the in vitro and in vivo effects of some antimicrobial agents on neutrophil locomotion and to show an approach (9) attempting to clarify the mechanism of antibiotic-induced inhibition of human PMN chemotaxis.

In Vitro Effect of Antibiotics on Locomotion

The in vitro effect of antibiotics on locomotion was evaluated both in the presence of drugs and after exposure of tested cells to the antibiotic for 30 minutes. Random migration and chemotaxis were determined according

Table 1. Migration Tests: Range of Normality[a]

Test	Mean	SD[b]	PT[c]
Random migration	34.49	11.98	11.01
Chemotaxis	98.67	11.14	76.84

to the method described by Wilkinson (16), using modified Boyden chambers. E. coli lypopolysaccharide-activated human serum or formyl-methionyl-leucyl-phenylalanine (FMLP) were used as chemotactic stimuli. Migration was evaluated by the "leading front method" (17), as the average distance in μm traveled in 90' by the two fastest cells in each of ten fields. Normal values for random migration and chemotaxis are presented in Table 1.

It is well known that β-lactam antibiotics are unable to penetrate into eukariotic cells (8). Many of them, in fact, did not affect either random or directed migration nor other neutrophil functions (6) even at concentrations higher than their therapeutically achieved levels (Table 2).

However, two third-generation cephalosporin derivatives, cefoperazone and ceftriaxone, irreversibly inhibited in vitro PMN chemotaxis (2,5). For both cephalosporins, the inhibition was evident in a range of concentrations readily achieved in treating patients ($\geq$ 5 μg/ml for cefoperazone; $\geq$ 40 μg/ml for ceftriaxone). No effect on random migration and other neutrophil functions was shown.

Rifamycins are molecules capable of penetrating mammalian cells, reaching intracellular concentrations effective against susceptible bacteria (2,8). Rifampicin and rifapentine irreversibly inhibited chemotaxis in the range of their therapeutic levels. In presence or after pretreatment of cells with 8-10 μg/ml of drug, neutrophil migration falls to about 50% of that obtained in cells not treated with the antibiotic (Figure 1). Also in this case no effect on random migration was shown.

Among some antimycotic agents (10) only amphotericin B showed an inhibitory effect on neutrophil chemotaxis at therapeutically achieved levels (Table 3). Finally no significant effect at therapeutic levels was demonstrated by some macrolide derivatives (Table 4), in spite of their effective penetration into phagocytes (1).

Table 2. In Vitro Effect of Beta-Lactam Antibiotics on Neutrophil Locomotion

A)	No effect on random migration and chemotaxis:	
	Ampicillin	Cefazolin
	Carbenicillin	Cefotaxime
	Piperacillin	Cefotetan
	Thienamycin	Ceftazidime
	Cephaloridine	Moxalactam
B)	Inhibition of chemotaxis:	
	Cefoperazone ($\geq$ 5 μg/ml)	
	Ceftriaxone ($\geq$ 40 μg/ml)	

Table 3. Effect of Amphotericin B on Neutrophil Chemotaxis[a]

μg/ml	0	0.6	1.25	2.50	5.00
in presence	91.2 ±9.9	76.8 ±5.5	39.8 ±5.4	48.0 ±5.8	34.3 ±8.5
after preincubation	91.3 ±6.7	79.2 ±6.7	50.3 ±7.85	53.5 ±5.1	41.2 ±8.1

[a]Chemotaxis is expressed as μm of "leading front."

Some important points arise from the above mentioned in vitro results. First of all no apparent correlation exists between the mechanism or the type of action of antibiotics and the effect on neutrophil functions. Moreover, the interference of chemotherapeutic drugs with chemotaxis does not relate exclusively to the capacity of the agent to penetrate phagocytic cells. In addition, unexplained differences in displaying this effect seem to exist among derivatives belonging to the same family of antibiotics.

Mechanisms by Which Antibiotics Inhibit PMN Chemotaxis

An important point in these studies concerns the mechanisms by which antibiotics affect PMN chemotaxis. The antibiotics may inhibit chemotaxis interfering with binding of chemotactic factors to specific receptors at the neutrophil surface, altering one of the mechanisms by which signal recognition is transmitted across the membrane and transduced into the intracellular effector mechanisms or directly affecting the effector mechanisms.

One of the first steps in the cellular activation following the exposure of neutrophils to chemoattractants is membrane potential changes (11-14).

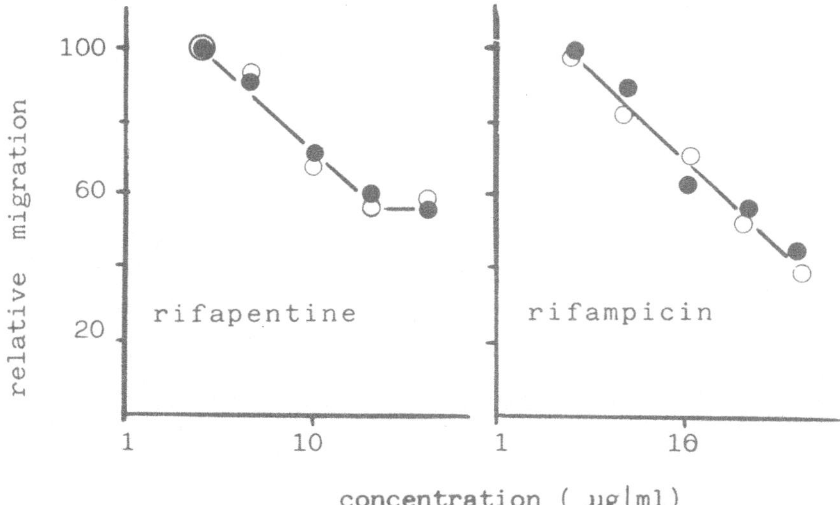

Figure 1. In vitro effect of rifamycins on human PMN chemotaxis. ●, in presence of antibiotics, O , after pretreatment with drugs.

Table 4. Effect of Macrolides on Random Migration and Chemotaxis

a)	Lack of effect at therapeutic levels:	
	Erythromycin	Macroflumycin
	Josamycin	RU 28965
b)	Irreversible inhibition of chemotaxis at high levels:	
	Macroflumycin ($\geq$ 50 μg/ml)	

Recently Sacchi and associates (9) utilizing a spectrofluorimetric assay that employs the fluorescent probe $DiOC_5$ sensitive to membrane potential changes, studied the effects of rifampicin, rifapentine, cefoperazone, ceftriaxone and amphotericin B on membrane potential changes.

They found that rifampicin, rifapentine, cefoperazone and ceftriaxone, which inhibited in vitro chemotaxis at therapeutic concentrations, had no effect on chemoattractant-induced membrane potential changes in PMNs at therapeutic or much higher concentrations. In contrast, amphotericin B irreversibly inhibited PMN membrane potential changes even at concentrations lower than the therapeutic levels. Nevertheless this antibiotic did not interfere with the binding of chemoattractants to their specific neutrophil membrane receptors.

<u>Ex Vivo Effects of Antibiotics on PMN Chemotaxis</u>

Finally the most important point that has to be taken into account concerns the in vivo significance of in vitro findings. We have investi-

Table 5. Serum Levels and Inhibition of Chemotaxis (CT) After Rifampicin Administration[a]

Subjects	Serum levels (μg/ml)	Relative chemotaxis ($CT_{90}{}^{b}/CT_{0}{}^{a}$,%)
1	1.04	103
2	2.81	103
3	2.95	130
4	3.08	98.3
5	3.3	101
6	3.3	99.1
7	3.4	100.9
8	3.7	99.7
9	3.81	70.2
10	4.31	38.1
11	4.35	57.4
12	5.62	32.29
13	6.64	55.9
14	7.63	59.9

[a]14 normal adult volunteers were given 600 mg of antibiotic orally every 24 hrs. The effect on neutrophil locomotion was investigated before[a] and 90[b] minutes after the drug administration.

gated the effects of ceftriaxone and rifampicin administration to normal volunteers on neutrophil chemotaxis. Ceftriaxone, also after repeated i.v. injections, did not produce any significant change in neutrophil migration in spite of its in vitro inhibition of chemotaxis at concentrations normally achieved in therapy (5). This ex vivo finding suggested that some phenomena observed in vitro may have little significance at clinical level, probably because of the presence of some protective factors of unknown origin.

In contrast, neutrophils from normal volunteers receiving 600 mg of rifampicin by oral route showed a reduced chemotactic activity. The chemotactic defect induced by rifampicin administration was related to the levels of antibiotic reached in serum after administration (Table 5). In fact, serum levels of rifampicin $\geq$ 4-5 µg/ml produced transient chemotactic defects, confirming the results obtained in vitro.

CONCLUSION

From these data it can be inferred that no definite conclusion on the possible influence of interactions between antimicrobial agents and neutrophil functions on the therapeutic efficacy of antibiotics is offered by findings derived from currently available data. Further studies on the possible mechanisms of synergistic or adverse effects and on the in vivo interference of antibiotics on host defense systems are necessary to obtain data useful in constructing rational therapeutic strategies for infections. However, clinicians should probably consider what is at the present time known on the interactions between drugs and host defense system when choosing chemotherapeutic agents in some particular situations, as in treating refractory, recurrent or life-threatening infectious diseases in patients with impaired host defense.

ACKNOWLEDGMENTS

The research discussed in this article has been support in part by the Italian Research Council grant N 84.00 602.44 (Progetto Finalizzato Oncologia) and grant N 844101862.52 (Progetto Finalizzato controllo malattie da infezione) and by Ministero Publica Istruzione (Rome, Italy). The authors wish to thank their collaborators particularly Patrizia Mangiarotti, Carla Bersani and Virginia De Rose.

REFERENCES

1. A. Fietta, C. Bersani, P. Mangiarotti, and G. Gialdroni Grassi, Lack of toxicity of macrolides on leukocyte functions, 4th Med. Congr. Chemother. Rhodos, Abs. 422 (1984).
2. A. Fietta, P. Mangiarotti and G. Gialdroni Grassi, Chemotherapeutic agents: aspects of their activity on natural mechanisms of defense against infections, Int. J. Clin. Pharmacol. Ther. Toxicol. 21:325 (1983).
3. A. Fietta, F. Sacchi, C. Bersani, F. Grassi, P. Mangiarotti and G. Gialdroni Grassi, Effect of β-lactam antibiotics on migration and bactericidal activity of human phagocytes, Anitmicrob. Agents. Chemother. 23:930 (1982).
4. A. Fietta, F. Sacchi, C. Bersani, P. Mangiarotti and V. De Rose, In vitro interaction between rifapentine (DL473), a semisynthetic rifamycin derivative, and human phagocytes, Proc. 13th Int. Congr. Chemother., P.S. 3 2/1-1, Vienna, Verlag H. Egerman.
5. G. Gialdroni Grassi, A. Fietta, F. Sacchi and V. De Rose, The influence of ceftriaxone on natural defense systems, Am. J. Med. 77:37 (1984).

6. G. Gialdroni Grassi and A. Fietta, Interference of antimicrobial agents with some reactions of host-defense system, Alabama J. Medical. Sciences 22:144 (1985).
7. G. D. Gray, C. W. Smith, J. C. Hollers, D. E. Chenoweth, V. D. Fiegel and R. D. Nelson, Rifampin affects polymorphonuclear leukocyte interactions with bacterial and synthetic chemotaxins but not interactions with serum-derived chemotaxins, Antimicrob. Agents Chemother. 24:777 (1983).
8. R. C. Prokesch and W. L. Hand, Antibiotic entry into human polymorphonuclear leukocytes, Antimicrob. Agents Chemother. 21:373 (1982).
9. F. Sacchi, N. H. Augustine, A. Fietta, G. Gialdroni Grassi and H. R. Hill, Amphotericin B completely prevents chemoattractant-induced mambrane potential changes in polymorphonuclear leukocytes, 85th Meeting ASM, Las Vegas, Abs. D 120 (1985).
10. F. Sacchi, A. Fietta, P. Mangiarotti, V. De Rose and C. Grassi, Interference between neutrophils and antimycotic agents, Proc. 13th Int. Congr. Chemother., S. E. 4 8/2-11, Vienna, Verlag H. Egerman (1983).
11. F. Sacchi and H. R. Hill, Defective membrane potential changes of neutrophils from human neonates, J. Exp. Med. 160:1247 (1984).
12. B. E. Seligman, E. K. Gallin, D. L. Martin, W. Shaim and J. I. Gallin, Evidence for membrane potential changes in human polymorphonuclear leukocytes during exposure to the chemotactic factor F-Met-Leu-Phe as the fluorescent dye dipentyloxacarbocyanine, J. Cell. Biol. 75:105 (1977).
13. B. E. Seligman and S. I. Gallin, Use of lipophilic probes of membrane potential to assess human neutrophil activation. Abnormality in chronic granulomatous disease, J. Clin. Invest. 66:493 (1980).
14. B. E. Seligman, E. K. Gallin, D. L. Martin, W. Shaim and J. I. Gallin, Interaction of chemotactic factors with polymorphonuclear leukocytes: studies using a membrane-potential sensitive dye, J. Membrane. Biol. 52:257 (1980).
15. R. Van Furth, Phagocytic cells in the defense against infections: introduction, Rev. Infect. Dis. 2:104 (1980).
16. P. C. Wilkinson, Neutrophil leukocyte function tests in: "Techniques in Clinical Immunology," R. A. Thompson, ed., Blackwell Scientific Publications, Oxford (1977).
17. S. M. Zigmond and S. G. Hirsch, Leukocyte locomotion and chemotaxis: new method for evaluation and demonstration of a cell-derived chemotactic factor, J. Exp. Med. 137:387 (1973).

INFLUENCE OF SUBINHIBITORY CONCENTRATIONS OF CLINDAMYCIN ON PHAGOCYTOSIS OF S.AUREUS

Etèl Veringa and J. Verhoef

Department of Medical Microbiology
Laboratory of Microbiology
Utrecht, The Netherlands

Human polymorphonuclear leucocytes (also called neutrophils or PMNs) serve as the cornerstone of defense against invading microorganisms, because of their ability to phagocytize and kill microorganisms. When bacteria invade the host, the outcome is determined by the function of the PMNs. This function depends on the integrity of the following processes: chemotaxis, opsonization, phagocytosis and killing.

After invasion of the tissue by microorganisms, the PMNs leave the circulation and move towards the vicinity of the invading microorganisms. This directional movement is called chemotaxis. Opsonization with serum complement or antibodies is a process which is absolutely necessary for optimal phagocytosis. Although opsonization with complement is primarily mediated through activation of complement via IgG at the bacterial cell surface, these factors may also become fixed to microorganisms without participation of antibody. In hyperimmune serum, IgG is the main opsonic source only amplified by complement, while in non-immune serum opsonization is primarily mediated by complement.

PMN receptors with specificity for activated complement components and for the Fc fragment of the antibody molecule have been described, and evidence suggests that these receptors play a major role in phagocytosis of staphylococci opsonized in normal serum. The process of phagocytosis has been separated into two distinct phases: attachment and ingestion. The attachment induces the formation of pseudopods that surround the particle. When the surrounding pseudopods meet and fuse, a phagocytic vacuole or phagosome, with the particle included, is formed. Then lysosomes fuse with the phagosomes and discharge their contents into the vacuole thus initiating the intracellular killing and digestion of the microorganisms.

During antimicrobial treatment, an important interaction may occur between the drug given and the defenses of the host to eradicate the invading bacteria. Besides a direct influence of antibiotics on bacteria, there may also be an indirect influence of antibiotics on the phagocytic process (7). It has already been shown that exposure to some antibiotics at concentrations lower than the minimal inhibitory concentration (MIC) not only induces morphological changes in bacteria (3), but also enhances the susceptibility of these bacteria to phagocytosis (1,2,4,6,8).

As opsonization of S. aureus is necessary for phagocytosis, this enhanced uptake after exposure to subMIC of antibiotics may be due to changes in the structure of antibody binding or complement activating sites (2,5). Therefore, the aim of our experiments was to study the influence of subMIC of clindamycin on opsonization and phagocytosis of S. aureus.

S. aureus was grown overnight in the presence or absence of one-quarter or one-half of the MIC of clindamycin. For phagocytosis studies, bacteria were radiolabeled by adding [^{3}H]-thymidine to the growth medium. For opsonization, the radioactive labeled bacteria were incubated in different concentrations of serum during various periods of time. The pre-opsonized bacteria were then incubated with PMNs, and after two, six and 12 minutes, respectively, phagocytosis was measured. The percentage of staphylococci taken up by the PMN was calculated from the uptake of radioactivity by the phagocytes and the total added radioactivity, determined in a separate vial. Radioactivity was then determined by liquid scintillation counting.

Using 5% normal human pooled serum as opsonic source during one, five and ten minutes, antibiotic-treated S. aureus was taken up faster than the control. Clindamycin at one-half of the MIC was more effective than at one-quarter of the MIC (Figure 1).

The difference in uptake rates between the control and the clindamycin treated bacteria was even more obvious when 1% serum was used as opsonic source (Figure 2). These results clearly reflect the opsonization kinetics. In normal serum opsonization is primarily mediated by complement, only amplified by antibodies. When only low concentrations of complement (and antibodies) are present (as in 1% serum), or when the opsonization time is short (for example, one minute), clindamycin treated S. aureus may bind complement (and antibodies) more readily than the control bacteria. Raising the serum concentration or extending the opsonization time, however, enables the control bacteria to activate the same amount of complement as the clindamycin treated bacteria (Figures 1 and 2). Because normal human pooled serum contains both complement and antibodies as opsonins, we are not able to really distinguish between opsonization mediated by the classic and the alternative complement pathway and by antibodies. Therefore, bacteria were opsonized in heated antiserum to inactivate the complement system and test the effect of antibodies alone, and bacteria were opsonized in serum of a patient with an antibody deficiency syndrome, to test the effect of complement alone.

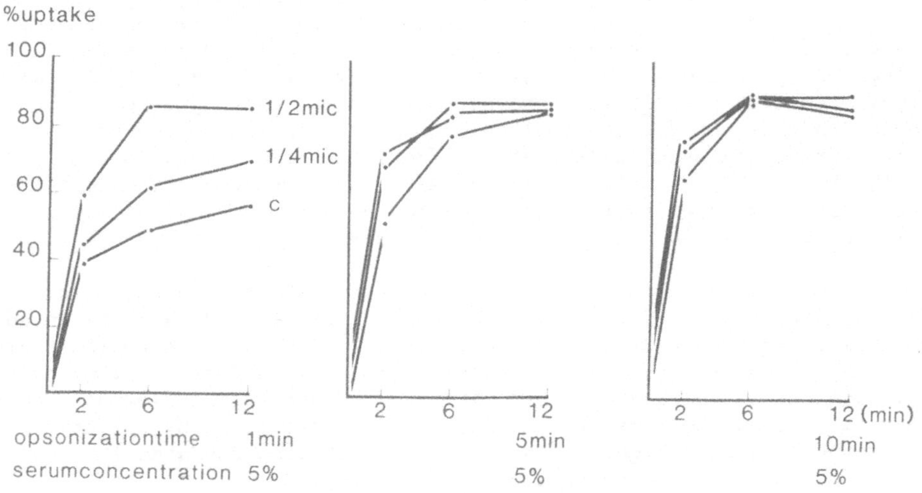

Figure 1. Clindamycin enhances uptake of S. aureus.

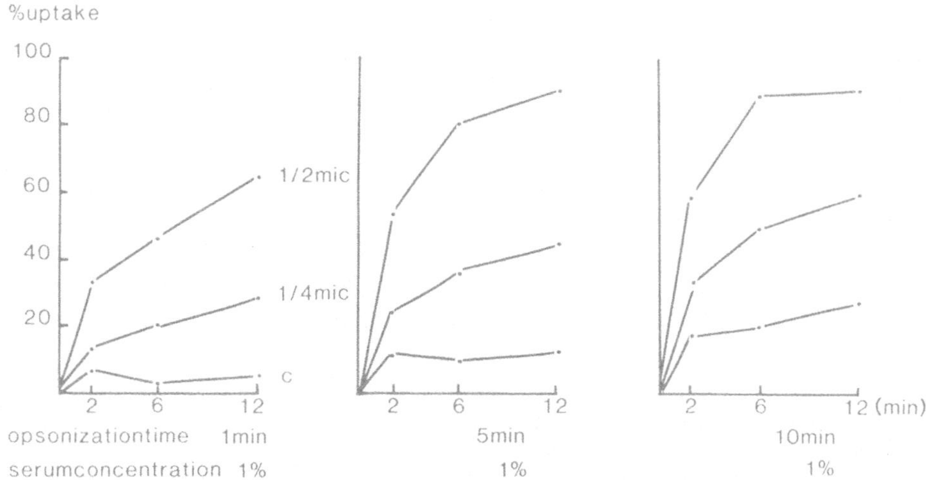

Figure 2. Clindamycin enhances uptake of S. aureus.

Using 1% heated antiserum as opsonic source during one, five and ten minutes, the clindamycin treated bacteria were taken up more readily than the control bacteria, indicating that clindamycin in subMIC enhances antibody dependent phagocytosis (Table 1). And when serum from a patient with agammaglobulinemia, which contains only complement as opsonic source, was used, it appeared that clindamycin also enhances complement dependent phagocytosis (Table 1).

To be sure that these enhanced uptake rates were not consequent of just enhanced attachment of the clindamycin treated bacteria to the granulocytes, we also performed killing experiments. After 12 minutes of phagocytosis, 0.1 ml samples were removed and diluted in 20 ml sterile water.

Table 1. Effect of Subinhibitory Concentrations of Clindamycin on Phagocytosis of S. aureus by PMN

	Opsonization time	Normal serum (1%)	Uptake % Antiserum (1%)	Agammaserum (10%)
S. aureus (control)	1 min.	5	30	30
	5	15	30	50
	10	25	30	50
S. aureus (1/4 MIC clindamycin)	1 min.	30	40	60
	5	45	55	85
	10	60	60	85
S. aureus (1/2 MIC clindamycin)	1 min.	65	50	85
	5	90	55	95
	10	90	55	95

Table 2. Effect of Subinhibitory Concentrations on Killing of S. aureus by PMN

	Killing %		
	normal serum (20%)	antiserum (5%)	antiserum (10%)
S. aureus (control)	96	88	96
S. aureus (1/4 MIC clindamycin)	99	98	99
S. aureus (1/2 MIC clindamycin)	99.9	99.5	99.5

water. The number of colony forming units (CFU) was determined by plating 1 ml of these diluted samples in agar. After incubation for 24 hours at 37°C the percentage viable bacteria in the granulocytes after 12 minutes phagocytosis was calculated from the amount of CFU on the agar plates and the total added amount of bacteria to the PMN. The results showed that the clindamycin treated bacteria were also better killed by the PMNs once they are ingested than were the control bacteria (Table 2).

So far we did all our experiments with the same strain, a clinical isolate of S. aureus. To see if we could obtain the same results with other strains, we performed the same experiments with different S. aureus strains. During these experiments, the results suggested that the enhancing effect of subMIC of clindamycin on phagocytosis was dependent on the presence of a certain amount of protein A on the bacterial cell surface.

Using S. aureus Cowan I, a laboratory strain, which contains a high amount of protein A, as target strain and 1% normal serum as opsonic source we found similar results as we obtained with our standard strain: the bacteria grown in subinhibitory concentrations of clindamycin were much better taken up than the control bacteria. However, when we performed the same experiment with S. aureus Cowan I NG, which is a protein A deficient mutant of S. aureus Cowan I, no such enhancement of phagocytosis was observed.

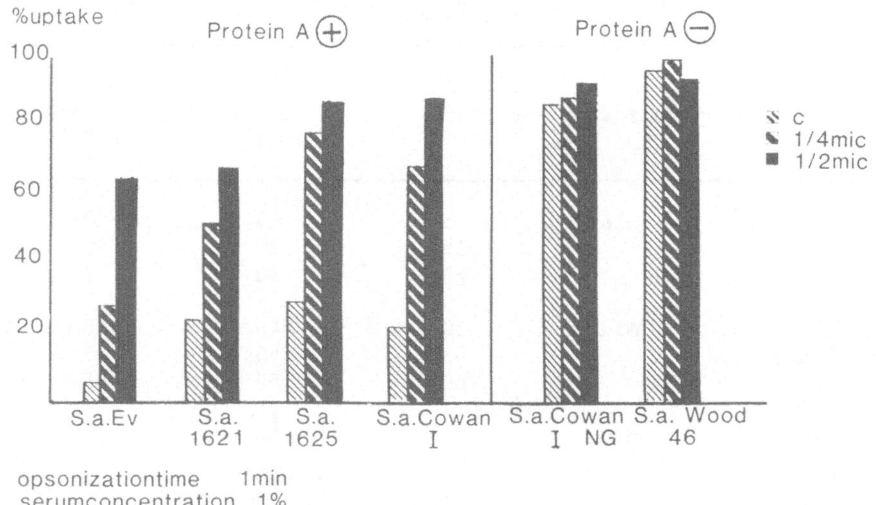

Figure 3. Clindamycin enhances uptake of protein A rich S. aureus.

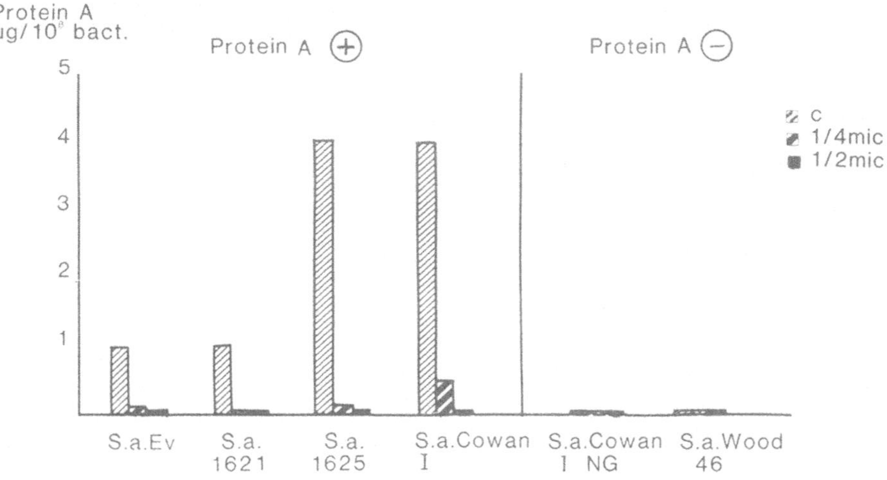

Figure 4. Clindamycin reduces the amount of protein A in S. aureus.

Figure 3 shows that these results also apply to other strains: enhancement of phagocytosis by clindamycin takes place in bacteria that are protein A rich, not in bacteria which are protein A poor strains. It is known, of course, that protein A, a component of the cell wall of S. aureus impairs opsonization by serum complement and by antibodies. Clindamycin in subMIC, however, enhances the uptake rates of the protein A rich strains. This enhancement of phagocytosis appears to be the outcome of an inhibition of protein A synthesis by clindamycin in subinhibitory concentrations. In clindamycin treated as well as untreated bacteria, the total amount of protein A was determined quantitatively by indirect haemagglutination with sheep red blood cells (SRBC) previously sensitized with a subagglutinating dose of IgG antibody against SRBC.

Figure 4 shows that in protein A rich strains the amount of protein A is reduced by subinhibitory concentrations of clindamycin. In protein A poor strains there was no protein A detectable, neither in the control, nor in the clindamycin treated bacteria. These results indicate that the enhanced phagocytosis of S. aureus treated with subMIC of clindamycin may be due to an inhibition of the protein A synthesis in S. aureus. Reduction of the amount of PA on the bacterial cell surface improves the possibilities for opsonization by serum complement and antibodies.

REFERENCES

1. H. Friedman and G. H. Warren, Enhanced susceptibility of penicillin-resistant staphylococci to phagocytosis after in vitro incubation with low doses of nafcillin, Proc. Soc. Exp. Biol. Med. 146:707 (1974).
2. C. G. Gemmell, Ph. K. Peterson, D. Schmeling, Y. Kim, J. Mathews, L. Wannamaker and P. Quie, Potentiation of opsonization and phagocytosis of Streptococcus pyogenes following growth in the presence of clindamycin, J. Clin. Invest. 67:1249 (1981).
3. V. Lorian, Some effects of subinhibitory concentrations of antibiotics on bacteria, Bull. of New York Acad. Med. 51:1046 (1975).
4. P. J. McDonald, B. L. Wetherall and H. Pruul, Postantibiotic leucocyte enhancement. Increased susceptibility of bacteria pretreated with antibiotics to activity of leucocytes, Rev. Inf. Dis. 3:38 (1981).

5. D. Milatovic, I. Braveny and J. Verhoef, Clindamycin enhances opsonization of Staphylococcus aureus, Antimicrob. Agents Chemother. 24:413 (1983).
6. D. Milatovic, Effect of subinhibitory concentrations on the phagocytosis of Staphylococcus aureus, Eur. J. Clin. Microbiol. 1:97 (1982).
7. D. Milatovic, Antibiotics and phagocytosis, Eur. J. Clin. Microbiol. 2:414 (1983).
8. D. Milatovic, Influence of subinhibitory concentrations of antibiotics on opsonization and phagocytosis of Pseudomonas aeruginosa by human polymorphonuclear leucocytes, Eur. J. Clin. Microbiol. 3:288 (1984).

ANTIBIOTIC-INDUCED CHANGES IN THE PATHOGENICITY OF BACTERIA AND THEIR INFLUENCE ON THE INTERACTION OF BACTERIA WITH PHAGOCYTIC CELLS IN VITRO AND IN VIVO

Curtis G. Gemmell

Department of Bacteriology, Medical School
University of Glasgow, Royal Infirmary
Glasgow, Scotland

The pathogenesis of bacteria for man is dependent upon a number of factors, some of which are engendered in the bacterial invader and others are based on the specific and non-specific defenses of the host. It is the outcome of the close interaction of these different factors which determines whether or not a life-threatening infection occurs. It is in exceptional circumstances when the specific strain of bacterial invader carries extraordinary virulence characteristics or when the host is immunocompromised that the balance becomes grossly disturbed in favor of the pathogen. The use of antibiotics in therapy becomes extremely important in this situation and this subject is addressed in several of the contributions to this volume. Some examples of the ways in which certain bacterial pathogens can avoid or overcome the serum-mediated or phagocytic cell-mediated defenses of the host are summarized in Tables 1 and 2.

The antibacterial activity of antibiotics is governed to some extent by their mechanism of action, e.g., inhibition of cell wall biosynthesis, inhibition of protein biosynthesis and interference with nucleic acid transcription and translation. Within these three biochemical target areas there exists important differences between various antibiotics. Their biological activity against a specific bacterium is measured in terms of their Minimum Inhibitory Concentration (MIC) or Minimum Bactericidal Concentration (MBC). To these we must now add Minimum Antibiotic Concentration (MAC) as defined by Lorian and de Freitas (20) as the lowest concentration of drug which causes some morphological change in the target bacterium. For a given antibiotic its MAC comes between its MBC and MIC.

This MAC concept has also been used to investigate the effect of various antibiotics on toxin and enzyme biosynthesis by various pathogenic bacteria (5,12,28). Their results and those of others are summarized in Table 3. In many cases the kinetics of expression of the virulence factors in artificial culture media were radically altered by growing the bacteria in the presence of the antibiotic at its MAC. For example _Staphylococcus aureus_ failed to elaborate much α- or δ- haemolysin, coagulase or DNAase when grown in the presence of 1/2 - 1/8 MIC clindamycin or lincomycin. In _Escherichia coli_ the elaboration of α-haemolysin was markedly inhibited by 1-2 mg/L clindamycin and streptomycin (3).

Table 1. Serum Defenses

	Mechanism	Example
Recognition by antibody	#1 antigenic heterogeneity	pili, capsules, lipopolysaccharide (LPS), M protein
	#2 masking of antigen	capsules, IgG binding proteins
	#3 destruction of antibody	Bacteroides sp. protease
	#4 antigenic variation	Borrelia sp.
Complement system	#1 failure to activate alternate pathway	sialic acid capsules (E. coli, group B streptococci)
	#2 inactivation of C components	Bacteroides sp. protease
	#3 resistance to bacteriolysis	Col V plasmid

Many of the toxins whose biosynthesis is impaired by low concentrations of antibiotics (i.e. sub-MIC) display important biological activity in the pathogenesis of infection by a direct action on the functions of the phagocytic cell system. Examples exist of toxins which can impair chemotaxis, phagocytic ingestion and killing and by so doing can impair the normal host response to the bacterial invader. It is likely that such antagonistic behavior is likely to be of direct benefit to the pathogen especially in the immunocompromised host. Impairment of their expression by the presence

Table 2. Phagocytic Defenses

Mechanism	Example(s)
# 1 inhibition of chemotaxis	Brucella, Salmonella, Neisseria cells
# 2 inhibition of attachment	capsules, M protein
# 3 inhibition of ingestion	protein A, fimbriae
# 4 inhibition of metabolic burst	Salmonella typhi (Vi antigen)
# 5 inhibition of degranulation	Mycobacterium sp.
# 6 resistance to cationic proteins	mucopeptide, lipopolysaccharide (LPS)
# 7 resistance to oxidative attack	catalase, superoxide dismutase, carotenoids
# 8 escape from phagosome	Mycobacterium sp., Legionella pneumophila
# 9 destruction of phagocyte	Streptococcus pyogenes, Pseudomonas aeruginosa
#10 intracellular multiplication	Brucella abortus, Neisseria meningitidis

Table 3. Toxins Whose Biosynthesis is Inhibited or Potentiated Presence of Antibiotics at Their Minimal Antibiotic Concentration

	Toxin	Organism	Antibiotic
Inhibition	α-toxin	Staph. aureus	clindamycin
	streptolysin O	Strep. pyogenes	clindamycin
	α-haemolysin	E. coli	streptomycin
	lipase	Propionibacterium acnes	tetracycline
	protease	Pseudomonas aeruginosa	tetracycline
Potentiation	cytotoxin	Clostridium difficile	clindamycin
	enterotoxin	E. coli	lincomycin
	pneumolysin	Strep. pneumoniae	penicillin

of antibiotics even at low concentrations becomes more significant under these circumstances.

For example Staphylococcus aureus owes its pathogenicity to the possession of α- and δ-haemolysins as well as leucocidin. Each of these toxins has been recognized to affect the structure and function of the mammalian leukocyte (10,16). At least in the case of DNAase and α-haemolysin, production of these toxins in experimental skin infections in mice has been shown to be impaired if the animals were receiving low doses of clindamycin intravenously or were infected with staphylococci grown previously in the presence of sub-MIC clindamycin (6,27). In these animal models of infection it was also recognized that modification of the clinical severity and histological appearance of the lesions occurred. It is possible also that such modified infections alter the normal immunological response because of the absence (or shortage) of the normal antigenic stimuli produced by the bacterial pathogen.

The antigenic mosaic carried by a pathogenic bacterium also be modified by prior exposure to low concentrations of an antibiotic. For example, in Streptococcus pyogenes which expresses M, T and R antigens, there is evidence available showing that growth in the presence of clindamycin or lincomycin reduces the amount of M and T antigen on the bacterial cell surface (R antigen was not measured). In these experiments the amount of antigen was measured serologically (5) but later it was shown (8) that reduced amounts of M antigen (partly compromising the electron-dense "fuzz" around the cell) were seen under the electron microscope. The loss of M antigen, known to act as an inhibitor of complement-mediated opsonization (1), potentiated opsonophagocytosis of the antibiotic-damaged bacteria by polymorphonuclear leukocytes and monocytes in vitro. At least two hours contact with 1/2 MIC clindamycin present in the culture medium was required before any stimulation of bacterial susceptibility to phagocytosis was measurable. Erythromycin and penicillin when used in the same way, were able to enhance opsonophagocytosis but did so without affecting M protein biosynthesis (11).

A wider range of antibiotics has been looked at in relation to their effect on the susceptibility of Staphylococcus aureus to phagocytosis. Phagocytosis of this bacterium is dependent upon adequate opsonization via activation of the alternative complement cascade: however, two cell components, namely protein A and capsule are known to impair this process

Table 4. Susceptibility of Antibiotic-exposed S. aureus to Serum Opsonization and Phagocytosis

Antibiotic exposure	Serum opsonization	Phagocytic ingestion	Phagocytic killing
Penicillin	-	+	+
Oxacillin	-	-	-*
Clindamycin	+	+	+
Fusidic acid	+	+	+
Pseudomonic acid	-	-	+

+ = potentiation; - = no effect; -* = impairment

(24,25). The β-lactam antibiotics cause the formation of thickened cross-walls which then fail to separate (18). Root et al. (26) showed that such cells failed to survive inside the polymorphonuclear leukocyte and increased killing rates were obtained when S. aureus was exposed to 1/2 MIC penicillin G. This enhanced susceptibility to killing by the phagocytic cells occurred even when phagosome formation was inhibited by the presence of cytochalasin B. In contrast, Lorian and Atkinson (19) showed that oxacillin exposed staphylococci were less susceptible to phagocytic killing. After 30 and 60 minutes incubation with polymorphonuclear leukocytes the killing rates for oxacillin-grown versus control staphylococci were 52 and 70% compared to 65 and 85%, respectively. Later studies have shown (17) that although the numbers of staphylococci killed by PMN following exposure to oxacillin was lower, the weight of staphylococcal cells killed was nevertheless greater. The difference was attributed to the marked morphological changes seen in the oxacillin-treated cells. When the processes of ingestion and killing of staphylococci by polymorphonuclear leukocytes were measured separately (7,22) only certain drugs were able to potentiate both processes (clindamycin and fusidic acid) whereas others were able to affect only phagocytic ingestion (doxycyline). The different effects reported for the action of antibiotics at low concentrations on the susceptibility of S. aureus to phagocytosis are summarized in Table 4. It is now known that those antibiotics which potentiate phagocytic ingestion do so through impairment of protein A biosynthesis and subsequent increased binding of complement as C3b on the bacterial cell surface (21). Short-term exposure of S. aureus to antibiotic concentrations greater than 1 x MIC also enhanced phagocytic ingestion and killing by alveolar macrophages (14).

Preliminary experiments with an encapsulated strain of S. aureus (M strain) and a strain of S. epidermidis possessing a slime layer, probably responsible for attachment to intravenous catheters (23), showed that their ability to stimulate particle-induced chemiluminescence by human polymorphonuclear leukocytes remains unaltered following exposure to various antibiotics. Thus there appears to be an important difference in antibiotic-induced damage to those bacteria with a proteinaceous surface component and those with a polysaccharide or glycoprotein surface determinant of pathogenicity in terms of their phagocytosis by PMN.

However, when one considers another encapsulated bacterium, namely Bacteroides fragilis, it is apparent that the degree of encapsulation of this organism is diminished when it is grown in the presence of low concentrations of clindamycin but not cefoxitin (13). In the latter case some enhancement of both encapsulation and filamentation of the individual

Table 5. Effect of U63196 E on Phagocytosis of Haemophilus influenzae by Human Polymorphonuclear Leukocytes

Drug Treatment	% Uptake* by PMN
none	31.2 + 1.8
1/2 MIC	41.5 + 6.1
1/4 MIC	49.7 + 9.2
1/8 MIC	28.8 + 7.5

* = mean of three experiments

bacilli was reported. The clindamycin-grown Bacteroides cells were slightly more sensitive to phagocytic ingestion by polymorphonuclear leukocytes but subsequent phagocytic killing was enhanced. Other studies (15) confirmed the finding that exposure of Bacteroides cells to clindamycin modified their susceptibility to phagocytic ingestion and killing. Little or no capsule was present on the surface of the antibiotic-damaged bacilli (13).

With Haemophilus influenzae also, there is circumstantial evidence that capsule formation is altered when the cells are exposed to 1/8 MIC ampicillin for three hours of 25 x MIC for ten minutes (2). After 60 minutes interaction of such drug-exposed bacteria with human PMN, there was significantly more killing of these bacteria (26 and 61%, respectively) compared to that of normal bacteria (1 and 38%, respectively). Preliminary studies from this laboratory have shown that bacterial ingestion is not potentiated by sub-MIC ampicillin. However, a new cephalosporin U63196E stimulated both ingestion and particle-induced chemiluminescence of H. influenzae by PMN (see Table 5).

Unfortunately most of the aforementioned studies have been conducted in vitro and the changes induced by antibiotics may be somewhat artificial since the experiments are carried out under almost ideal experimental conditions where known numbers of bacteria come into contact with the chosen antibacterial agent in the absence of any host factors such as serum or cells of the reticuloendothelial system. Then they are opsonized in normal serum before being interacted with normal polymorphonuclear leucocytes or macrophages. In reality it is more likely that in vivo the bacteria will be growing more slowly in a non-ideal environment where nutrients may be limited. In addition, for the antibiotic to exert its damage on the bacterial cells in a focus of infection the drug must be able to penetrate and slowly accumulate in an active form within the lesion. The finding that various antibiotics can be concentrated with the PMN or macrophage (e.g., ciprofloxacin, clindamycin, erythromycin and rifampicin) adds a new dimension to the bacterium-antibiotic-phagocytic cell interaction.

It is thus not surprising that hitherto few studies have been directed towards the measurement of antibiotic action in relation to host response in vivo. Even in those reports where low concentrations of drugs were administered to the experimental animal during infection or where antibiotic-damaged bacteria were inoculated there is only presumptive evidence that the host response and hence the severity of the infection in mice or quinea pigs was modified by the presence of antibiotics known to affect the expression of structural and soluble bacterial virulence factors. We shall have to await more discriminative experimentation before any firm conclusion can be drawn as to the relative efficacy of various antibacterial agents in the treatment of infection through modification of the host-parasite relationship. In summary, therefore we can list a number of possible consequences of the interaction between antibiotic-damaged bacteria and the cells of the reticuloendothelial system as follows:

1. Increase or decrease of yields of various exotoxins which have an action on PMN function;
2. Alterations in cell morphology resulting in filamentation or additional cell walls or thickened cell walls;
3. Loss of surface antigen(s) or exposure of hidden antigens;
4. Increase or decrease in expression of chemotaxin(s);
5. Altered requirements for serum opsonins;
6. Altered rates of phagocytic ingestion and killing;
7. Variable release of antigen from phagocytic cell;
8. Variable activation of macrophage and presentation of antigen to B lymphocytes; and
9. Variable antibody response

On the basis of the experiments reported so far any fears that antibiotic-damaged bacteria produced through exposure to antibiotics at their MAC would adversely affect the host's immune response have not been substantiated. On the contrary certain aspects of the host response are potentiated.

REFERENCES

1. A. L. Bisno, Alternate complement pathway activation by Group A streptococci: role of M protein, Infect. Immun. 25:1172 (1979).
2. K. L. Cates and L. Caparas, Neutrophil (PMN) killing of *Haemophilus influenzae* b; effect of pretreatment with ampicillin and chloramphenicol, Abstract no. 658, in: "21st Interscience Conference on Antimicrobial Agents and Chemotherapy," American Society of Microbiology, Washington, D.C. (1981).
3. E. P. Dellinger, Clindamycin inhibition of growth and hemolysin production by *Escherichia coli*, in: "Clindamycin and Modulation of Host Defense," J. Verhoef, ed., Excerpta Medica, Princeton, N.J. (1984).
4. C. G. Gemmell and M. K. A. Amir, Antibiotic-induced changes in streptococci with respect to their interaction with human polymorphonuclear leukocytes, in: "Current Chemotherapy and Infectious Disease," J. D. Nelson and C. Grassi, eds., American Society of Microbiology, Washington, D.C. 2:810 (1980).
5. C. G. Gemmell and M. K. A. Amir, Effects of certain antibiotics on the formation of cellular antigens and extracellular products by group A streptococci, in: "Pathogenic Streptococci," M. T. Parker, ed., Reedbooks, Chertsey, England (1979).
6. C. G. Gemmell, Effect of sub-growth inhibitory concentrations of antibiotics on experimental pyogenic infections in mice, in: "Current Chemotherapy," W. Siegenthaler and R. Luthy, eds., American Society of Microbiology, Washington, D.C. (1978).
7. C. G. Gemmell and A. O'Dowd, Regulation of protein A biosynthesis in *Staphylococcus aureus* by certain antibiotics: its effect on phagocytosis by leukocytes, J. Antimicrob. Chemother. 12:587 (1983).
8. C. G. Gemmell, P. K. Peterson, D. Schmeling, Y. Kim, J. Mathews, L. W. Wannamaker and P. G. Quie, Potentiation of opsonization and phagocytosis of *Streptococcus pyogenes* following growth in the presence of clindamycin, J. Clin. Invest. 67:1249 (1981).
9. C. G. Gemmell, P. K. Peterson, D. Schmeling, J. Mathews and P. G.

Quie, Drug-induced modification of Bacteroides fragilis and its susceptibility to phagocytosis by human polymorphonuclear leukocytes, Eur. J. Clin. Microbiol. 2:327 (1983).

10. C. G. Gemmell, P. K. Peterson, D. Schmeling and P. G. Quie, Effect of staphylococcal α-toxin on phagocytosis of staphylococci by human polymorphonuclear leukocytes, Infect. Immun. 38:975 (1982).
11. C. G. Gemmell, P. K. Peterson, D. Schmeling and P. G. Quie, Studies on the potentiation of phagocytosis of Streptococcus pyogenes by treatment with various antibiotics, Drugs Exptl. Clin. Res. 8:235 (1982).
12. C. G. Gemmell and A. M. A. Shibl, The control of toxin and enzyme biosynthesis in staphylococci by antibiotics, in: "Staphylococci and Staphylococcal Infections," J. Jeljaszewicz, ed., G. Fischer, Stuttgart (1976).
13. C. G. Gemmell, T. Spear and P. K. Peterson, Morphological changes in Bacteroides fragilis and Klebsiella pneumoniae attributable to growth in the presence of various antibiotics, Eur. J. Clin. Microbiol. 2:1 (1983).
14. W. L. Hand, N. L. King-Thompson and J. D. Johnson, Influence of bacterial-antibiotic interactions on subsequent antimicrobial activity of alveolar macrophages, J. Infect. Dis. 149:271 (1984).
15. R. J. Howard and D. M. Soucy, Potentiation of phagocytosis of Bacteroides fragilis following incubation with clindamycin, J. Antimicrob. Ag. Chemother. 12(Suppl.):63 (1983).
16. A. W. Jackson and R. M. Little, Leukocidal effect of staphylococcal δ-lysin, Canad. J. Microbiol. 3:101 (1957).
17. V. Lorian, Changes in bacterial cell mass after incubation with β-lactam antibiotics, in: "The Influence of Antibiotics on the Host Parasite Relationship," G. Gillissen, H. Hahn and W. Opferkuch, eds., Springer Verlag, Berlin (1985).
18. V. Lorian and B. Atkinson, Effects of subinhibitory concentrations of antibiotics on cross walls of cocci, Antimicrob. Ag. Chemother. 9:1043 (1976).
19. V. Lorian and B. Atkinson, Killing of oxacillin-exposed staphylococci in human polymorphonuclear leukocytes, Antimicrob. Ag. Chemother. 18:807 (1980).
20. V. Lorian and C. C. de Freitas, The minimum antibiotic concentrations (MACs) of aminoglycosides and beta-lactam antibiotics for some gram-negative bacilli and gram-positive cocci, J. Infect. Dis. 139:599 (1979).
21. D. Milatovic, I. Braveny, and J. Verhoef, Clindamycin enhances opsonization of Staphylococcus aureus, Antimicrob. Ag. Chemother. 24:413 (1983).
22. D. Milatovic, Effect of subinhibitory antibiotic concentrations on the phagocytosis of Staphylococcus aureus, Eur. J. Clin. Microbiol. 1:97 (1982).
23. G. Peters, R. Locci and G. Pulverer, Adherence and growth of coagulase-negative staphylococci on surfaces of intravenous catheters, J. Infect. Dis. 146:479 (1982).
24. P. K. Peterson, J. Verhoef, D. Schmeling and P. G. Quie, Effect of protein A on staphylococcal opsonization, Infect. Immun. 15:760 (1977).
25. P. K. Peterson, B. J. Wilkinson, Y. Kim, D. Schmeling and P. G. Quie, Influence of encapsulation on staphylococcal opsonization and phagocytosis by human polymorphonuclear leukocytes, Infect. Immun. 19:943 (1978).
26. R. K. Root, R. Isturiz, A. Molavi, J. A. Metcalfe and H. L. Malech, Interaction between antibiotics and human neutrophils in the killing of staphylococci: studies with normal and cytochalasin-B-treated cells, J. Clin. Invest. 67:247 (1981).

27. A. M. A. Shibl, The effect of antibiotics on enzyme and toxin production by *Staphylococcus aureus*, Ph. D. Thesis, University of Glasgow (1977).
28. A. M. A. Shibl and C. G. Gemmell, Effect of four antibiotics on haemolysin production and adherence to human uroepithelial cells by *Escherichia coli*, *J. Med. Microbiol*. 16:341 (1983).

A MODEL FOR IN VITRO TESTING OF DRUG EFFECTS ON NEUTROPHIL FUNCTION

Lionel A. Mandell

McMaster University
Hamilton, Ontario, Canada

INTRODUCTION

In recent years, there has been a great deal of interest in the effects of antimicrobial drugs on host defense mechanisms, particularly phagocytic cells. Several reviews of this area have recently been published (18,31). While the studies are interesting and provide insight into understanding the neutrophil and its functions, variations in methodology and design of experiments have sometimes resulted in conflicting data making it difficult at times to draw firm conclusions. Even more difficult is the assignment of any definite clinical relevance to the data. Generally, one is dealing with in vitro experiments that may have little to do with what is happening in vivo.

In dealing with infections, one of the most difficult situations the physician must face is infection in the cancer patient. This is especially true for patients with hematologic malignancies undergoing myelosuppressive chemotherapy who develop bacterial infections (4). Typically, antibiotic combinations are used in the hope of providing broad coverage for suspected pathogens and additive or synergistic therapy directed against aerobic gram-negative rods (20,33).

With respect to neutrophils, such patients have obvious quantitative problems but may also have qualitative defects resulting from the presence of chemotactic inhibitors in their serum (7,15,21,28,30).

A recently completed clinical trial done under the auspices of the National Cancer Institute of Canada provided clinical efficacy data for ticarcillin/tobramycin (tic/tob) versus ticarcillin/moxalactam (tic/mox) in the treatment of febrile neutropenic patients (7). Having this clinical data and using sera from leukemic patients containing chemotactic inhibitors, the effects of these drug combinations on PMN (polymorphonuclear neutrophil) chemotaxis were tested using an in vitro system that more closely approximated the in vivo situation.

In this chapter is a report of some of our earlier results dealing with drug effects on neutrophil function as well as the results of our combination drug studies in the presence of chemotactic inhibitors.

MATERIALS AND METHODS

Antimicrobials

The antimicrobials studied were: clindamycin phosphate (Upjohn Co., Canada), sodium penicillin G (Glaxo Laboratories, Toronto), sodium cephalothin (Eli Lilly, Canada), erythromycin gluceptate (Eli Lilly, Canada), chloramphenicol succinate (Pentagone Labs, Toronto), gentamicin sulphate (Schering, Canada), vancomycin hydrochloride (Eli Lilly, Canada), tetracycline hydrochloride (Lederle Products, Cyanamid of Canada), rifampin (Dow Pharmaceuticals, Richmond Hill), 5-fluorocytosine (Hoffmann-LaRoche, Quebec) and adenine arabinoside (Parke-Davis, Canada).

Combinations of ticarcillin disodium (Beecham Laboratories, Quebec) and tobramycin sulfate (Eli Lilly, Canada) and ticarcillin disodium and moxalactam disodium (Eli Lilly, Canada) were also tested. Fresh stock solutions were prepared for each drug using normal saline or distilled water according to instructions from the parent company for reconstitution of the drugs. The concentrations of each drug used were determined by reference to standard therapeutic levels (14). For testing of single drug effects, three concentrations were used for each drug so as to incorporate low and high levels within the therapeutic range as well as a level well above that normally obtainable in serum. The final concentrations for each drug were adjusted according to drug assay values supplied by the parent company. For tic/tob and tic/mox combinations, low and high concentrations within the therapeutic range were used. The drugs and their concentrations are listed in Table 1.

Table 1. Concentrations of Antimicrobial Drugs

	High Concentration (μg/ml)	Therapeutic Concentration (μg/ml)	Low Concentration (μg/ml)
Single Drugs			
Clindamycin	15	10	5
Erythromycin	9	3	1
Penicillin G	800	400	1
Cephalothin	400	200	6.25
Chloramphenicol	32	16	4
Tetracycline	15	5	1
Vancomycin	21	14	2
Gentamicin	36	12	3
Rifampin	16	8	4
5-Fluorocytosine	45	22	11
Adenine arabinoside	1.0	0.5	0.25
Drug Combinations			
Ticarcillin	225		50
Tobramycin	5.5		2.0
Ticarcillin	225		50
Moxalactam	200		50

Phagocytosis and NBT Reduction

Phagocytosis was measured by quantifying the uptake of diisodecyl phthalate Oil Red O particles by human PMNs as described previously (19,26). After mixing with *E. coli* lipopolysaccharide, the particles were opsonized using pooled human serum. PMNs from normal human volunteers were incubated with the test drug for 30 minutes at 37°C and then washed and resuspended in Hank's balanced salt solution (HBSS). The preopsonized particles were then incubated with the washed PMNs with the final incubation mixture containing 10 million cells in 0.8 ml HBSS plus 0.2 ml preopsonized particles. At three time points, 5, 8 and 12 minutes, the reaction was stopped by the addition of ice cold 1 mM N-ethylmaleimide. The tubes were vortexed to disrupt the cell pellets and the dye was extracted with dioxane and read using a spectrophotometer. By use of a predetermined formula, the optical density reading at 525 nM was converted to mg phthalate/10^7 cells.

The NBT reduction assay was a measure of the reduction of NBT to formazan and has also been described in detail elsewhere (19,26). It was essentially the same as the phagocytosis assay except that 0.4 ml of NBT in balanced salt solution were included in the incubation mixture. NBT reduction was measured at the five minute point only. The formazan produced as a result of the NBT reduction was extracted from the cells using dioxane and heating to 90°C for 15 minutes. The optical density of the formazan was then read at 580 nM using a spectrophotometer. Use of a predetermined formula allowed expression of the final results as μg formazan/10^7 cells.

In all of these experiments, control cells exposed to saline instead of to drugs formed the basis of comparison with our test cells. Additional controls to ensure the validity of the assay results included measuring phagocytosis: at 0°C, in the presence of cytochalasin B, and while altering particle/cell ratios and testing NBT reduction using cells from a patient with chronic granulomatous disease.

Chemotaxis

The modified method of chemotaxis under agarose was used (6,22). Pretreated glass microscope slides were covered with an agarose gel solution (1% agarose, 0.25% gelatin). After cooling and hardening, two parallel rows of five holes per row were punched in the agarose to provide wells for PMNs and chemotactic factors. The latter consisted of C5a and *Escherichia coli* bacterial filtrate (BF). The C5a was donated to us by Dr. Peter Ward. The BF was prepared from one loopful of *E. coli* (ATCC) incubated overnight at 37°C in a peptone broth, then passed through a Seitz filter.

There were essentially three types of experiments carried out involving chemotaxis:

1. Measurement of drug effects on chemotaxis;
2. Measurement of inhibition of chemotaxis by serum from cancer patients; and
3. Measurement of effects of drug combinations on chemotaxis in the presence of known chemotactic inhibitors

Measurement of Drug Effects on Chemotaxis. The PMNs were incubated with a specific drug or drug combination for 30 minutes at 37°C and then washed. Ten microliters of the washed cells (5 x 10^7 cells/ml) were then added to one row of wells while 10 microliters of C5a and bacterial filtrate were each added in duplicate to wells in the opposite row. HBSS was added to the fifth well, thereby providing a control for random migration.

The slides were then incubated at 37°C for 3 hours in 5% CO_2. Karnovsky's fixative was added, the agarose was stripped and the slides were washed with methyl alcohol and stained with Giemsa. Using a microprojector, the chemotactic index (CI) was determined.

$$CI = \frac{\text{Directed migration (chemotaxis)}}{\text{Random migration}}$$

The linear distance the cells had migrated from the margin of the well toward the chemoattractant represented chemotaxis. The furthest point of migration was defined as that point at which three cells were aligned in the same plane parallel to the margin of the well. Random migration was represented either by linear distance travelled by the cells toward the well containing HBSS or by the distance travelled from the side of the well opposite the chemoattractant.

Measurement of Inhibition of Chemotaxis by Sera from Cancer Patients. Sera from patients with a variety of neoplasms were tested. These included carcinoma of the lung, carcinoma of breast, leukemia and lymphoma. The patients must not have received antineoplastic chemotherapy within two weeks prior to testing their serum. Tests for chemotactic factor inhibitors (CFI) and cell directed inhibitors (CDI) were done.

CFI. Serum samples from test cases were incubated with C5a or BF as 40% and 50% solutions respectively at 37°C for 30 minutes. Ten microlitres of the C5a or BF solutions were then put into the appropriate wells. Ten microliters of untreated PMNs from normal human volunteers were put into the opposite wells. Incubation for 3 hours was followed by fixing and staining of the cells. Chemotaxis was then measured.

CDI. Serum samples from test cases were incubated with PMNs from normal human volunteers in a 1 to 1 ratio by volume at 37°C for 30 minutes. The cells were then washed and resuspended in HBSS and 10 microliters of the cell suspension were then added to each of the appropriate wells. C5a and BF were added to the opposite wells. After 3 hours incubation, the cells were fixed and stained and chemotaxis was measured.

Measurement of Effects of Drug Combinations on Chemotaxis in the Presence of Known Chemotactic Inhibitors. Using pooled serum from leukemia patients known to contain cell directed inhibitors, PMNs were incubated with either patient serum or control serum plus drug combination (tic/tob or tic/mox) at 37°C x 30 minutes. The cells were then washed and put into the appropriate wells with C5a and BF added to the opposite wells. Following incubation, the cells were fixed and stained and chemotaxis was measured.

Statistical Considerations

To minimize "within experiment" and "between experiment" error, duplicate measurements were carried out on five separate occasions for phagocytosis and NBT experiments and on three separate occasions for chemotaxis experiments.

Direct drug effects on PMN function were analyzed using two-way analysis of variance. Three statistical questions were of primary interest:

1. Was there any evidence to show that phagocytosis, NBT reduction or chemotaxis were different across the treatment groups?
2. Was there any evidence to show that the average therapeutic response was different from control?
3. Was there any evidence to suggest a dose response relationship among the drug treated groups?

Table 2. Effects of Antimicrobial Drugs on Phagocytosis and NBT Reduction

	Potentiating Effect	Inhibiting Effect	No Effect
Phagocytosis	Erythromycin Chloramphenicol Penicillin G Cephalothin Tetracycline Vancomycin 5-Fluorocytosine Adenine arabinoside	Gentamicin Rifampin	Clindamycin
NBT Reduction			All drugs tested

The data for inhibitors and for drug effects on chemotaxis in the presence of inhibitors were analyzed using one-way analysis of variance and the Student's t test. P values of less than 0.05 were considered to be statistically significant.

RESULTS

Phagocytosis and NBT Reduction

A composite mean made up of duplicate daily results determined for five separate days was calculated and used in the analysis of the data. Figure 1 shows the results plotted for erythromycin effects on phagocytosis. The vertical axis represents phagocytic capacity and the horizontal

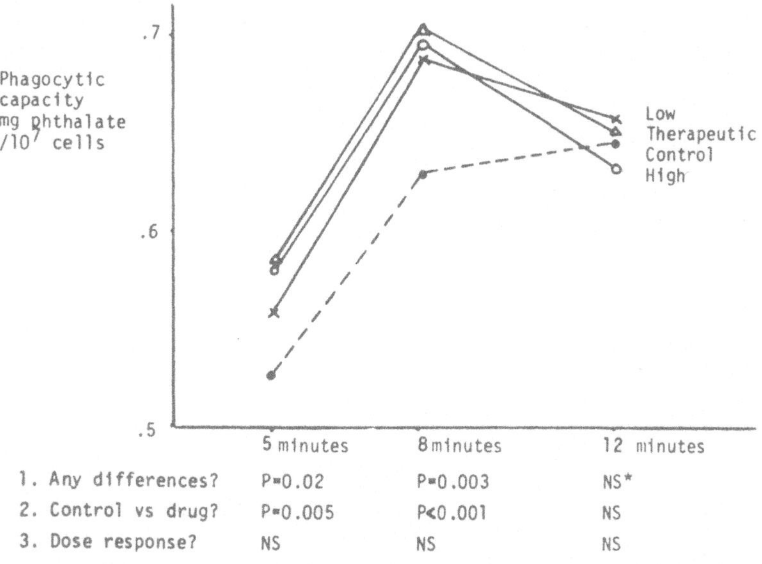

Figure 1. Effects of erythromycin on phagocytosis. (NS = not significant.)

Table 3. Specificity of Chemotactic Inhibition by Antimicrobial Drugs

Specific Effects C5a	Specific Effects BF	Nonspecific Effects	No Effect
Erythromycin	Vancomycin	Tetracycline	Clindamycin
Chloramphenicol		Penicillin	Gentamicin
5-Fluorocytosine		Cephalothin	
		Rifampin	
		Adenine arabinoside	

axis represents time. Underneath are tabulated at each of the three measured timepoints the P values associated with the three statistical questions of interest. With erythromycin, there was strong evidence in favor of real differences in phagocytic activity at 5 and 8 minutes, but these differences were not sustained at 12 minutes. There also appeared to be a general elevation in the three drug treated groups above control at 5 and 8 minutes, but this increase was not dose related. No effects on NBT reduction were seen with erythromycin or any of the other drugs tested. Results for these experiments have been reported in detail elsewhere (19). The results are summarized in Table 2.

Chemotaxis

Drug Effects on Chemotaxis - Single Drugs. Figure 2 shows the results for vancomycin effects on PMN chemotaxis in response to C5a and BF. The vertical axis represents the chemotactic index while the various drug concentrations are listed on the horizontal axis. The P values for the three statistical questions of interest are listed under the headings C5a and BF. It is clear that with C5a as the attractant, no statistically significant effects were seen. With BF as the attractant, however, there was a very clear inhibitory effect noticeable with good evidence for a dose response relationship as well. None of the drugs tested affected random motility. These data have been reported in detail (6,19). The results are summarized in Table 3.

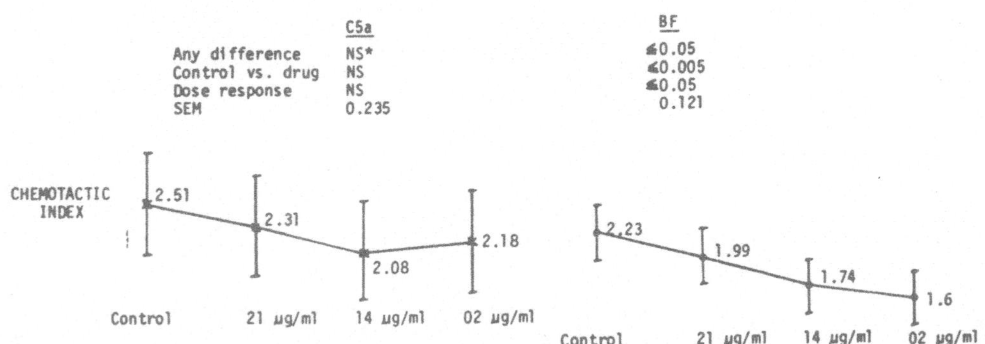

Figure 2. Effects of vancomycin on chemotaxis with C5a and bacterial filtrate (BF) as chemoattractants. (NS = not significant; SEM = standard error of the mean for chemotactic indices.)

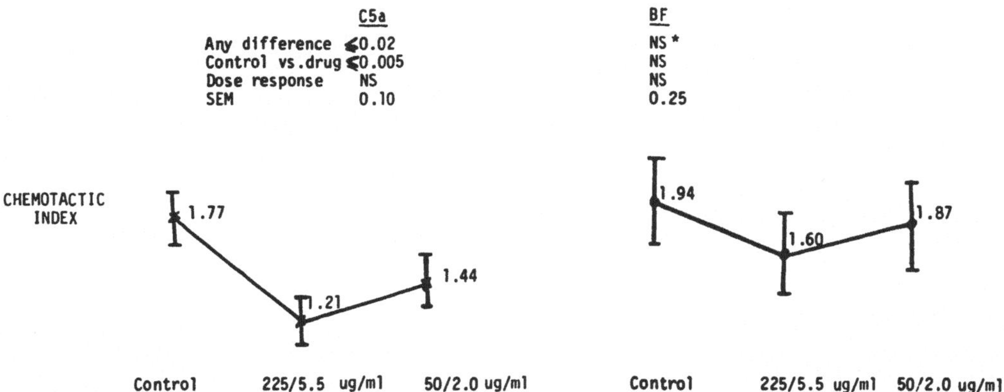

Figure 3. Effects of ticarcillin/tobramycin on chemotaxis with C5a and bacterial filtrate (BF) as chemoattractants. (NS = not significant, SEM = standard error of mean for chemotactic indices.)

Drug Effects on Chemotaxis - Combination Drugs. Figures 3 and 4 show the results plotted for effects of tic/tob and tic/mox respectively on PMN chemotaxis. With tic/tob there appeared to be a statistically significant difference across the groups and between the control and drug-treated groups when C5a was the attractant. No differences were seen, however, when BF was the attractant. When tic/mox was incubated with the PMNs, no statistically significant effects on chemotaxis were found regardless of the chemoattractant used.

Inhibition of Chemotaxis by Serum from Cancer Patients. Some of the results of studies with chemotactic inhibitors have been reported previously (21). They showed that both the type and specificity of chemotactic inhibitor present in serum varies with the underlying neoplasm. The CFI were specific for C5a in lung cancer (P<0.001) and leukemia (P<0.005) but

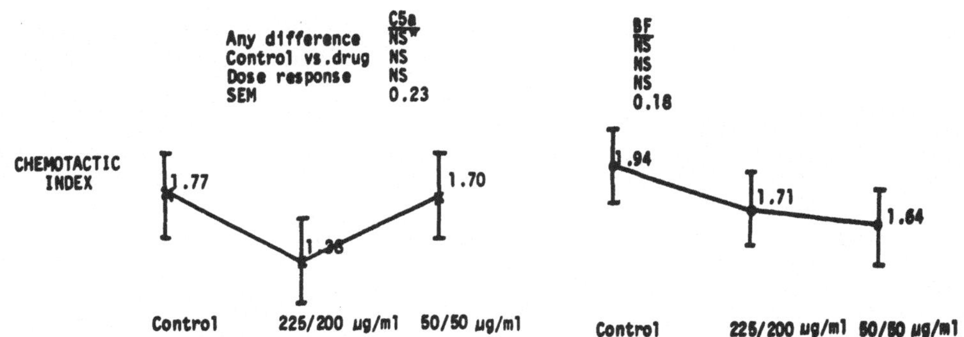

Figure 4. Effects of ticarcillin/moxalactam on chemotaxis with C5a and bacterial filtrate (BF) as chemoattractants. (NS = not significant, SEM = standard error of mean for chemotactic indices.)

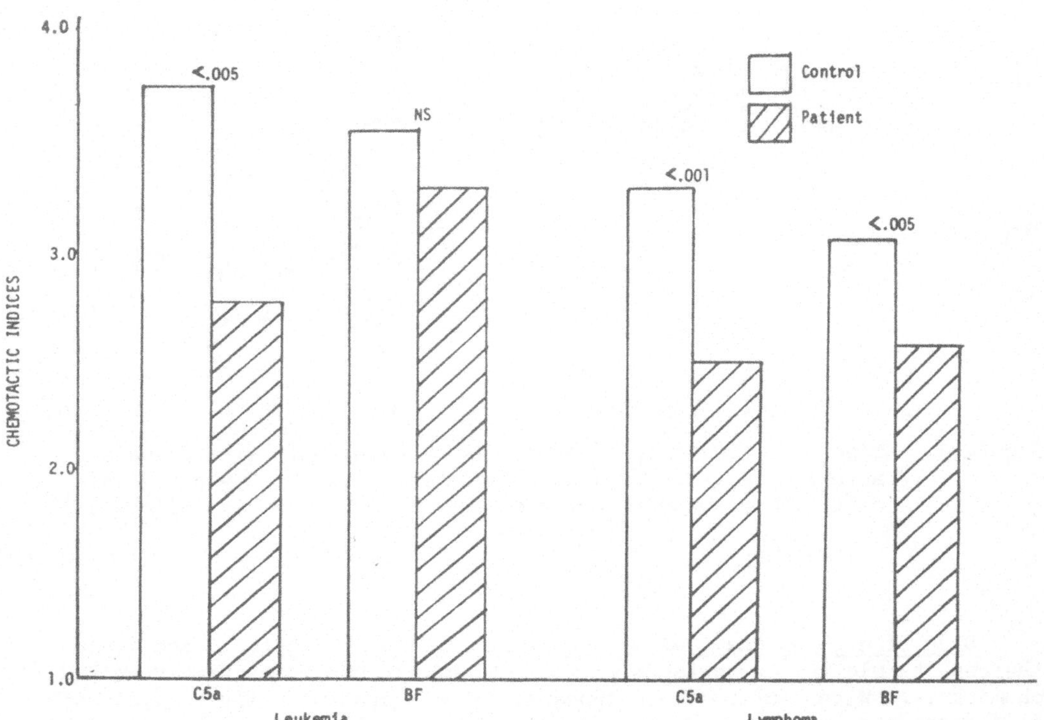

Figure 5. Chemotactic indices for PMNs with control and patient serum.

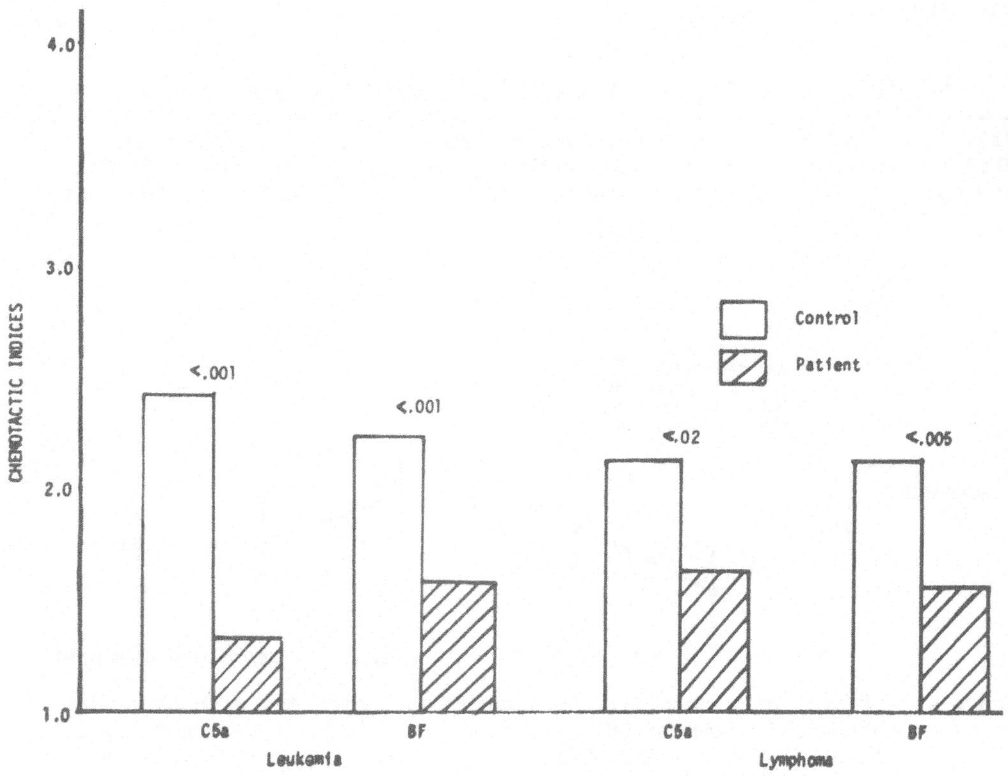

Figure 6. Chemotactic indices for PMNs with control and patient serum.

for BF in breast cancer (P<0.025). Nonspecific inhibition of the chemotactic factors was found in lymphoma patients (P<0.005). Nonspecific CDI were found with leukemia and lymphoma patients (P<0.001) but with lung cancer, the inhibition could be overcome with BF as the attractant (P=0.18). No CDI were detected in the serum of patients with breast carcinoma. Figures 5 and 6 show CFI and CDI data respectively for leukemia and lymphoma patient sera. The P values displayed in these figures represent the results of statistically comparing effects of control and patient serum on chemotaxis toward either C5a or BF.

Drug Effects on Chemotaxis in the Presence of Chemotactic Inhibitors. Table 1 lists the drug concentrations used when combinations of tic/tob and tic/mox were tested. The data are plotted in histogram form in Figure 7. Comparison of the mean chemotactic index when BF was the attractant with the mean index with C5a as the attractant shows that overall there was greater migration in response to BF (P<0.003) regardless of the drug combinations used. In direct comparisons of tic/tob and tic/mox for each of the situations (C5a: low drug concentration, high drug concentration; BF: low drug concentration, high drug concentration) no statistically significant differences were found except at the lower drug concentrations with C5a as the attractant. Although not statistically significant, it appeared that there was a trend toward greater inhibition of chemotaxis with increasing concentrations of tic/mox with both C5a and BF as the attractants. Increasing tic/tob concentrations appeared to have no significant effects on cell migration when results for C5a and BF were examined separately. Using the technique of analysis of variance, there were no differences among chemotactic indices found across all four groups with either C5a or BF.

DISCUSSION

In a review dealing with effects on human cells of drugs whose concentrations were within the therapeutic range, it was concluded that none of

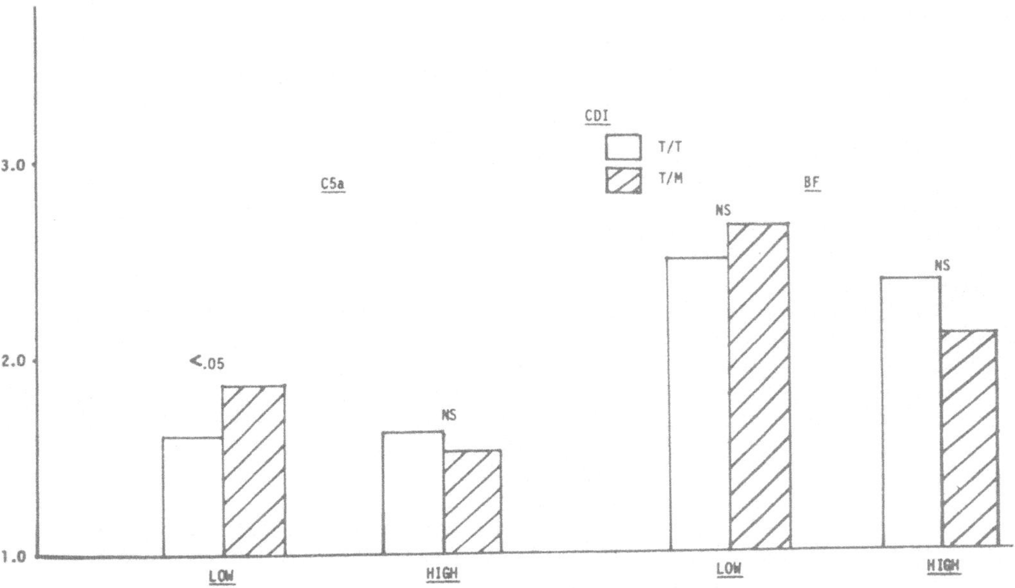

Figure 7. Chemotactic indices for PMNs + cell directed inhibitor + drugs. (T/T = ticarcillin/tobramycin, T/M = ticarcillin/moxalactam)

the bactericidal drugs tested adversely affected phagocytic function but that certain bacteriostatic drugs did (18). Tetracycline and sulfonamides inhibited phagocytosis and microbicidal activity respectively. Our own data showed potentiation of phagocytosis with all of the drugs tested with the exception of clindamycin, gentamicin and rifampin. Our findings with tetracycline differ from the results reported by Munoz (23) and Forsgren (8) but concur with those of Hoeprich (13). None of the drugs tested in this study affected NBT reduction.

Our chemotaxis data are of interest in that the results show both specific and nonspecific inhibition of chemotaxis. It appears that certain antimicrobial drugs not only inhibit chemotaxis but may do so by altering the cell's ability to respond to a specific chemoattractant. The human PMN has receptors on its surface capable of interacting with C5a or the small molecular weight peptides found in bacterial filtrate (32). Inhibition of chemotaxis in response to a specific chemoattractant suggests possible interference with receptor-mediated mechanisms. For example, erythromycin might interfere with C5a receptor-mediated mechanisms while vancomycin might alter BF receptor interaction. Such findings are supported by a study (1) in which the antibiotics gramicidin S, tyrocidine and bacitracin containing Leu-Phe or Ile-Phe sequences interact with receptors for synthetic peptides on PMNs (1). In the case of both our phagocytosis and chemotaxis experiments, following incubation of the cells with the drugs the cells were washed thereby ensuring that any observed effects would be due solely to drug effects on the cells themselves and not on particles or chemoattractants.

Since the PMN plays a critical role in host defense, inhibition of PMN function may alter the cell's ability to deal with invading pathogens. The process of chemotaxis ensures that the cells arrive at the site of infection where they can then ingest and kill the infecting organisms. A variety of factors including complement-related fragments, endogenous enzymes, bacterial factors and lymphokines to name only a few are able to act as chemoattractants (25). As a result of interactions between the PMN and these attractants, a number of changes take place including cationic fluxes (24), activation of intracellular enzymes (2,29) and activation of secondary biochemical events (10,12) resulting in a cell that is hyperadherent, metabolically active and motile (25).

Chemotactic factors play a central role in modulating inflammatory reactions in vivo. Chemotaxis is also regulated to some extent however, by chemotactic inhibitors normally present in serum in small amounts (3,17) or induced by various disease states possibly as acute phase reactants (16,27, 30). Chemotactic inhibitors may also be produced by human PMNs themselves and may serve in the localization and augmentation of the inflammatory response by concentrating PMNs at the inflammatory focus (5,9,11).

Some of our data on chemotactic inhibitors have been reported previously (21). Our hypothesis in the original inhibitor experiments had stated that heterogeneous factors exist in the serum of patients with neoplastic disease that are capable of inhibiting the chemotactic response of the human PMN. Our experimental design allowed us to test this hypothesis using both C5a and BF as chemoattractants. These specific attractants were chosen since it was felt that in the infected patient both C5a and _E. coli_ BF would be commonly encountered chemoattractants.

The results showed that in fact both types of inhibitors (CFI & CDI) were present in serum of cancer patients and that the type of inhibitor as well as its specificity for the chemoattractant (C5a or BF) varied with the underlying neoplasm.

Having determined the presence of such chemotactic inhibitors, it was then possible to measure drug effects on chemotactic function in a manner that more closely approximated in vivo conditions. Drug combinations used in our clinical trial (7) were studied in vitro with PMNs from normal donors thereby precluding the possibility that any intrinsic PMN defects might account for alterations in chemotaxis.

In the experiments testing effects of the drug combinations (tic/tob, tic/mox) in an inhibitor-free system, significant inhibition of chemotaxis was seen when tic/tob was used and C5a was the attractant.

When the inhibitor was present however, despite the fact that a number of changes were seen as discussed in the results section of this paper, there were in fact no significant differences between the tic/tob and tic/mox effects with the exception of the difference noted when low concentrations of the drugs were tested in the presence of C5a (Figure 7).

The greater migration seen toward BF in the presence of chemotactic inhibitors is in fact in keeping with our original observations of inhibitors in the serum of leukemia patients in which BF appears to be a more potent chemoattractant than C5a.

If drug effects on PMN function had in fact been significant enough to impair the cell's ability to respond to chemoattractants to such an extent that it was clinically important, one would expect such an effect to show up in a therapeutic trial. In fact, the results of the clinical study showed that there were no statistically significant differences in the outcome measures tested, i.e. clinical response, response by site of infection and response by pathogen (7). By testing drug effects in the presence of chemotactic inhibitors, we found results that correlated with clinical outcome in infected patients treated with these same drugs.

REFERENCES

1. S. Aswanikumar, E. Schiffmann, and B. A. Corcoran, Antibiotics and peptides with agonist and antagonist chemotactic activity, _Biochem. Biophys. Res. Commun._ 80:464 (1978).
2. E. L. Becker, The relationship of the chemotactic behavior of the complement-derived factors C3a, C5a and C567, and a bacterial chemotactic factor to their ability to activate the proesterase I of rabbit polymorphonuclear leukocytes, _J. Exp. Med._ 135:376 (1972).
3. J. L. Berenberg and P. A. Ward, Chemotactic factor inactivator in normal human serum, _J. Clin. Invest._ 52:1200 (1973).
4. A. E. Brown and D. Armstrong, "Infectious Complications of Neoplastic Disease. Controversies in Management," York Medical Books, New York, N.Y. (1985).
5. J. P. Brozna, R. M. Senior and D. L. Kreutzer, Chemotactic factor inactivators of human granulocytes, _J. Clin. Invest._ 60:1280 (1977).
6. D. E. Chenoweth, J. G. Rowe and T. E. Hugli, A modified method for chemotaxis under agarose, _J. Immunol. Methods_, 25:337 (1979).
7. R. Feld, T. J. Louie, L. Mandell, H. Robson, A. Chow, A. Belch, G. Goldsand and J. Pater, A multicentre comparative trial of tobramycin and ticarcillin versus moxalactam and ticarcillin in febrile neutropenic patients, _Arch. Intern. Med._ (in press).
8. A. Forsgren, D. Schmeling and P. G. Quie, Effect of tetracycline on the phagocytic function of human leukocytes, _J. Infect. Dis._ 130:412 (1974).

9. E. J. Goetzl and K. F. Austen, A neutrophil-immobilizing factor derived from human leukocytes. I. Generation and partial characterization, J. Exp. Med. 136:1564 (1972).
10. E. J. Goetzl and K. F. Austen, Stimulation of human neutrophil leukocyte aerobic glucose metabolism by purified chemotactic factors, J. Clin. Invest. 53:591 (1974).
11. E. J. Goetzl, I. Gigli, S. Wasserman and K. F. Austen, A neutrophil immobilizing factor derived from human leukocytes. II. Specificity of action on polymorphonuclear leukocyte mobility, J. Immunol. 111:938 (1973).
12. I. M. Goldstein, D. Roos, H. B. Kaplan and G. Weissmann, Complement and immunoglobulins stimulate superoxide production by human leukocytes independently of phagocytosis, J. Clin. Invest. 56:1155 (1975).
13. P. D. Hoeprich and C. H. Martin, Effect of tetracycline, polymyxin B and rifampin on phagocytosis, Clin. Pharmacol. Ther. 11:418 (1970).
14. A. Kucers and N. McK. Bennett, "The Use of Antibiotics: A Comprehensive Review with Clinical Emphasis, 3rd edition," Wm. Heinemann Medical Books Ltd., London (1979).
15. E. G. Maderazo, T. F. Anton and P. A. Ward, Serum-associated inhibition of leukotaxis in humans with cancer, Clin. Immunol. Immunopathol. 9:166 (1978).
16. E. Maderazo, P. A. Ward and R. Quintiliani, Defective regulation of chemotaxis in cirrhosis, J. Lab. Clin. Med. 85:621 (1975).
17. E. G. Maderazo, P. A. Ward, C. L. Woronick and R. Quintiliani, Partial characterization of a cell-directed inhibitor of leukotaxis in human serum, J. Lab. Clin. Med. 89:190 (1977).
18. L. A. Mandell, Effects of antimicrobial and antineoplastic drugs on the phagocytic and microbicidal function of the polymorphonuclear leukocyte, Rev. Infect. Dis. 4:683 (1982).
19. L. A. Mandell, The effects of antibacterial, antiviral and antifungal drugs on the phagocytic, microbicidal and chemotactic function of the human polymorphonuclear leukocyte, in: "The Influence of Antibiotics on the Host Parasite Relationship," H. U. Eickenberg, H. Hahn and W. Opferkuch, eds., Springer-Verlag Press, Heidelberg (1982).
20. L. A. Mandell, Management of the febrile neutropenic patient, Can. Med. Assoc. J. 128:915 (1983).
21. L. A. Mandell, Modulators of host defense in malignancy, in: "Proceedings of 2nd International Symposium on Infections in the Immunocompromised Host," C. S. F. Easmon and H. Gaya, eds., Academic Press, London (1983).
22. L. A. Mandell, The effects of antibacterial drugs on neutrophil function, in: "Proceedings of Symposium on Clindamycin and Modulators of Host Defense," J. Verhoef, ed., Excerpta Medica, The Netherlands (1984).
23. J. Munoz and R. Geister, Inhibition of phagocytosis of aureomycin, Proc. Soc. Exp. Biol. Med. 75:367 (1950).
24. P. H. Naccache, H. J. Showell, E. L. Becker and R. I. Sha'afi, Transport of sodium, potassium and calcium across rabbit polymorphonuclear leukocyte membranes. Effect of chemotactic factor, J. Cell. Biol. 73:428 (1977).
25. J. T. O'Flaherty and P. A. Ward, Chemotactic factors and the neutrophil, Semin. Hematol. 16:163 (1979).
26. T. P. Stossel, Evaluation of opsonic and leukocyte function with a spectrophotometric test in patients with infection and with phagocytic disorders, Blood 42:121 (1973).
27. D. E. Van Epps, R. G. Strickland and R. C. Williams, Jr., Inhibitors of leukocyte chemotaxis in alcoholic liver disease, Am. J. Med. 59:200 (1975).

28. D. E. Van Epps and R. C. Williams, Jr., Suppression of leukocyte chemotaxis by human IgA myeloma components, J. Exp. Med. 144:1227 (1976).
29. P. A. Ward and E. L. Becker, The deactivation of rabbit neutrophils by chemotactic factor and the nature of the activatable esterase, J. Exp. Med. 127:693 (1968).
30. P. A. Ward and J. L. Berenberg, Defective regulation of inflammatory mediators in Hodgkin's disease. Supernormal levels of chemotactic-factor inactivator, N. Engl. J. Med. 290:76 (1974).
31. E. L. Yourtee and R. K. Root, Antibiotic-neutrophil interactions in Microbial killing, in: "Advances in Host Defense Mechanisms, Vol. 1," J. I. Gallin and A. S. Fauci, eds., Raven Press, New York (1982).
32. S. H. Zigmond, Chemotaxis by polymorphonuclear leukocytes, J. Cell. Biol. 77:269 (1978).
33. The EORTC International Antimicrobial Therapy Project Group: Three antibiotic regimens in the treatment of infection in febrile granulocytopenic patients with cancer, J. Infect. Dis. 137:14 (1978).

EFFECT OF β-LACTAM ANTIBIOTICS ON THE BACTERICIDAL ACTIVITY OF POLYMORPHONUCLEAR LEUKOCYTES AGAINST *ESCHERICHIA COLI*

Axel Dalhoff

Institute for Chemotherapy
Bayer AG
Wuppertal, F.R.G.

INTRODUCTION

Opsonization of bacteria with antibodies as well as phagocytosis and intracellular killing of the pathogens are important factors contributing to host resistance to bacterial infections. Numerous data have been accumulated indicating that antimicrobial agents may affect polymorphonuclear leukocyte (PMN) function (1,2,34).

Similarly, antibiotic exposed bacteria have been shown to undergo morphologic and biochemical changes (2,26,27), including changes in surface properties (23,45). Surface adhesions mediate the binding of *E. coli* to epithelial cells and PMN (3,4,36,42). Thus, anti-adhesive effects of antibiotics may result in a dual mode of interaction with host defense mechanisms. Subinhibitory concentrations of various antibiotics including β-lactams causing filamentation of the bacteria were found to suppress expression of surface adhesions and thereby impaired the ability of *E. coli* and Streptococci respectively to adhere to eucaryotic cells (9-11,37,41,46). On the other hand, however, it appears that β-lactams in general render *E. coli*, *Staph. aureus*, Streptococci and *P. aeruginosa* more susceptible to leukocyte killing (1,5,6,12-15,17,19,29,30,35,38,40,44). These discrepancies may either be due to the variety of mechanisms of pilus mediated adhesions of *E. coli* to eukaryotic cells (21,22,32,39) or to the widely different methods used to quantitate phagocytosis and/or adhesion. Furthermore, it is difficult to foresee the clinical relevance of the above mentioned data as they all were obtained by adopting specific in vitro systems. The aims of this study were firstly to assess the effect of β-lactam antibiotics on phagocytosis and intracellular killing in an experimental system resembling the complex in vivo conditions in the infected host most closely; secondly, by adopting the same system, the attempt should be made to examine the mechanism underlying the β-lactam promoted increase in intracellular killing of *E. coli*.

MATERIALS AND METHODS

Antimicrobial Agents

Cefoxitin and lamoxactam were obtained from Eli Lilly (Giessen, FRG) ticarcillin from Beecham-Wulfing (Neuss, FRG) piperacillin from Cyanamid-

Lederle (Wolfratshausen, FRG) and mezocillin from Bayer AG (Leverkusen, FRG).

Bacteria

Isogenic E. coli strains differing in their O- and K-antigens respectively were used throughout this study: F492 = 08^+: $K27^+$; F639 = 08^-; $K27^+$; F459 = 08^+; $K27^-$; F470 = 08^-; $K27^-$. Strains were precultivated in Mueller Hinton broth under static conditions at 37°C for 18 hrs. Prior to infection of the explants, strains were diluted tenfold into fresh medium supplemented with Hanks buffered salt solution and incubated at 37°C for 1 hr; 0.5 ml of this bacterial culture was used to inoculate the explants. These strains express mannose sensitive pili on their outer membrane.

Intracellular Killing Activity of Rat PMN.

Killing of E. coli by rat-PMN was studied by using a modified rat polyvinyl sponge model as described recently (7). Briefly, sponges presoaked with heat killed bacteria were implanted subcutaneously on both sides between the shoulders of female wistar rats weighing 120-160g; 24 hrs later sponges were removed aseptically. During this period in time an inflammatory exudate as well as 10^9 PMN/1 sponge fluid invaded into the explants. Following explantation sponges were inoculated with a 0.5 ml of the corresponding bacterial culture to which the antibiotic or other chemicals were added; the ratio of bacteria to PMN was 10:1. The explants were then placed in a humid chamber and incubated under static conditions at 37°C. The number of colony forming units (CFU/ml) was determined by squeezing the sponges thoroughly in ice-cold distilled water followed by an immediate dilution into physiological saline. An irreversible binding of bacteria to the sponge matrix can be excluded due to the data reported by Isenberg et al. (20). All experiments were repeated twice; the standard deviation from the mean was less than 4%.

In parallel to the determination of viable counts the length of an individual bacterium was determined. Bacteria were separated from PMN by differential centrifugation. Immediately afterwards they were examined by phase contrast microscopy at a magnification of x 1,000. A series of photographs was taken for every drug and sampling time; the length of at least 100 bacteria per drug and sampling time was measured and the length of an individual bacterium was calculated from the arithmetic mean of these measurements.

A comparison of the bactericidal activities of rat PMN (rat polyvinyl sponge model) and human PMN (prepared by sedimentation through amipaque and albumin) respectively against three different clinical isolates of P. aeruginosa was performed. Data summarized in Figure 1 showed that engulfment and intracellular killing of three clinical isolates of Ps. aeruginosa either by human PMN suspended in the homologous serum obtained from healthy volunteers or by the ex-vivo system were highly similar for two of the three strains tested. Following an incubation period of 90 min 70-80% of the initial inoculum was killed by human and rat PMN. Pretreatment of these strains with subinhibitory azlocillin concentrations resulted in a highly significant increase in intracellular killing irrespective of whether the bacteria were exposed to either human or rat PMN (Figure 1).

Free Flow Electrophoresis

Free flow electrophoresis (FFE) of intact bacteria and/or heparinized guinea pig blood was carried out in Desaga "FF48 Free Flow Electrophoretic Separator." Blood was obtained by direct heart puncture of female guinea pigs. The bacteria used for the FFE were isolated from the explants by differential centrifugation after an incubation period of 1 hr at 37°C. The sediment was resuspended in heparinized blood to yield a final bacterial count of 10^8 CFU/ml. This suspension was slightly agitated for 15 min. An aliquot of the suspension was electrophoretically separated thereafter in an 0.0114M phosphate-sucrose-glucose buffer.

The following buffer-stock solutions (bss) were prepared: i. 9.078 g/l KH_2PO_4; i.i. 11.876 g/l Na_2HPO_4; i.i.i. 10% sucrose; and i.v. 5% glucose. In order to yield the separation buffer 12 ml of bss 1, 131 ml of bss 2, 857 ml of bss 3 and 40 ml of bss 4 were mixed; the electrode buffer was obtained by adding 1,680 ml bss 1 to 4,320 ml bss 2. The run was done at 165 mA, 600 V/cm at a temperature of 5°C. The pump settings were 3 and 5 respectively for sample injection and for buffer flow in the separation chamber. Equal volumes of the separated material were collected in 48 fractions and the bacterial counts in every second fraction were determined by plating aliquots of serial dilutions onto Mueller Hinton agar.

RESULTS

Effect of β-Lactam Antibiotics on Killing of E. coli by PMN.

Of the six β-lactams tested, only the penicillins mezlocillin (1 mg/l), piperacillin (1 mg/l) and ticarcillin (2 mg/l) augmented within the 3 hr incubation period the intracellular killing of all four isogenic *E. coli* strains as compared to the drug free controls (Figure 2). Among the cefalosporins lamoxactam (0.25 mg/l) was marginally effective whereas cefoxitin (4 mg/l) was completely ineffective; cefotaxime (0.06 mg/l) caused an increase in intracellular killing of the capsule-defective mutants only. The antibiotic concentrations applied in these tests correspond to the individual minimal inhibitory concentrations. In order to evaluate if the increase in intracellular killing was due to an uptake of the β-lactams simultaneously with engulfment of the bacteria followed by an intracellular

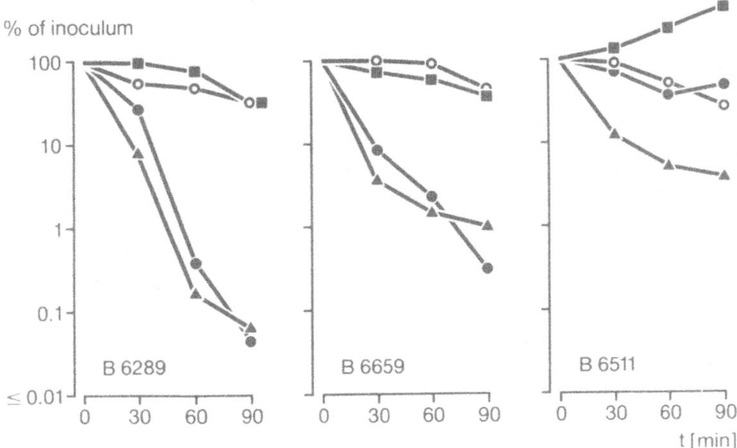

Figure 1. Antimicrobial action of human PMN (O) and rat PMN (■, rat polyvinyl sponge model) against three clinical isolates of *Ps. aeruginosa* and effect of pretreatment of these strains with subinhibitory azlocillin concentrations on their susceptibility to activity of human PMN (▲) and rat PMN (●). Human PMN were obtained from a healthy volunteer and suspended in homologous serum.

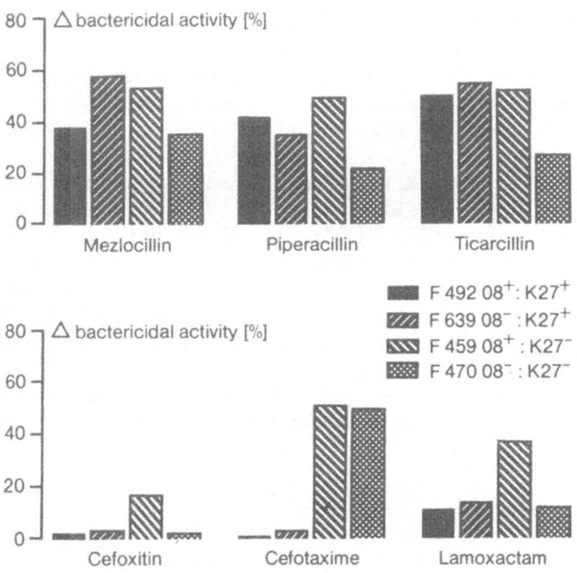

Figure 2. Effect of β-lactam antibiotics on killing of E. coli by PMN.

bactericidal action of the drugs, phenylbutazone (5mM) was added to the explants either simultaneously with inoculation or 15 min afterwards. In any case, neither drug reduced the viable counts of the four E. coli strains; viable counts remained constant during the 3 hr incubation period in the presence of phenylbutazone (data not shown).

To determine whether the mezlocillin mediated increase in intracellular killing can be inhibited by mannose or its derivatives, 50mM of either α-methylmannoside or α-methylglucoside were added simultaneously with mezlocillin onto the explants. Data summarized in Figure 3 clearly indicate that the presence of α-methylmannoside could not render the four isogenic E. coli strains more susceptible to leukocyte killing whereas α-methylglucoside had no antagonistic effect. The sugars on their own did not affect the bactericidal activity of the PMN (data not shown).

Free Flow Electrophoretic Separation of Mezlocillin-Treated Bacteria and Erythrocytes

The electrophoretic distribution profiles of E. coli F492 and erythrocytes respectively are shown in Figure 4; erythrocytes peaked in fraction 12 and the untreated bacteria peaked in fraction 25. However, the majority of bacteria having been exposed to mezlocillin were collected from fractions 12 to 16. Following simultaneous incubation of E. coli F492 with α-methylmannoside and mezlocillin respectively, the peak shifted back to fraction 22. In contrast, α-methylglucoside did not affect the distribution profile of the mezlocillin treated bacteria; they, too, peaked in fractions 12 to 16. Thus, mezlocillin-mediated comigration of bacteria with erythrocytes can be inhibited by α-methylmannoside.

Correlation Between Bacterial Length and Susceptibility to Leukocyte Killing

In parallel to the determination of viable counts in the course of the experiments on intraleukocyte killing the length of an individual bacterium was determined also. Data summarized in Figure 5 illustrate the results obtained with E. coli F459 as in contrast to the other three isogenic E. coli strains cefataxime and lamoxactam as well as the three penicillins rendered this strain more susceptible to leukocyte killing. Incubation of E.coli F459 in the presence of the β-lactams tested resulted in a time dependent increase in the length of an individual bacterium whereas the shape of the drug free controls remained unchanged. Obviously, the degree of filamentation was directly correlated to the increased susceptibility to leukocyte killing as compared to the corresponding drug free controls (Figure 5). In general, analogous data were obtained with the other three isogenic E. coli strains having been exposed to the three penicillins tested (data not shown).

DISCUSSION

In agreement with previously published data (summary in 34) the results of this study indicate firstly, that the penicillins tested rendered the

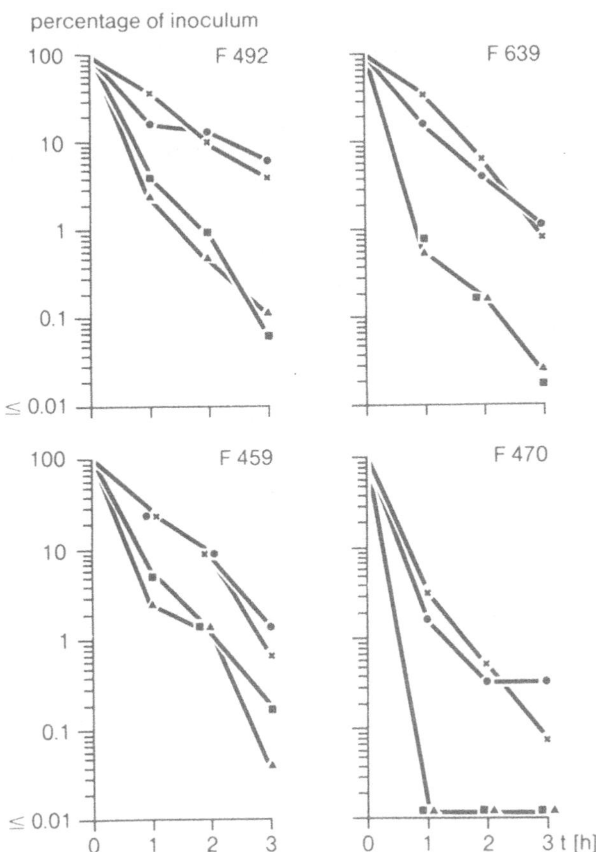

Figure 3. Effect of α-methylmannoside (●) and α-methylglucoside (■) on mezlocillin-mediated increase in bactericidal activity of PMN against four isogenic E. coli strains. (▲) mezlocillin alone, (x) drug free control.

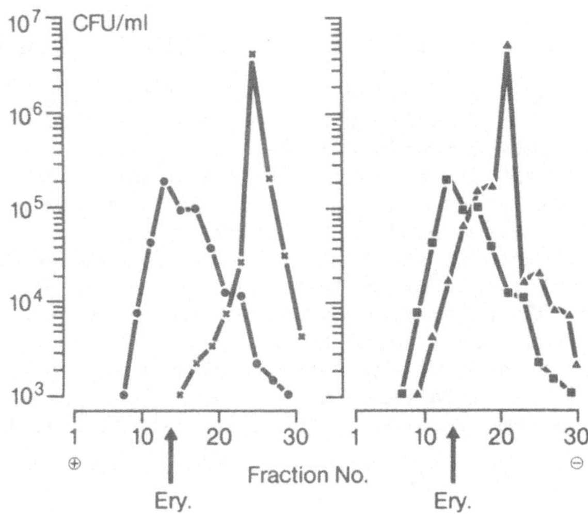

Figure 4. Free flow electrophoretic separation of E. coli F492 in the presence of guinea pig erythrocytes (Ery.). (X) drug free control, (●) mezlocillin alone, (■) mezlocillin plus α-methyl-glucoside, (▲) mezlocillin plus α-methylmannoside.

four isogenic E. coli strains more susceptible to leukocyte killing, whereas this effect was significantly less marked in case of the cefalosporins examined. Secondly, the penicillins do not only evolve these effects in the specific in vitro test systems as reported by others (34) but also under the complex conditions adopted in this study, resembling the in vivo situation in the infected host more closely. Thirdly, O- and K-antigens respectively did not affect the penicillin mediated increase in leukocyte killing

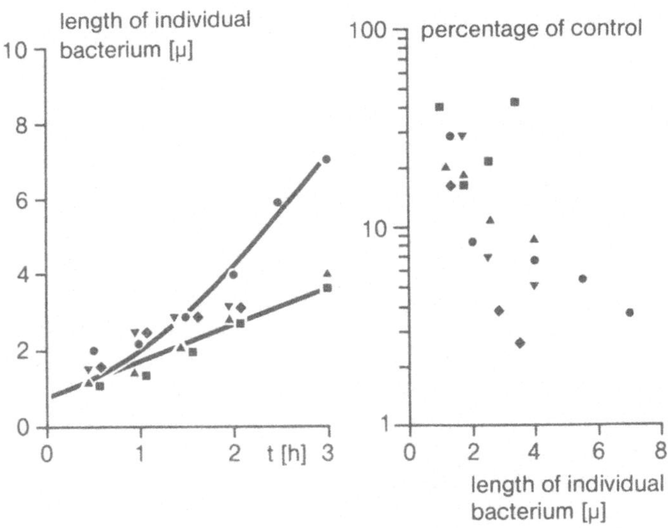

Figure 5. Effect of various β-lactams on the shape of E. coli F459 (left) and increase in bactericidal activity of PMN against these β-lactam induced filaments (right). (●) = mezlocillin; (▲) - piperacillin; (▼) = lamoxactam; (■) = ticarcillin; (◆) = cefotaxime.

of these four isogenic E. coli strains. Fourthly, the enhanced susceptibility to leukocyte killing in the presence of the penicillins is not due to an increased antibacterial action of the β-lactams in the presence of PMN. An addition of phenylbutazone which has been found to inhibit both engulfment and intracellular killing of E. coli without affecting viability of intraphagocytic bacteria (43) caused an immediate cessation of bactericidal activity. Thus, the marked increase in leukocyte killing of E. coli being exposed to mezlocillin is either due to an immunomodulating effect of mezlocillin or the drug renders the bacterium more susceptible to leukocyte killing. Based on recently published data (8) it can be excluded that mezlocillin exhibit an immunomodulating effect on PMN function. However, it was reported that several cefalosporins, including cefoxitin and lamoxactam, produced a dose related reduction in mononuclear leukocyte- or PMN-function (18,25,31,47). These findings may explain the differences between the penicillin on the one hand and the cefalosporins on the other hand with respect to their effect on the bactericidal activity of PMN as illustrated in Figure 1. Thus, it seems to be conceivable that mezlocillin may induce changes in the surface properties of the test strains. Since the early years of penicillin research it is well known that β-lactams turn gram negative bacilli into filaments (16). However, there was little evidence to show that they are more susceptible than individual bacilli to opsonization and phagocytosis. Data summarized in Figure 5 clearly indicate that the degree of filamentation due to the exposure to various β-lactams is directly correlated to the increased intraleukocyte killing of E. coli. As demonstrated in Figures 4 and 5, this effect is antagonized by α-methylmannoside, thus indicating that mezlocillin interferes with the mannose sensitive (MS) adhesions of E. coli. Similarly, Klein and Opferkuch (24) described that exposure of E. coli to subinhibitory concentrations of various β-lactams resulted in an increased hemagglutination provided MS-strains were used; this effect could not be demonstrated in mannose resistant strains. Silverblatt et al. (42) reported that MS carrying strains are more susceptible to phagocytosis than are non-fimbriated strains. The increased intraleukocyte killing caused by mezlocillin may thus reflect filamentation of the test strains during exposure to the antibiotic. Assuming that the surfaces of a bacterium of normal shape and filament respectively are equally fimbriated as reported by Klein and Opferkuch (24), it seems logical that a filament which is larger than a normal bacterium should exhibit increased adhesiveness to PMN, followed by phagocytosis and intracellular killing.

Filamentation of bacteria in the course of antibacterial chemotherapy has been demonstrated to be of clinical relevance. During ampicillin treatment filaments of E. coli and Salmonella spp. respectively were detected in the clinical specimens (27). Filaments of Pseudomonas aeruginosa as well as Klebsiella pneumoniae were observed in the sputum or the spinal fluid of patients who were treated with carbenicillin or cefazolin (28,33). Thus, filamentation may, on one hand, indicate either sublethal antibiotic concentration at the site of infection or an inadequate dosage. On the other hand, however, filamentation may be beneficial as it renders the bacteria more susceptible to phagocytosis and intracellular killing.

REFERENCES

1. J. W. Alexander and R. A. Good, Effect of antibiotics on the bactericidal activity of human leukocytes, J. Lab. Clin. Med. 71:971 (1968).
2. B. A. Atkinson and L. Amaral, Sublethal concentrations of antibiotics, effects on bacteria and the immune systems, CRC Critical Reviews in Microbiology 9:101 (1982).
3. Z. Bar-Shavit, R. Goldman, I. Ofek, N. Sharon and D. Mirelman, Mannose-residues on phagocytes as receptors for the attachment of Escherichia coli and Salmonella typhi, Biochem. Biophys. Res. Commun. 78:455 (1977).

4. Z. Bar-Shavit, I. Ofek, R. Goldmann, D. Mirelman and N. Sharon, Mannose-binding activity of Escherichia coli: A determinant of attachment and ingestion of the bacteria by macrophages, Infect. Immun. 29:417 (1980).
5. M. Bassler, H. Blaschke, M. Just and F. D. Daschner, Effect of ceftriaxone on Pseudomonas aerugionosa and Staphylococcus aureus in broth, serum, and in combination with human polymorphonuclear leukocytes, Chemotherapy 28:390 (1982).
6. M. Bassler, W. Depuis, C. Utz, H. M. Just and F. D. Daschner, Interaction of azlocillin and piperacillin in subinhibitory and inhibitory concentrations on Staphylococcus aureus and Pseudomonas aeruginosa in broth, serum and in the presence of human polymorphonuclear leukocytes, Eur. J. Clin. Microbiol. 2:439 (1983).
7. A. Dalhoff, Synergy between acylureidopenicillins and immunoglobulin G in experimental animals, Am. J. Med. 76:91 (1984).
8. D. Duncker and U. Ullmann, Einfluss von Antibiotika auf die Phagozytose humaner Granulozyten gemessen mit der Chemilumineszenz, FAC 3:263 (1984).
9. B. I. Eisenstein, I. Ofek and E. H. Beachey, Interference with the mannose binding and epithelial cell adherence of Escherichia coli by sublethal concentrations of streptomycin, J. Clin. Invest. 63:1219 (1979).
10. B. I. Eisenstein, E. H. Beachey and I. Ofek, Influence of sublethal concentrations of antibiotics on the expression of the mannose-specific ligand of Escherichia coli, Infect. Immun. 28:154 (1980).
11. B. I. Eisenstein, I. Ofek and E. H. Beachey, Loss of lectin-like activity in aberrant type I fimbriae of Escherichia coli, Infect. Immun. 31:792 (1981).
12. G. R. Elliot, P. K. Peterson, H. A. Verbrugh, M. R. Freiberg, J. R. Hoidal and P. G. Quie, Influence of subinhibitory concentrations of penicillin, cephalothin and clindamycin on Staphylococcus aureus growth in human phagocytic cells, Antimicrob. Agents Chemother. 22:781 (1982).
13. H. Friedman and G. H. Warren, Enhanced susceptibility of penicillin resistant staphylococci to phagocytosis after in vitro incubation with low doses of nafcillin (38177), Proc. Soc. Exp. Biol. Med. 146:707 (1974).
14. H. Friedman and G. H. Warren, Antibody-mediated bacteriolysis: enhanced killing of cyclacillin-treated bacteria, Proc. Soc. Exp. Biol. Med. 153:301 (1976).
15. H. Friedman and G. H. Warren, Increased phagocytosis of Escherichia coli pretreated with subinhibitory concentrations of cyclacillin or ampicillin (41347), Proc. Soc. Exp. Biol. Med. 169:301 (1982).
16. A. D. Gardner, Morphological effects of penicillin on bacteria, Nature (Land) 146:857 (1940).
17. C. G. Gemell, P. K. Peterson, D. Schmeling and P. G. Quie, Studies on the potentiation of phagocytosis of Streptococcus pyogenes by treatment with various antibiotics, Drugs Exptl. Clin. Res. 8:235 (1982).
18. G. Gillissen, Non-specific influence of antibiotics on the course of infectious processes, Infection 10:128 (1982).
19. D. Horne and A. Tomasz, Hypersusceptibility of penicillin treated group B streptococci to bactericidal activity of human polymorphonuclear leukocytes, Antimicrob. Agents Chemother. 19:745 (1981).
20. H. D. Isenberg, S. L. Wiener, G. A. Isenberg, J. Sampson Schere, M. Urivetzky and M. Berkman, Rat polyvinyl sponge model for the study of infections: factors and microbial proliferation, Infect. Immun. 14:490 (1976).
21. K. Jann, G. Schmidt, E. Blumenstock and K. Vosbeck, Escherichia coli adhesion to Saccharomyces cerevisiae and mammalian cells: role of

piliation and surface hydrophobicity, Infect. Immun. 32:484 (1981).
22. K. Jann, B. Jann and G. Schmidt, SDS polyacrylamide gel electrophoresis and serological analysis of pili from Escherichia coli of different pathogenic origin, FEMS Microbiol. Lett. 11:21 (1981).
23. A. S. Klainer and R. L. Perkins, Surface manifestations of antibiotic-induced alterations in protein synthesis in bacterial cells, Antimicrob. Agents Chemother. 1:164 (1972).
24. U. Klein and W. Opferkuch, The effect of subinhibitory concentrations of antibiotics on the adherence of E. coli, Zbl. Bakt. Hyg. I. Abt. Orig. A 253:442 (1983).
25. S. E. Larson, G. J. DaMart, C. Collins-Lech and P. G. Sohnle, Direct stimulations of lymphokine production by cephalothin, J. Infect. Dis. 142:265 (1980).
26. V. Lorian, B. Atkinson and W. H. Ewing, Agglutination with O antisera of salmonella exposed to antibiotics, Am. J. Clin. Pathol. 66:1004 (1976).
27. V. Lorian, Effects of subminimum inhibitory concentrations of antibiotics on bacteria, in: "Antibiotics in Laboratory Medicine," V. Lorian, ed., Williams and Wilkins, Baltimore (1980).
28. V. Lorian, A. Waluschka and Y. Kim, Abnormal morphology of bacteria in the sputa of patients treated with antibiotics, J. Clin. Microbiol. 16:382 (1982).
29. V. Lorian, B. Atkinson and Y. Kim, Phagocytosis of filaments of Escherichia coli produced with mezlocillin, J. Antimicrob. Chemother. 11:Suppl. C., 71 (1983).
30. P. J. McDonald, B. L. Wetherall and H. Pruul, Postantibiotic leukocyte enhancement, increased Susceptibility of bacteria pretreated with antibiotics to activity of leukocytes, Rev. Infect. Dis. 3:38 (1981).
31. J. P. Manzella and J. K. Clark, Effects of moxalactam and cefuroxime on mitogen-stimulated human mononuclear leukocytes, Antimicrob. Agents Chemother. 23:360 (1983).
32. H. Mett, L. Kloetzlein and K. Vosbeck, Properties of pili from Escherichia coli SS142 that mediate mannose-resistant adhesion to mamalian cells, J. Bacteriol. 153:1038 (1983).
33. J. Middleton and H. Cheuel, Aberrant forms of Pseudomonas aeruginosa in sputum and cerebrospinal fluid causing infection in a compromised host, J. Clin. Pathol. 31:351 (1978).
34. D. Milatovic, Antibiotics and phagocytosis, Eur. J. Clin. Microbiol. 2:414 (1983).
35. M. Nishida, Y. Mine, S. Nonoyama and Y. Yokota, Effects of antibiotics on the phagocytosis and killing of Pseudomonas aeruginosa by rabbit polymorphonuclear leukocytes, Chemotherapy 22:203 (1976).
36. I. Ofek, D. Mirelman and N. Sharon, Adherence of Escherichia coli to human mucosal cells mediated by mannose receptors, Nature 265:623 (1977).
37. I. Ofek, E. H. Beachey, B. I. Eisenstein, M. L. Alkan and N. Sharon, Suppression of bacterial adherence by subminimal inhibitory concentration of β-lactam and aminoglycoside antibiotics, Rev. Infect. Dis. 1:832 (1979).
38. H. Ohnishi, H. Kosuzume, H. Inabe, M. Okura, H. Mochizuki, Y. Suzuki and R. Fujii, Effects of AC-1370, a new semisynthetic cephalosporin, on phagocyte function, Antimicrob. Agents Chemother. 23:874 (1983).
39. S. H. Parry, S. N. Abraham and M. Sussman, Adhesion of urinary strains of Escherichia coli, J. Med. Microbiol. 13:6 (1980).
40. J. C. Petit and G. L. Daguest, Enhanced killing of Pseudomonas aeruginosa by human polymorphonuclear leukocytes in the presence of subinhibitory concentrations of carbenicillin and ticarcillin, Biomedicine 34:29 (1981).
41. T. Sandberg, K. Stengvist and C. Svanborg-Eden, Effect of subminimal inhibitory concentrations of ampicillin, chloramphenicol, and

nitrofurantoin on the attachment of Escherichia coli to human epithelial cells in vitro, Rev. Infect. Dis. 1:838 (1979).
42. F. J. Silverblatt, J. S. Dreyer and S. Schauer, Effect of pili on susceptibility of Escherichia coli to phagocytosis, Infect. Immun. 24:218 (1979).
43. R. R. Strauss, B. B. Paul and A. J. Sbarra, Effect of phenylbutazone on phagocytosis and intracellular killing by guinea pig polymorphonuclear leukocytes, J. Bacteriol. 96:1982 (1968).
44. G. Stübner and A. Dalhoff, Effect of subinhibitory β-lactam concentration on intracellular killing of Ps. aeruginosa by human polymorphonuclear granulocytes, 13th International Congress of chemotherapy, Vienna, Proceedings part 53, SE 3.2./1 (1983).
45. I. J. Sud and D. S. Feingold, Detection of agents that alter the bacterial cell surface, Antimicrob. Agents Chemother. 8:34 (1975).
46. K. Vosbeck, H. Handschin, E. B. Menge and O. Zak, Effects of subminimal inhibitory concentrations of antibiotics on adhesiveness of Escherichia coli in vitro, Rev. Infect. Dis. 1:845 (1979).
47. W. D. Welch, D. Davis and L. D. Thrupp, Effect of antimicrobial agents on human polymorphonuclear leukocyte microbicidal function, Antimicrob. Agents Chemother. 20:15 (1981).

PHAGOCYTOSIS OF E. COLI, K. PNEUMONIAE AND S. AUREUS BY HUMAN GRANULOCYTES

P. M. Shah, C. Thomas, J. Rower, R. Schattschneider and H. Rogge

Infektiologie, Zentrum der Inneren Medizin
Klinikum der J. W. Goethe-Universität
Frankfurt, F.R.G.

INTRODUCTION

Many authors have studied the phagocytosis of mono-cultures by leucocytes (1,2,3,5). In a clinical setting infections caused by mixed culture could occur. We were thus interested in studying phagocytic activity of human granulocytes against cultures containing gram-negative and gram-positive organisms.

MATERIAL AND METHODS

Polymorphonuclear cells were harvested from fresh blood of human volunteers by sedimentation of cells in colloidal silica (Percoll) as described by Pertoft and Laurent in 1969. These cells were washed twice in saline at room temperature. The number of cells per ml was determined by counting the cells in Fuchs-Rosenthal chamber.

Bacteria

Escherichia coli C 10 was given to us by Dr. Metzger, Bayer AG, Wuppertal. *Klebsiella pneumoniae* 4601 and *Staphylococcus aureus* S 301 are from our collection.

Antibiotic

Mezlocillin was supplied by Bayer AG, Leverkusen.

Bacteria were pre-incubated at 37°C for 4 hours in nutrient broth, centrifuged and the pellet was washed twice before the organisms were resuspended in active serum (same serum from which the granulocytes were harvested). Granulocytes were added to give a final ratio bacteria: granulocytes = 1:10 in all instances. In parallel experiments *E. coli*, *K. pneumoniae* and *S. aureus* were exposed to granulocytes in mono-cultures and in cultures containing *E. coli* + *S. aureus* and *K. pneumoniae* + *S. aureus*. Phagocytic activity was measured by determining the surviving number of bacteria at different time intervals (killing curves) by plating aliquots on agar plates which were incubated at 37 °C overnight.

We also studied the behavior of *K. pneumoniae* and *S. aureus* when exposed to granulocytes and mezlocillin. All experiments were run three times and mean values were calculated.

Table 1. Colony Forming Units in % of Inoculum Surviving When Exposed to Granulocytes

Time (hr)	*E. coli* mono culture	*E. coli* mixed with *S. aureus*	*S. aureus* mono culture	*S. aureus* mixed with *E. coli*
0.25	- 61	- 66	- 45	- 26
0.5	- 271	+ 100	+ 48	- 69
1	- 233	+ 233	+ 7	- 33
2	- 253	- 333	- 30	- 26
5	- 22869	- 33	- 462	- 2700

Average of 3 determinations are given.

RESULTS

Figure 1 shows the killing curves for *E. coli* without granulocytes. *E. coli* C 10 grew in serum, whether in mono or mixed culture. When granulocytes were present there was a reduction in number of viable *E. coli* cells over the 5 hour period. Table 1 gives the number of colony forming units determined.

The killing of *S. aureus* by granulocytes was less in mono cultures and enhanced in mixed culture (Figure 2).

Figure 3 shows the results for *K. pneumoniae*. In mixed culture with *S. aureus* there was a reduction in *K. pneumoniae* at 1 hour but then the

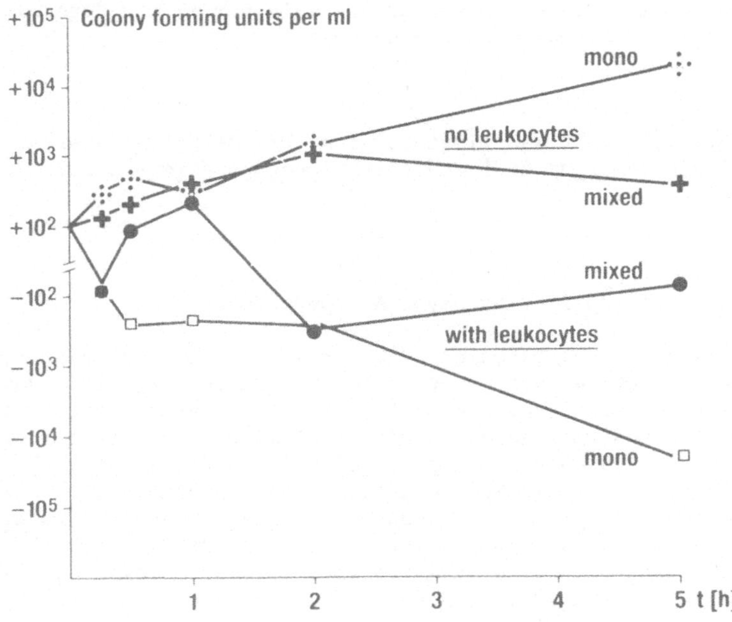

Figure 1. Killing of *E. coli* C 10 by granulocytes in mono and mixed culture with *S. aureus* S 301.

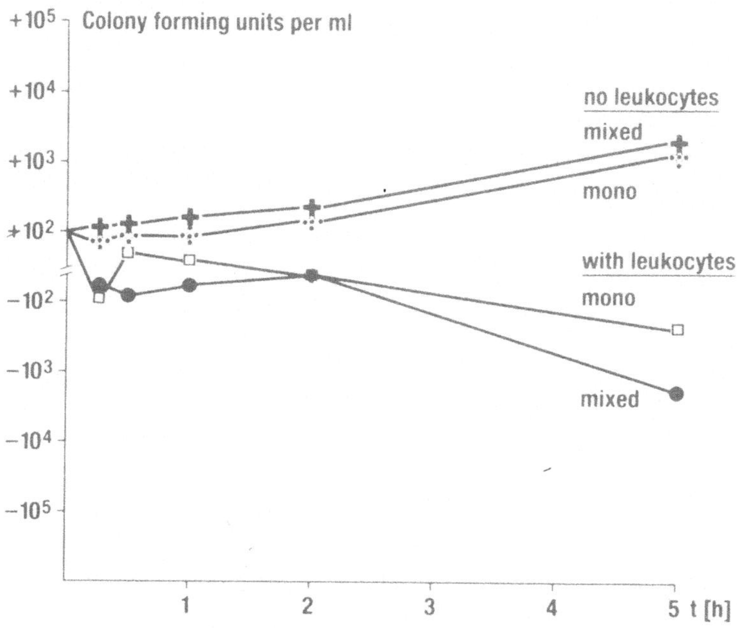

Figure 2. Killing of S. aureus S 301 by granulocytes in mono and mixed culture with E. coli C 10.

number grew to 10^3% of inoculum. Mezlocillin 8 mcg/ml initially had negative effect (= increase in colony forming units of K. pneumoniae) but from the second hour onward there was a rapid killing. Mezlocillin reversed the negative effect of S. aureus on phagocytosis of K. pneumoniae.

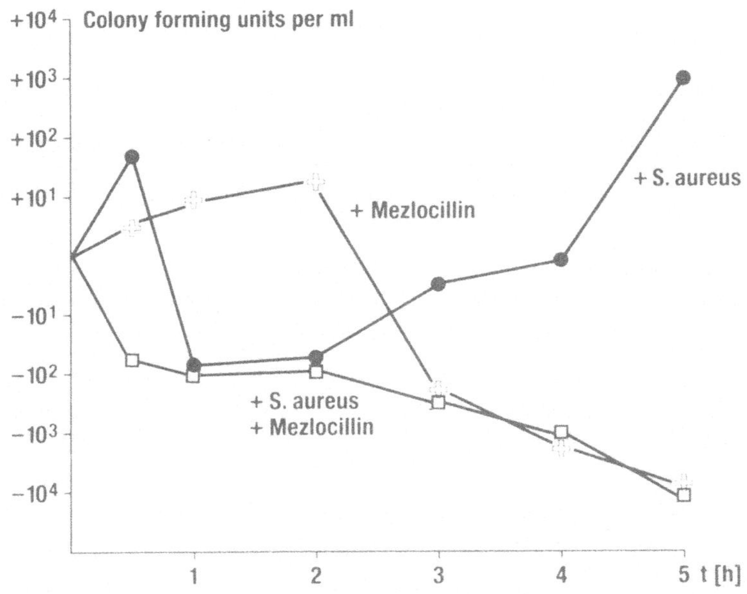

Figure 3. Killing of K. pneumoniae 4601 by granulocytes when incubated with mezlocillin (8 µg/ml) with S. aureus S 301, and with S. aureus + mezlocillin.

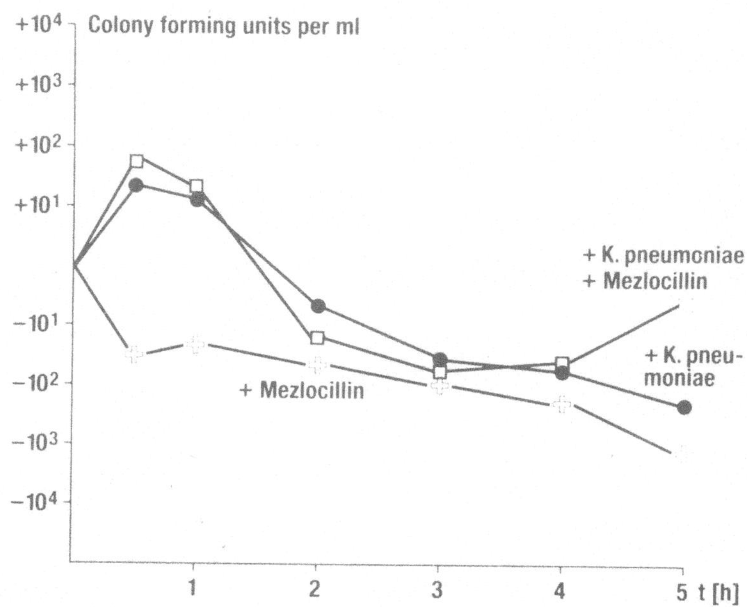

Figure 4. Killing of S. aureus S 301 by granulocytes when incubated with mezlocillin (8 mg/ml), with K. pneumoniae 4601, and with K. pneumoniae and mezlocillin.

Phagocytic activity against S. aureus was less pronounced. During the first hour there was an increase in number of S. aureus and after that they gradually decreased to -10% in mixed culture with K. pneumoniae. Mezlocillin, together with granulocytes, had a better killing activity (Figure 4).

DISCUSSION

As mentioned in the introduction, many authors have studied the phagocytic activity of granulocytes against pure cultures of either gram-negative or gram-positive bacteria. No information is available on phagocytic behavior on mixed cultures of gram-negative and gram-positive bacteria. Jones and Gemmell (4) reported of reduced phagocytosis in mixed cultures of Bacteroides species and Enterobacteriaceae.

The results shown here show that in the presence of S. aureus the rate of phagocytosis and killing of both E. coli and K. pneumoniae was markedly reduced. When no S. aureus were present in the culture media granulocytes reduced the number of viable E. coli by 3 log, but when S. aureus was present, the killing was reduced to only 1 log in the fifth hour. A similar negative effect of S. aureus was also seen in the case of K. pneumoniae. This negative effect of S. aureus was reversed when mezlocillin was added to the test tubes.

The preferred phagocytosis of S. aureus was observed in phase contrast microscopy and has been documented on video (copies are available on request to the author). The reason for this is at present not understood. It could be due to better chemotaxis by S. aureus than the gram-negative organisms investigated here.

REFERENCES

1. D. Adam, W. Schaffert and W. Marget, Enhanced in vitro phagocytosis by human monocytes in the presence of ampicillin, tetracyclin and chloramphenicol, Infect. Immun. 9:811 (1974).
2. A. Forsgren, G. Banck, H. Beckmann and A. Bellahsene, Antibiotic-host defense interactions in vitro and in vivo, Scand. J. Infect. Dis. (Suppl. 10):195 (1980).
3. C. G. Gemmell, P. K. Peterson, D. Schmeling, Y. Kim, J. Mathews, L. Wanamaker and P. G. Quie, Potentiation of opsonization and phagocytosis of Streptococcus pyogenes following growth in the presence of clindamycin, J. Clin. Invest. 67:1249 (1981).
4. G. R. Jones and C. G. Gemmell, Impairment of Bacteroides species of opsonization and phagocytosis of enterobacteria, J. Med. Microbiol. 15:351 (1982).
5. D. Milatovic and I. Braveny, Wechselwirkung zwischen Antibiotika und Phagozytose, Dtsch. Med. Wschr. 107:1975 (1982).
6. H. Pertoft and T. C. Laurent, The use of gradients of colloidal silica for the separation of cells and subcellular particles, in: "Modern Separation Methods of Macromolecules and Particles," T. Gerritsen, ed., Wiley (Interscience), New York (1969).

ANTIBACTERIAL ACTIVITY OF MONOCYTES AND MACROPHAGES AGAINST STAPHYLOCOCCUS AUREUS AND KLEBSIELLA PNEUMONIAE IN COMBINATION WITH LATAMOXEF

H.-M. Just[1], M. T. Ramos Carneiro Leao, F. D. Daschner, and R. Andreesen[2]

Department of Hospital Epidemiology[1]
Department of Haemathology and Oncology[2]
University Hospital of Freiburg, F.R.G.

INTRODUCTION

There are mainly two functional morphologically different phagocytic cell populations in human peripheral blood, responsible for the defense mechanism against infections, polymorphonuclear leukocytes and monocytes, both deriving from precursor cells in the bone marrow. To transform monocytes into macrophages, monocytes have been cultured on artificial membranes (7), showing properties of typical macrophages during a period of eight to 12 days (4,20). Our initial objective was to determine the effect of different stages of maturity of Teflon membrane cultivated mononuclear cells, on the killing-rate of Staphylococcus aureus and Klebsiella pneumoniae. Furthermore, the influence of normal and heat-inactivated human pooled serum, the effect of latamoxef, and the variability between individuals in the function of mononuclear phagocytes were evaluated.

MATERIALS AND METHODS

Bacterial Strains

Staphylococcus aureus ATCC 25923 and Klebsiella pneumoniae, a clinical isolate, were used as test strains throughout the study. Both strains were resistant to lysis by serum of each of the individuals investigated. Maintained on nutrient agar slope and subcultured weekly, the bacteria were incubated overnight at 37°C before being used for the experiments. After centrifugation at 2.500 g for 10 min the pellet was washed twice in normal saline and then resuspended in 3 ml Hank's balanced salt solution (HBSS, pH 7.4) without Ca^{++} and Mg^{++} but enriched with 0.1 % gelatin. The resulting suspension was adjusted with a Coleman junior photometer to the final concentration of 5 x 10^4 bacteria/ml in the test tubes.

Mononuclear Cell Isolation

Blood was obtained from healthy volunteers without any medication. Mononuclear cells were separated from heparinized buffy coat by Ficoll-Hypaque Centrifugation (Ficoll-Paque[R], Pharmacia, Fine Chemicals Inc., Uppsala, Sweden) as described by Territo and Cline (19). Monocytes separated from lymphocytes by adherence to plastic were cultured in

Table 1. Summary of Experiments

Antibacterial Activity	HBSS-gel (ml)	Buffer (ml)	Pooled Serum (ml)	Mononuclear cells (ml)	Bacteria (ml)	Antibiotic (ml)
Mononuclear cells in normal serum	-	(0.02)	0.06 (normal)	0.1	0.02	0.02
Mononuclear cells in inactivated	-	(0.02)	0.06 (inactivated)	0.1	0.02	0.02
Mononuclear cells in HBSS-gel	0.06	(0.02)	-	0.1	0.02	0.02
Control	0.16	(0.02	-	-	0.02	0.02

( ) = buffer used in experiments without antibiotic.

different Teflon bags (Biofolie 25, W. C. Heraeus, Hanau, F.R.G.) in RPMI 1640 (Grand Island Biological Co., Grand Island, N. Y.) supplemented with 5 x 10^{-5} M 2 mercaptoethanol, antibiotics, and 15% human AB-group serum pooled from selected donors. The precultivated cells were then washed and adjusted to final concentrations of 5 x 10^5 cells/ml. The viability of the macrophages, determined by the ability to ingest 0.1% trypan blue dye, was greater than 95%.

Experimental Protocol

The experimental protocol is outlined in Table 1. Two different ratios of bacteria to mononuclear cells (100:1 and 1:1) were used. Stock solutions of latamoxef-dinatrium (Moxalactam^R; Eli Lilly GmbH, Giessen, FRG) were stored at -20°C and diluted to the required concentrations of 1/4, 1 and 4 x MIC immediately before use. The MIC of latamoxef for the _Klebsiella pneumoniae_ strain was 0.06 mg/l and 4 mg/l for the _Staphylococcus aureus_. For control Dulbeco's phosphate buffer saline (PBS) without Ca^{++} and Mg^{++} (Gibco Ltd., Paisley Scotland) was used. Immediately after the mononuclear cells and the antibiotic were added to the microtiter plates, and 60, 120 and 180 min. thereafter, the solution was gently mixed, 5 µl aliquots were plated on nutrient DST agar (Oxoid Ltd., Basingstoke, Hants, England) and incubated overnight at 37°C. The number of colony forming units (cfu) was counted and expressed as the percentage of viable cfu/ml. For bacterial opsonization, human pooled serum was used.

RESULTS

The antibacterial effect of blood-born monocytes in normal human serum at the first day of culture, compared to that after incubation on Teflon membrane bags, for up to 15 days demonstrates the activity-dependence of the maturity stage. Against _Staphylococcus aureus_, monocytes had a demonstrable bacteriostatic effect whereas macrophages (after 5 to 15 days of cultivation) showed a significant bacterial killing, compared to control (p-0.05) (Figure 1). Against _Klebsiella pneumoniae_, however, monocytes had no antibacterial effect within three hours of incubation, but macrophages were highly effective (p-0.01) (Figure 2). Within the 15 days of incubation, monocytes showed increasing antibacterial activity in serum. Table 2 details the mean values of surviving _Klebsiella pneumoniae_ (cfu x 10^4/ml) at 60, 120 and 180 min when incubated with monocytes and macrophages at different maturity stages. The inoculum at the beginning of the experi-

Table 2. Number of Klebsiella pneumoniae ($x10^4$/ml) after Incubation for 3 Hrs. with Monocytes and Macrophages of Different Maturity Stages

Time/maturity	Monocytes	Macrophages		
day	1 (n=26)	5 (n=5)	7 (n=12)	10-12 (n=14)
60 minutes	2.15 ± 0.19	1.71 ± 0.37	1.59 ± 0.51	0.94 ± 0.70
120 minutes	2.64 ± 0.18	1.00 ± 0.58	0.64 ± 0.50	0.26 ± 0.39
180 minutes	2.81 ± 0.19	0.51 ± 0.55	0.23 ± 0.24	0.02 ± 0.06

ments was about 5 x 10^4 cfu/ml. There is a significant difference between the activity of monocytes and macrophages after 10 to 15 days of cultivation for all three times measured (p-0.0001). In order to determine whether the phagocytic activity of mononuclear cells is dependent on the ratio of bacteria to cells, we added Staphylococcus aureus and Klebsiella pneumoniae to cells in two different proportions bacteria per phagocyte cells, i.e., 100 to 1 and 1 to 1. In suspensions containing monocytes or macrophages from the same individual the results obtained for Staphylococcus aureus and Klebsiella pneumoniae as well showed no significant differences when comparing the two concentrations of bacteria.

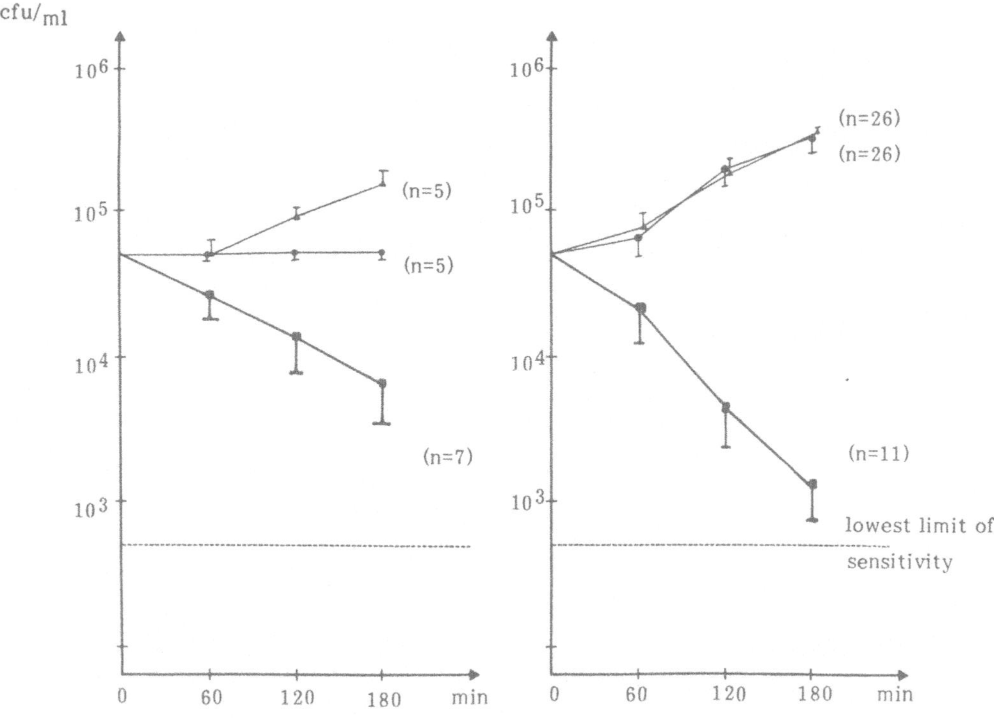

Figure 1. Antibacterial activity in normal serum against Staphylococcus aureus of monocytes (●) and macrophages (■); controls (▲).

Figure 2. Antibacterial activity in normal serum against Klebsiella pneumoniae of monocytes (●) and macrophages (■); controls (▲).

Incubated in human serum, monocytes were bacteriostatic against Staphylococcus aureus but not against Klebsiella pneumoniae (Figure 3, A & B). The antibacterial activity of latamoxef alone in either concentration was not significantly different from the antibacterial activity of latamoxef in combination with monocytes. With macrophages, however, the activity of latamoxef against Klebsiella pneumoniae was significantly increased even in subinhibitory concentrations (p-0.01) as shown in Figure 3, D. The increasing activity of 1 x MIC latamoxef alone could not be demonstrated in combination with macrophages. No bacteria, however, could be grown after three

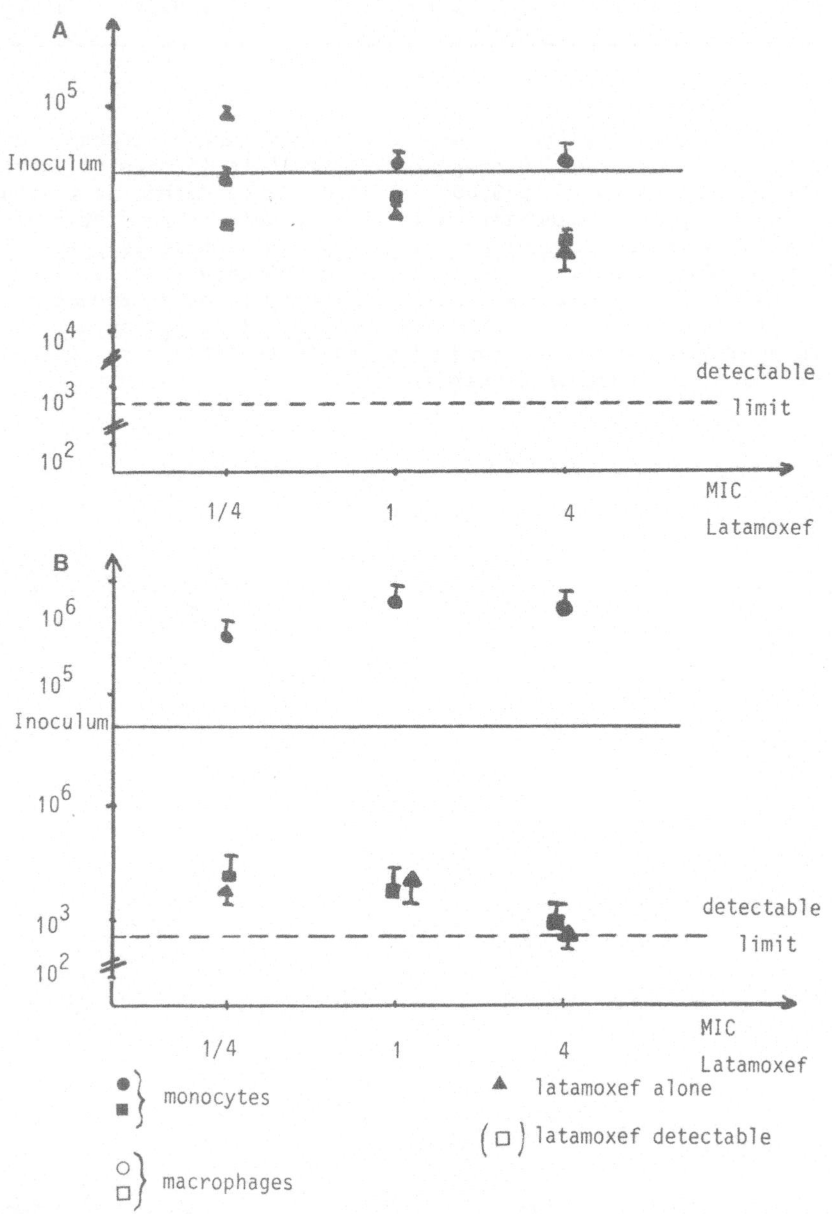

Figure 3. Effect of Latamoxef on the antibacterial activity of human monocytes (A,B) and macrophages (C,D) for 3 hrs against Staphylococcus aureus (A,C) and Klebsiella pneumoniae (B,D).

hours of incubation of the macrophages with 4 x MIC. Against <u>Staphylococcus aureus</u> the significantly better activity of macrophages compared to monocytes could not be further enhanced by subinhibitory or inhibitory concentrations of latamoxef (Figure 3). Comparing the antibacterial activity of latamoxef in combination with monocytes or macrophages in normal human pooled serum with the results of the same experiments in heat-inactivated serum and in HBSS-gel, there was no difference in the bactericidal effect of latamoxef at any concentration.

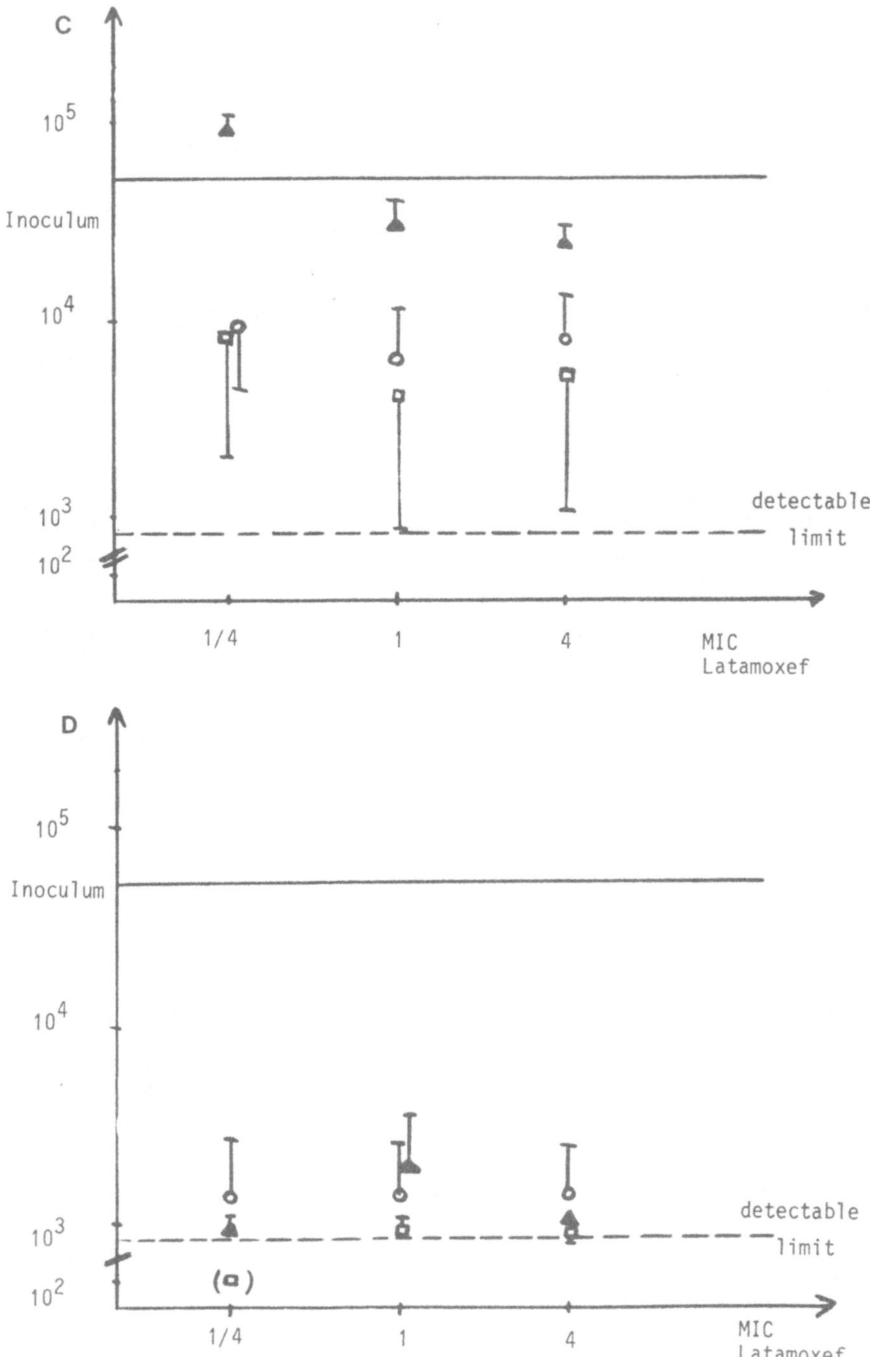

Figure 3. C and D (see opposite page for legend).

DISCUSSION

The ability of polymorphonuclear cells and mononuclear phagocytes to phagocytize and kill bacteria are two important functions of the human defense system against infection. It is known that defects in these functions can lead to recurrent infections in the host, and that these cell functions may also be influenced by the use of corticosteroids (16), tetracyclines (10), or by very high concentrations of cigarette smoke (12). Furthermore, this system is subject to the action of various substances, e.g., phenylbutazone, which can prevent intracellular killing by both monocytes and neutrophils (21). Mononuclear phagocytes have been obtained readily from different anatomical locations (tissue macrophages) and isolated from whole blood and used for studies of different functions (21,23,-24). Munder et al. (15) provided a new approach to monolayer cell culture, developing the use of Teflon membranes for cell cultures, which are biologically inert and gas permeable. This method, later used by van der Meer et al. (20), and recently by Andreesen et al. (3), allowed us to recover macrophages at any stage of maturation for our experimental purposes.

In our experiments, blood-born monocytes, incubated on Teflon membranes, underwent transformation into macrophages in a period of four to eight days, which in each experiment was confirmed by parallel macrophage surface marker determinations, cytochemistry and antitumor activity by one of the authors (R. Andreesen). When cells were examined until the 15th day of culture, monocytes killed a significantly smaller proportion of each of the two bacterial strains investigated than did monocyte-originated macrophages obtained from the same individuals. These results correlate well with those of Cohen and Cline (8), who cultivated human alveolar macrophages for up to 50 days. They observed that cells that underwent transformation had more than thirty times the phagocytic capacity as the same cells after one day of culture in vitro.

The ability to kill bacteria seems to develop during the macrophage maturation. Some of the macrophage populations, however, had no or a significantly lower antibacterial activity, suggesting that some monocytes underwent transformation into macrophages, or only part of them underwent transformation. This could represent the presence of a heterogeneous population of cells, which has been recently described also in vivo (22). We would like to point out that tests with the same macrophage culture yielded quite reproducible results, when cells were tested on the same day against the same bacterial suspensions.

Comparing the killing-rate of bacteria that had been incubated in the presence of 8% normal human pooled serum, heat-inactivated serum, or HBSS-gel without serum, most rapid antibacterial killing was observed by mature macrophages when normal serum was used as opsonin. The killing activity of bacteria opsonized without serum, however, was well preserved, although at somewhat lower rates. This could be attributed to heat-labile factors, that might accelerate the rate of phagocytosis of bacteria by macrophages (13). While the antibacterial activity of monocytes was not significantly improved by serum, macrophages need serum for efficient killing of *Staphylococcus aureus*, but apparently not of *Klebsiella pneumoniae*. The latter is contrary to the results of Ehrenkranz et al. (9) showing that monocyte killing of gram negative bacteria but not of *Staphylococcus aureus* was serum-dependent.

There are many studies in the literature about the interaction of antibiotics with granulocyte functions (2,14,17,18) but very few reports exist about the influence of antibiotics on monocyte or macrophage function. Adam et al. (1) studied the phagocytic activity of human macrophages grown from blood monocytes in the presence of ampicillin, tetracycline and chloramphenicol: subinhibitory amount of the antibiotics enhanced the phagocytic activity significantly.

Friedman and Warren (11) demonstrated increased susceptibility of Staphylococcus aureus to phagocytosis by mice peritoneal exsudate macrophages, when cells were previously exposed to subinhibitory doses of nafcillin. It was supposed that antibiotics exert nonlethal changes in the bacterial membrane, leading these organisms to be more susceptible to the action of host factors such as serum and antibodies.

In our studies we found no significant effect of any concentration of latamoxef on monocytes function, but a significant improved killing of Staphylococcus aureus and Klebsiella pneumoniae by macrophages, already with 1/4 x MIC of latamoxef, which could not be improved by 1 x MIC or 4 x MIC. This corresponds to results obtained in our laboratory with polymorphonuclears and various antibiotics (6,11). Neither the replacement of normal human pooled serum with heat-inactivated pooled serum nor the replacement with Hank's balanced salt solution enriched with gelatin had any effect on the bactericidal activity of latamoxef.

The origin of the tissue macrophage is yet subject of discussion, but it seems evident that the circulating monocyte is capable of such a grade of transformation, after a few days of incubation in vitro, that they are capable to show killing activity similar to that of human tissue macrophages.

The assays described in this report provide a relatively simple and potentially useful means of studying mononuclear phagocyte activity, making use of Teflon membranes for cell cultivation. The method, however, does not distinguish between phagocytosis and inhibition of bacteria growth by macrophage-secreted substances of killing by inhibitors present at the solution. Further studies of factors that influence the phagocytic function of cells in order to rule out the possibility of attachment of bacteria to cell surfaces, the influence of other factors produced by macrophages, and studies of cells in selected patient populations are recommended.

REFERENCES

1. D. Adam, W. Schaffert and W. Marget, Enhanced in vitro phagocytosis of Listeria monocytogenes by human monocytes in the presence of ampicillin, tetracycline and chloramphenicol, Infect. Immun. 9:811 (1974).
2. J. W. Alexander and R. A. Good, Effect of antibiotics on the bactericidal activity of human leukocytes, J. Labor. Clin. Med. 71:979 (1968).
3. R. Andreesen, J. Osterholz, K. J. Bross, A. Schulz and G. A. Luckenbach, Cytotoxic effector cell function at different stages of human monocyte-macrophage maturation, Cancer Res. 43:5931 (1983).
4. R. Andreesen, J. Picht and G. W. Lohr, Primary cultures of human blood-born macrophages grown on hydrophobic Teflon membranes, J. Immunol. Meth. 56:295 (1983).
5. M. Bassler, W. Depuis, E. Utz, H -M. Just and F. Daschner, Effect of azlocillin and piperacillin in subinhibitory and inhibitory concentrations on Staphylococcus aureus and Pseudomonas aeruginosa in broth, in serum and in the presence of human polymorphonuclear leukocytes, Eur. J. Clin. Microbiol. 2:439 (1983).
6. M. Bassler, L. Dieterle, M. Drechsler, H -M. Just and F. Daschner, Die Wechselwirkung von Cefmenoxim mit Faktoren der körpereigenen Abwehr (Serum, polymorphkernige Granulozyten), Fortschr. Antimikr. Antineoplast. Chemother. 2:271 (1983).

7. T. Brücher, A. Dill and M. Gräber, Untersuchungen über Gewebsmakrophagen, Acta. Haematol. 41:76 (1969).
8. A. B. Cohen and M. J. Cline, The human alveolar macrophage: isolation, cultivation in vitro and studies of morphologic and functional characteristics, J. Clin. Invest. 50:1390 (1971).
9. N. J. Ehrenkranz, D. F. Elliott and R. Zarco, Serum bacteriostasis of Staphylococcus aureus, Infect. Immun. 3:664 (1971).
10. A. Forsgren, D. Schmeling and P. G. Quie, Effect of tetracycline on the phagocytic function of human leukocytes, J. Infect. Dis. 130:412 (1974).
11. H. Friedman and G. H. Warren, Enhanced susceptibility of penicillin-resistant staphylococci to phagocytosis after in vitro incubation with low doses of nafcillin, Proc. Soc. Exper. Biol. Med. 146:707 (1974).
12. W. L. Hand, R. M. Boozer and N. L. King-Thompson, Antibiotic uptake by alveolar macrophages of smokers, Antimicrob. Agents Chemother. 27:42 (1985).
13. R. J. Lehrer and M. J. Cline, Interaction of Candida albicans with human leukocytes and serum, J. Bacteriol. 98:996 (1969).
14. D. Milatovič, Antibiotics and phagocytosis, Eur. J. Clin. Microbiol. 2:414 (1983).
15. P. G. Munder, M. Modolell and D. F. H. Wallach, Cell propagation on films of polymeric fluorocarbon as a means to regulate pericellular pH and pO_2 in cultured monolayers, FEBS Lett. 15:191 (1971).
16. J. J. Rinehart, A. L. Sagone, S. P. Balcerzak, G. A. Ackerman and A. F. LoBuglio, Effects of corticosteroid therapy on human monocyte function, N. Engl. J. Med, 292:236 (1975).
17. R. K. Root, R. Isturiz, A. Molavi, J. A. Metcalf and H. L. Malech, Interactions between antibiotics and human neutrophils in the killing of staphylococci, J. Clin. Invest. 67:247 (1981).
18. C. D. Solberg, Effect of antibiotics on the bactericidal activity of human leukocytes, Infection 6:116 (1978).
19. M. C. Territo and M. J. Cline, Monocyte function in man, J. Immunol. 118:187 (1977).
20. J. M. M. van der Meer, J. S. van de Gevel, A. Blussé van Oud Alblas, J. A. Kramps, T. L. van Zwet, P. C. J. Leijh and R. van Furth, Characteristic of human monocytes cultured in the Teflon culture bag, Immunol. 47:617 (1982).
21. R. van Furth, Origin and kinetics of monocytes and macrophages, Sem. Hematol. 7:125 (1970).
22. R. van Furth, Current view on the mononuclear phagocyte system, Immunobiol. 161:178 (1982).
23. H. A. Verbrugh, R. Peters, P. K. Peterson and J. Verhoef, Phagocytosis and killing of staphylococci by human polymorphonuclear and mononuclear leukocytes, J. Clin. Pathol. 31:539 (1978).
24. R. van Furth, T. L. van Zwet and J. A. Raeburn, Characteristics of human mononuclear phagocytes, Blood 54:485 (1979).

INFLUENCE OF ANTIBIOTICS ON PHAGOCYTOSIS OF *KLEBSIELLA PNEUMONIAE* BY GUINEA PIG ALVEOLAR MACROPHAGES

Horst Schroten, Christian Undeutsch and Helmut Brunner

Institute for Medical Microbiology and Virology
University of Düsseldorf, F.R.G.

INTRODUCTION

Phagocytosis and intracellular killing of invasive microorganisms by alveolar macrophages is the first and most important line of defense in the respiratory tract (4,12,16,19). Together with other local mechanisms of resistance, the activity of alveolar macrophages usually results in bacterial clearance from the lung. Therefore, functional impairment of alveolar macrophages often leads to severe acute or chronic progressive inflammatory lung diseases.

Klebsiella pneumoniae is a frequently occurring pathogen of the human respiratory tract, especially in hospitalized patients, who are often compromised in their resistance against infections. Antimicrobial chemotherapy is to be started as early as possible if a patient suffers from pneumonia. In Klebsiella infections aminoglycosides are frequently used.

It has been shown in recent years, that some antibiotics can stimulate or suppress immune functions (2,9,15,28,29,33). On the other hand, it was demonstrated that subinhibitory concentrations of antibiotics which do not kill the bacteria, may increase the susceptibility of the microorganisms to phagocytosis (1,5,11,14). Because gentamicin is often administered in severe respiratory tract infections, we considered it worthwhile to study the interaction of alveolar macrophages with *K. pneumoniae* in the presence of this antibiotic. Human lung macrophages are usually not available in sufficient numbers. Thus, guinea pigs were used, because 1 to 2 x 10^7 macrophages can be obtained from a single animal by lung lavage without stimulation (25).

MATERIALS AND METHODS

Bacteria

An encapsulated strain of *K. pneumoniae* in the late logarithmic growth phase was used. The strain was virulent for outbred mice CFW1, LD50 1 x 10^7 colony forming units (CFU) per mouse after intraperitoneal injection.

Antibiotic and Bacterial Susceptibility Testing

Gentamicin-sulfate (Merck, AG, Darmstadt, F.R.G.) was used. Antibiotic susceptibility testing was performed according to Ericsson and Sherris (7).

The minimal inhibitory concentration (MIC) for the K. pneumoniae organism used was 0.15 μg/ml, the minimal bactericidal concentration (MBC) was 1.2 μg/ml.

Guinea Pigs

Randomly selected adult guinea pigs of both sexes were used. The animals came from a local source.

Isolation and Cultivation of Alveolar Macrophages

The procedure for isolation and cultivation of lung lavage cells from guinea pigs has been described in detail previously (32). Briefly, lung lavage was performed in guinea pigs under pentobarbital anaesthesia by injection of 10 ml of sterile Hanks' balanced salt solution, prewarmed to 37°C. This procedure was repeated six times and yielded 1 to 2 x 10^7 viable cells (85% glass adherent macrophages, 10% lymphocytes and 5% polymorphonuclear leukocytes). Viability of the cells was tested by trypan-blue exclusion. The number of viable cells usually exceeded 95%. Since contamination of the culture with upper respiratory tract flora of the animals was a rather cumbersome problem, the cells were exposed to streptomycin (100 μg/ml) for 5 hrs during the adherence process. The cells were washed three times with culture-medium to remove non-adherent cells and streptomycin. The cells were then cultured for 24 hrs in Eagle's MEM, supplemented with glutamine and 10% heat inactivated (56°C, 30 min) fetal calf serum (FCS) without antibiotics, before phagocytosis experiments were performed (20,23).

Phagocytosis and Intracellular Killing

For phagocytosis, the medium was removed and 4 x 10^6 CFU of K. pneumoniae per 4 x 10^5 macrophages, i.e. > 10 bacteria per macrophage, were added. Phagocytosis was allowed to proceed for 1 hr at 37°C. After washing, fixing and staining (May-Grünwald-Giemsa stain) the number of bacteria per 100 macrophages was calculated by counting the bacteria in 200 macrophages in each tube by two investigators independently. In separate experiments the cells were lysed and the number of CFU was determined by plating tenfold dilutions of the bacterial suspension on Muller-Hinton agar, incubation at 37°C, and counting of colonies.

Opsonization

Rabbit antiserum against phenol-water extracts of K. pneumoniae was used for opsonization (34). The ELISA-test for determination of antibodies has been described previously (24).

Spleen Cells

Autologous spleen cells were used. Spleens were removed aseptically and single cell-suspensions were prepared during the 5 hr period, while alveolar macrophages attached to glass. After pressure of the spleen through a metal sieve of 0.8 mm pore size, a suspension of predominantly single cells was obtained. After lysis of erythrocytes by ammoniumchloride, damaged cells were removed, according to a method described by von Boehmer and Shortman (3).

To achieve isoosmotic conditions with guinea pig serum, 52.46 g/l of sorbitol and 51.88 g/l of glucose were mixed (personal communication, K. Burow, Zentralinstitut für Versuchstierkunde, Hannover, F.R.G.). After 10 min of incubation, damaged and dead cells had clumped. Clumps of cells were retained by filtration through a cotton wool column. Subsequently, macrophages were removed by a column of glass wool. Cells in the effluent were resuspended in Eagles' MEM with 10% FCS but without antibiotics. This cell suspension contained less than 5% macrophages as shown by specific macrophage staining procedures.

Determination of Nonspecific Esterase and Acid Phosphatase

Nonspecific esterase and acid phosphatase were determined by standard procedures (31).

Identification of B- and T-Lymphocytes

B-lymphocytes were quuantitated after determination of surface immunoglobulins via indirect immunofluorescence (30). Forty per cent of guinea pig spleen cells were B-lymphocytes. This is in accordance with a personal communication by D. Thomas and J. E. Niederhuber, Department of Surgery, University of Michigan, Ann Arbor, MI. T-lymphocytes were identified by the rosette-forming reaction using rabbit erythrocytes as described by Kaplan and Clark in 1974. Rabbit erythrocytes were pretreated with S-(2-aminoethyl)isothiouronium-hydrobromide, AET (Serva, Heidelberg). Phagocytozing cells were identified by phase-contrast microscopy after uptake of latex particles (36).

Statistical Analysis

Two-way analysis of variance and student's t-test were used for the analysis of the data.

RESULTS

Macrophages

As can be seen in Figure 1, a rather pure culture of alveolar macrophages was obtained after lung lavage and adherence for five hours to glass. The typical morphological appearance of macrophages is evident.

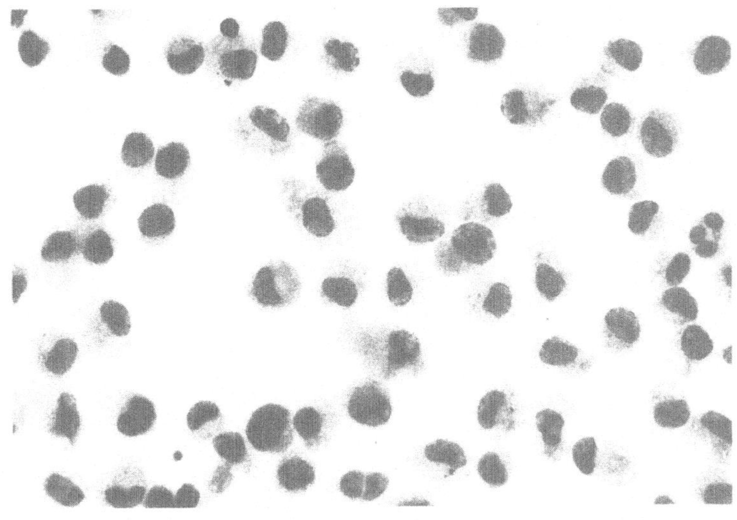

Figure 1. Culture of alveolar macrophages of guinea pigs 36 hrs after lung lavage (May-Grünwald-Giemsa stain, magnification approximately 500-fold). Reprinted from (32) with permission.

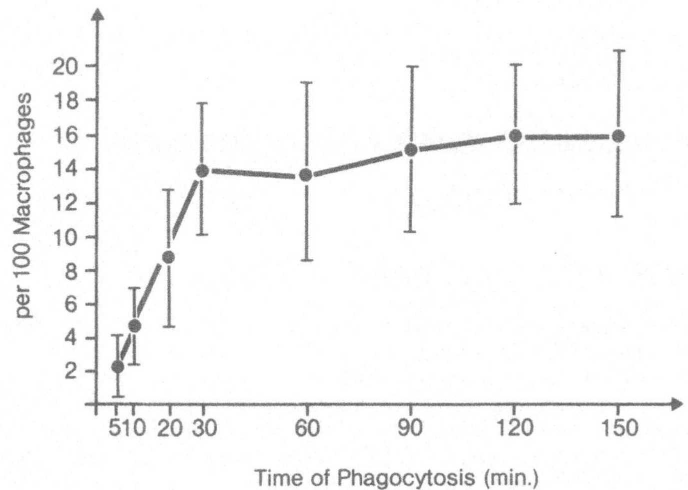

Figure 2. Kinetics of the uptake of unopsonized K. pneumoniae by alveolar macrophages. Reprinted from (32) with permission.

Uptake of Unopsonized K. pneumoniae

When ten bacteria per macrophage were added to the cells, and uptake was determined at various times thereafter, the number of ingested bacteria increased with time reaching a maximum after 30 min (Figure 2). The number of ingested bacteria did not decrease for two hours afterwards. In subsequent experiments phagocytosis was therefore terminated after 60 min. Great care was taken to remove bacteria which adhered to macrophages, but

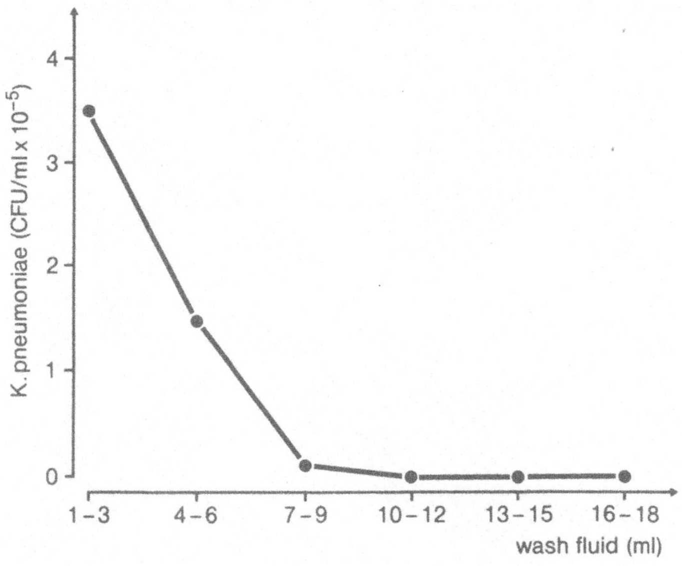

Figure 3. Colony forming units of K. pneumoniae in portions of 3 ml of wash-fluid from macrophage monolayers after 1 hr of phagocytosis.

had not been ingested. This was achieved by washing of the cell monolayer six times with portions of three ml of medium (Figure 3). As can be seen, viable bacteria cannot be detected in wash fluid already after four consecutive washing steps.

Uptake of Opsonized K. pneumoniae

When rabbit antiserum (ELISA-titer 1:20480) to phenol-water extracts of K. pneumoniae were present during phagocytosis, a significant increase in the number of bacteria taken up by the macrophages was seen (Figure 4). Heat inactivation (56°C, 30 min) of the antiserum did not decrease the opsonizing capacity, indicating that the contribution of complement to opsonization played a minor role in this system. Preimmunization-serum contained antibodies, detectable by ELISA (titer 1:320). It was thus not surprising that rabbit serum, prior to immunization, also enhanced phagocytosis (Figure 4).

Phagocytosis in Combined Cultures of Macrophages and Splenic Lymphocytes

In further experiments, the influence of spleen lymphocytes on macrophages in the absence of antibodies was studied. Macrophages were mixed with different numbers of lymphocytes and incubated for 24 hrs at 37°C. Thereafter, lymphocytes were removed by decantation of the medium from the macrophage-monolayer and subsequent washing of the alveolar macrophages with six times three ml of medium. After addition of bacteria for 1 hour to the macrophages, the number of ingested bacteria was determined. Results of representative experiments are shown in Figures 5, 6 and 7. As can be seen in Figures 5 and 6, a significant ($p < 0.05$) increase in the uptake of bacteria could be seen, when the proportion of macrophages to lymphocytes was 1:4. This was observed in either the absence or the presence of phenol-water extract of the bacteria during the 24 hrs incubation period before

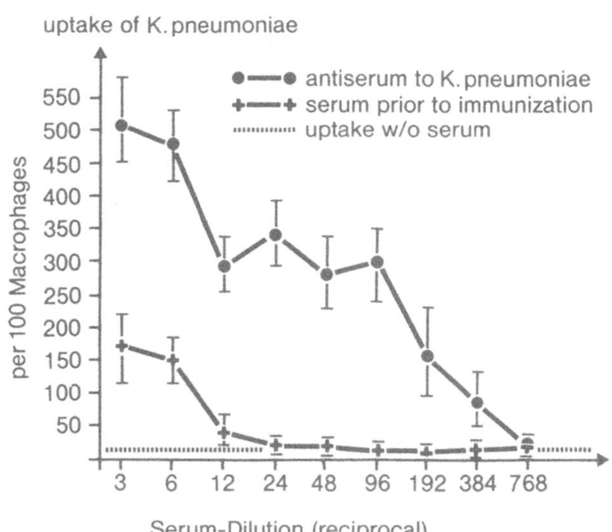

Figure 4. Phagocytosis of K. pneumoniae in the presence of various dilutions of rabbit-antiserum (ELISA titer 1:20480) to phenol-water extracts of the bacteria. For comparison, data with various dilutions of preimmunization serum (ELISA titer 1:320) are also shown.

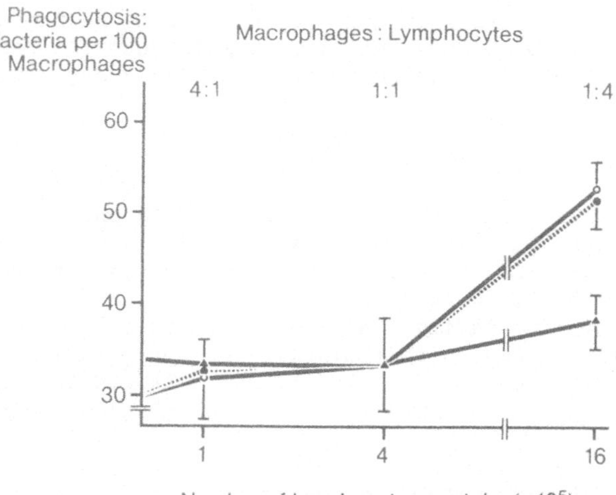

Figure 5. Ingestion of K. pneumoniae by alveolar macrophages of an unimmunized guinea pig in the presence of various number of autologous lymphocytes. Serum antibody titer 1:192 by ELISA. O—O macrophages and lymphocytes incubated 24 hrs together, removal of lymphocytes, thereafter addition of bacteria and phagocytosis for 1 hr. ●···● macrophages, lymphocytes and phenol-water extract (100 µg/ml of bacteria). ▲—▲macrophages and lymphocytes were cultivated for 24 hrs separately, incubated together for the 1 hr phagocytosis period only.

phagocytosis, and thus, could not be further enhanced by the addition of bacterial antigens.

Even after immunization of guinea pigs with phenol-water extracts of K. pneumoniae, an additional increase in the rate of phagocytosis was not observed, although the animals had developed a more than four-fold increase

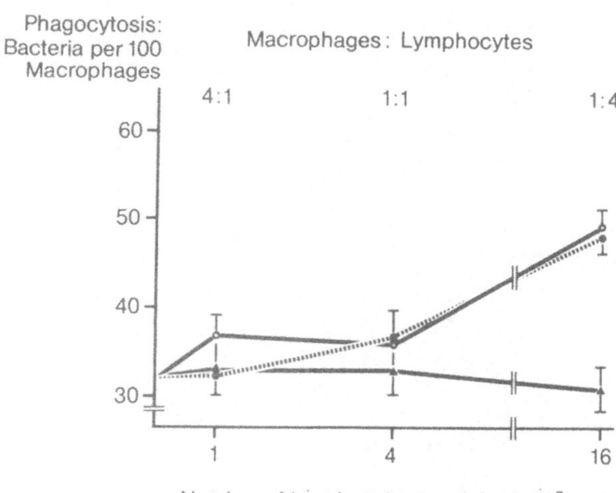

Figure 6. Ingestion of K. pneumoniae by alveolar macrophages of immunized animals. Serum antibody titer to phenol-water extract of K. pneumoniae (ELISA) was 1:840. See Figure 5 for legend.

in the titer of specific antibodies, as shown by ELISA (Figure 6). The increase in uptake of bacteria was not seen when lymphocytes were added to macrophages for the 1 hr phagocytosis period only. When the proportion of macrophages was varied over a wide range, an influence of lymphocytes on phagocytosis during the short (1 hr) incubation period was not seen (Figure 7). This was seen in immunized as well as in unimmunized animals.

Influence of Gentamicin on Phagocytosis of Opsonized Bacteria

When various concentrations of gentamicin were added to macrophages in the presence of opsonized bacteria during the one hour of phagocytosis, a significant decrease in the number of visible intracellular bacteria was observed at antibiotic concentrations above 12.8 µg/ml (Table 1). The number of surviving bacteria within macrophages was reduced at gentamicin concentrations of 0.05 µg/ml or higher (Table 1).

Effect of Gentamicin on Mixed Cultures of Lymphocytes and Macrophages

In further experiments, gentamicin, at various concentrations, was added to the culture of macrophages and lymphocytes (at optimal proportions, 1:4) for 24 hrs. Subsequently, lymphocytes and gentamicin were washed away and bacteria were added to the macrophages in the absence of antibiotics. A reduction in the number of visible bacteria within macrophages at antibiotic concentrations above 2.9 µg/ml was seen (Figure 8).

DISCUSSION

Alveolar macrophages serve important functions in host defense because many pathogens enter the body via the respiratory tract. Our studies provid-

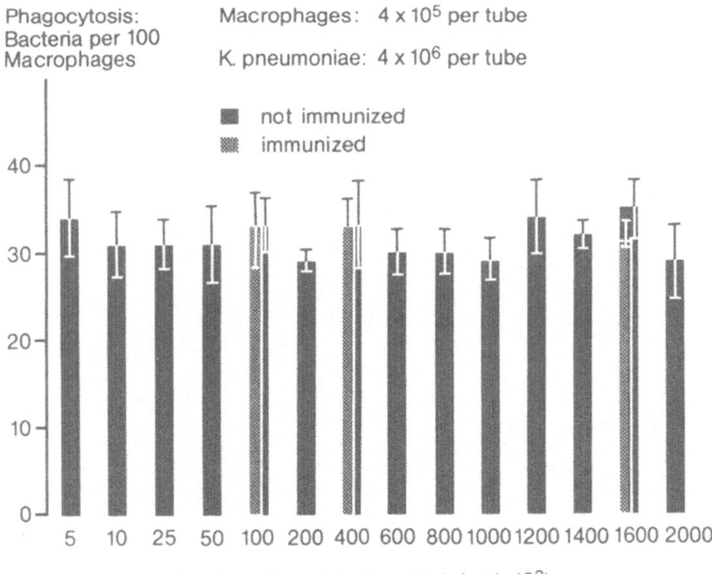

Figure 7. Number of visible intracellular K. pneumoniae after 1 hr of phagocytosis in presence of various numbers of lymphocytes.

Table 1. Visible Bacteria and Intracellular Survivors of Opsonized K. pneumoniae in Guinea Pig Alveolar Macrophages in the Presence of Variable Concentrations of Gentamicin[a]

Gentamicin (µg/ml)	Visible bacteria (%) Mean	S.D.	Intracellular survivors (%) Mean	S.D.
none	100	13	100	18
0.003	109	14	89	12
0.013	105	14	91	15
0.05	105	14	44	7
0.2	101	13	36	6
0.8	104	13	36	8
3.2	93	17	30	8
12.8	63	13	33	6
51.2	48	14	13	4
204.8	43	13	16	5
819.2	37	13	16	5
3276.8	31	13	24	3

[a]Gentamicin and opsonized bacteria were added simultaneously and incubated for 1 hour together with the macrophages.

ed evidence that alveolar macrophages, obtained by lung lavage from guinea pigs, could ingest and kill virulent, encapsulated K. pneumoniae without opsonization. Furthermore, we have confirmed that phagocytosis by these macrophages is increased considerably in the presence of specific antibodies to surface components of the bacteria (4,12,14,16,19,26).

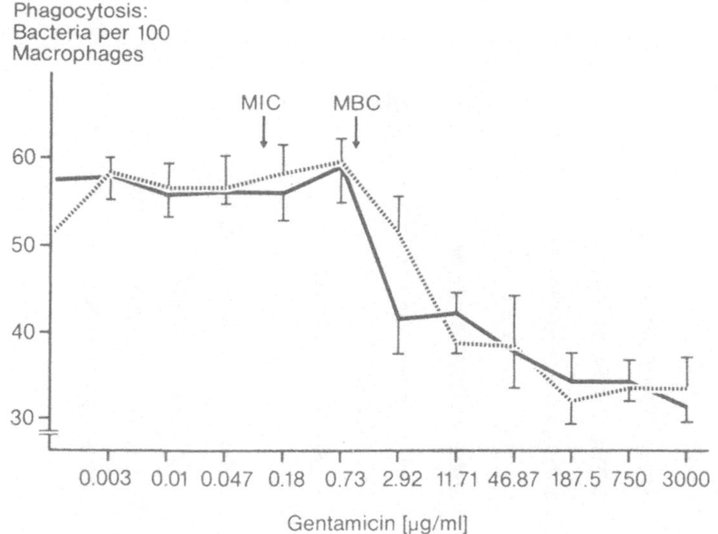

Figure 8. Number of visible intracellular K. pneumoniae after incubation of macrophages with lymphocytes. (1:4) in presence of various concentrations of gentamicin for 24 hrs. Lymphocytes and antibiotic were then removed and bacteria added for 1 hr. —— immunized; --- unimmunized.

In addition, we provide evidence for enhanced uptake of the bacteria after co-cultivation of the macrophages with autologous lymphocytes prior to phagocytosis. This occurred although the lymphocytes were no longer present during uptake of bacteria by macrophages (10,13,17,22,27). It is unlikely, that specific antibodies have contributed considerably to this increase in phagocytosis, because such antibodies could not be detected in the supernatants of lymphocytes by the sensitive ELISA-technique. The enhanced ingestion of bacteria was correlated with the number of lymphocytes present requiring a minimal number of four lymphocytes per macrophage. The increased ingestion of bacteria by alveolar macrophages after co-cultivation with autologous lymphocytes can be explained by the release of mediators from the lymphocytes, together with direct contact of lymphocytes with macrophages, which led to the activation of the macrophages. Opsonization of K. pneumoniae by specific antibodies to phenol-water extracts of the bacteria resulted in a more than 30-fold increase in uptake of bacteria by the alveolar macrophages. As expected, a similar degree of ingestion was never obtained when macrophages had been preincubated with spleen lymphocytes in the absence of detectable antibodies.

When gentamicin was added to the macrophages, a significant decrease in the number of visible bacteria in macrophages was seen at antibiotic concentrations of 12.8 μg/ml and above. In addition, it was observed that the number of viable bacteria within the alveolar macrophages already decreased at antibiotic concentrations of 0.05 μg/ml, i.e. at one third of the MIC (Table 1). In further experiments gentamicin in various concentrations was added to mixtures of lymphocytes and macrophages for 24 hrs. Prior to phagocytosis, gentamicin and lymphocytes were removed. Under these conditions, the number of visible bacteria within macrophages were reduced beginning at gentamicin concentrations of 2.9 μg/ml (Figure 8). These observations can be explained in three ways.

First, when gentamicin was present during the one hour phagocytosis period, the bacteria could be rendered more susceptible to killing within the macrophages already at antibiotic concentrations below the MIC (1,5,11,14).

Second, when gentamicin was present for 24 hrs prior to phagocytosis, penetration of the antibiotic into macrophages might play a significant role in the reduction of visible bacteria observed in our experiments (6). In human alveolar macrophages a rather poor uptake of gentamicin was reported by Hand and associates (18).

Third, it has been described by several investigators, that aminoglycosides might impair the function of eukaryotic cells including phagocytes and lymphocytes (2,8,29,33,35). It is thus possible, that gentamicin in concentrations of 2.9 μg/ml and above impairs the function of guinea pig lymphocytes and/or macrophages.

It is obvious that conclusions for the use of these antibiotics in the clinic cannot be drawn from these preliminary results, since many questions remain unanswered and the difficulties of transferring results obtained in animals to the human situation also have to be mentioned. The results, nevertheless, emphasized the usefulness of drug monitoring during treatment of severe infections by aminoglycosides.

The results have been presented in part at the annual meeting of the Deutsche Gesellschaft für Hygiene und Mikrobiologie, Bonn. Abstract Zbl. Bakt. Hyg. I. Abt. Orig. A 256:418 (1984). Please address requests for reprints to Prof. Dr. H. Brunner, Institute for Chemotherapy, Bayer AG, Wuppertal, F.R.G.

REFERENCES

1. D. Adam, P. Philipp and B. H. Belohradsky, Studies on the influence of host defense mechanisms on antimicrobial effect of chemotherapeutic agents. Effects of antibiotics on phagocytosis of mouse peritoneal macrophages in vitro, Ärztl. Forsch. 25:181 (1971).
2. G. Banck and A. Forsgren, Antibiotics and suppression of lymphocyte function in vitro, Antimicrob. Agents Chemother. 16:554 (1979).
3. H. von Boehmer and K. Shortman, The separation of different cell classes from lymphoid organs. IX. A simple and rapid method for removal of damaged cells from lymphoid cell suspensions, J. Immunol. Methods. 2:293 (1973).
4. J. D. Brain, D. W. Golde, G. M. Green, D. J. Massaro, P. A. Valberg, P. A. Ward and Z. Werb, Biologic potential of pulmonary macrophages, Am. Rev. Resp. Dis. 118:435 (1978).
5. H. Brunner and Ch. Undeutsch, Effect of cephalothin and gentamicin on phagocytosis of Klebsiella pneumoniae by guinea pig alveolar macrophages, in: "The Influence of Antibiotics on the Host-Parasite Relationship," H. U. Eickenberg, H. Hahn and W. Opferkuch, eds., Springer-Verlag, Berlin (1982).
6. C. S. F. Easmon, The effect of antibiotics on the intracellular survival of Staphylococcus aureus in vitro, Br. J. Exp. Pathol. 60:24 (1979).
7. H. M. Ericsson and J. C. Sherris, Antibiotic sensitivity testing. Report of an international collaborative study, Acta Pathol. Microbiol. Scand. B Suppl. 271 (1971).
8. F. A. Ferrari, A. Pagani, M. Marconi, R. Stefanoni and A. G. Siccardi, Inhibition of candidacidal activity of human neutrophil leukocytes by aminoglycoside antibiotics, Antimicrob. Agents Chemother. 17:87 (1980).
9. A. Forsgren, D. Schmeling and P. G. Quie, Effect of tetracycline on the phagocytic function of human leukocytes, J. Infect. Dis. 130:412 (1974).
10. R. E. Fowles, I. M. Fajardo, J. L. Leibowitch and J. R. David, The enhancement of macrophage bacteriostasis by products of activated lymphocytes, J. Exp. Med. 138:952 (1973).
11. H. Friedman and G. Warren, Muramyl dipeptide-induced enhancement of phagocytosis of antibiotic pretreated Escherichia coli by macrophages, Proc. Soc. Exp. Biol. Med. 176:366 (1984).
12. R. van Furth, Current view on the mononuclear phagocyte system, Immunobiol. 161:178 (1982).
13. R. Ganguly and R. H. Waldman, Respiratory tract cell-mediated immunity, Bull. Eur. Physiopathol. Respir. 13:95 (1977).
14. C. G. Gemmell, P. K. Peterson, D. Schmeling, Y. Kim, J. Mathews, L. Wannamaker and P. G. Quie, Potentiation of opsonization and phagocytosis of Streptococcus pyogenes following growth in the presence of clindamycin, J. Clin. Invest. 67:1249 (1981).
15. G. Gillissen, Non-specific influence of antibiotics on the course of infectious processes, Infection 10:128 (1982).
16. K. M. Green and E. H. Kass, The role of the alveolar macrophage in the clearance of bacteria from the lung, J. Exp. Med. 119:167 (1964).
17. H. Hahn and S. H. E. Kaufmann, The role of cell-mediated immunity in bacterial infections, Rev. Inf. Dis. 3:1221 (1981).
18. W. L. Hand, R. W. Corwin, T. H. Steinberg and G. D. Grossman, Uptake of antibiotics by human alveolar macrophages, Am. Rev. Respir. Dis. 129:933 (1984).
19. W. G. Hocking and D. W. Golde, The pulmonary alveolar macrophage, N. Engl. J. Med. 301:580, 639 (1979).
20. P. G. Holt, Alveolar macrophages. I. A simple technique for the preparation of viable alveolar macrophages from small laboratory animals, J. Immunol. Methods 27:189 (1979).

21. M. E. Kaplan and C. Clark, An improved rosetting assay for detection of human T-lymphocytes, J. Immunol. Methods 5:131 (1974).
22. P. E. Lipski and A. S. Rosenthal, Macrophage-lymphocyte interaction. I. Characteristics of the antigen-independent-binding of guinea pig thymocytes and lymphocytes to syngeneic macrophages, J. Exp. Med. 138:900 (1973).
23. K. W. Maxwell, T. Dietz and S. Marcus, An in situ method for harvesting guinea pig alveolar macrophages, Amer. Rev. Resp. Dis. 89:579 (1964).
24. S. Meyer and H. Brunner, Enyzme-Immuno-Assay in listeriosis: Detection of antibody and antigen, Zbl. Bakt. Hyg. I. Abt. Orig. A. 248:469 (1981).
25. Q. N. Myrvik, E. S. Leake and B. Farris, Studies on pulmonary alveolar macrophages from the normal rabbit: a technique to produce them in a high state of purity, J. Immunol. 86:128 (1961).
26. H. Y. Reynolds, J. A. Kazmicrowski and H. H. Newball, Specificity of opsonic antibodies to enhance phagocytosis of Pseudomonas aeruginosa by human alveolar macrophages, J. Clin. Invest. 56:376 (1975).
27. S. Riisgaard, J. M. Rhodes and J. Bennedsen, Macrophage activation by lymphokines and after direct contact with sensitized lymphocytes: Histocompatibility requirements and the effect of inhibitors, Scand. J. Immunol. 7:209 (1978).
28. W. Roszkowski, H. L. Ko, K. Roszkowski, J. Jeljaszewicz and G. Pulverer, Antibiotics and immunomodulation: Effects of cefotaxime, amikacin, mezlocillin, piperacillin and clindamycin, Med. Microbiol. Immunol. 173:279 (1985).
29. M. M. Seklecki, R. Quintiliani and E. G. Maderazo, Aminoglycoside antibiotics moderately impair granulocyte function, Antimicrob. Agents Chemother. 13:552 (1978).
30. M. Seligmann, J. L. Preud'Homme and J. -C. Brouet, B and T cell markers in human proliferative blood diseases and primary immuno-deficiencies with special reference to membrane bound immunoglobulins, Transplant Rev. 16:85 (1973).
31. A. E. Stuart, J. A. Habeshaw and A. E. Davidson, Phagocytes in vitro, in: "Handbook of Experimental Immunology," D. M. Weir, ed., Vol. 2, Blackwell Scientific Publication, Oxford (1978).
32. C. Undeutsch and H. Brunner, Influence of antibodies on the phagocytosis of Klebsiella pneumoniae by alveolar macrophages, Zbl. Bakt. Hyg. I. Abt. Orig. A 249:43 (1981).
33. P. Vaudaux and F. A. Waldvogel, Gentamicin antibacterial activity in the presence of human polymorphonuclear leukocytes, Antimicrob. Agents Chemother. 16:743 (1979).
34. O. Westphal, O. Luderitz and F. Bister, Über die Extraktion von Bakterien mit Phenol/Wasser, Z. Naturforsch. 76:148 (1952).
35. J. M. Wilhelm, S. E. Pettitt and J. J. Jessop, Aminoglycoside antibiotics and eukaryotic protein synthesis: Structure-function relationships in the stimulation of misreading, Biochemistry 17:1143 (1978).
36. A. B. Wilson, D. G. Haegert and R. R. A. Coombs, Increased sensitivity of the rosette-forming reaction of human T-lymphocytes with sheep erythrocytes afforded by papain treatment of the sheep cell. Clin. Exp. Immunol. 22:177 (1975).

SECTION V
ANTIMICROBIAL EFFECTS ON HUMORAL AND CELLULAR LYMPHOCYTE RESPONSES

INFLUENCE OF THE QUINOLONES AND TETRACYCLINE ON SPECIFIC T-CELL-ANTIGEN INTERACTIONS IN VITRO AND ON DELAYED TYPE HYPERSENSITIVITY TO SRBC IN MICE

Helmut Hahn, Beate Wos, Andreas Press and Uwe Sperling

Department of Medical Microbiology
Freie Universität Berlin
Berlin, F.R.G.

INTRODUCTION

The decision for the application of antimicrobial drugs should not only be based on the activity of the drug on the microorganism itself, but must take into consideration the reciprocal effects between agent and host organism (2,9). In particular, possible influences on the immune system should be considered - either on components of the immune system directly or indirectly via alterations of the bacteria which might result in a different handling by the immune system.

In 1982, a first meeting with international attendance was held in Munich which was entirely devoted to this subject (2). There are now many published studies which report on various antimicrobial drugs having various influences on the immune system. For instance, tetracyclines are reported to negatively influence phagocytosis (6) chemotaxis (4,5), antibody formation (1), and specific interactions between T cells and antigens (8). Others, such as β-lactam antibiotics have so far been shown to exert no, or minor, effects on the immune system (2).

Being of particular interest to us, we investigated possible influences antimicrobials might exert on specific immune reactions relevant to the defense of bacterial diseases. Since interactions between antigen-presenting macrophages and specific T cells represent a key function in T cell-dependent immunity to facultatively intracellular bacteria, we have started to investigate aspects of these interactions in vitro (8), likewise the effects antimicrobial substances might have in vivo appeared of similar interest.

Two recently developed Quinolones, Ciprofloxacin and Ofloxacin, Doxycyclin, a Tetracycline derivative, and HR 221, a newly developed β-lactam antibiotic were chosen as test substances. These were assayed with respect to their influence on the following immune parameters: (a) specific interaction of T cells with antigen presented by macrophages in vitro and/or (b) delayed type hypersensitivity to sheep red blood cells in mice.

MATERIALS AND METHODS

Antibiotics

Ciprofloxacin (laboratory standard) was a gift from Bayer AG, Leverkusen; Ofloxacin and HR 221 were gifts from Hoechst AG, Hoechst, and Doxycyclin was a gift from Pfizer GmbH, Karlsruhe. Solutions were freshly prepared for each experiment by dissolving the agents in RPMI 1640 medium supplemented with 5% FCS and 2 mM L-glutamine for in vitro experiments, and in physiological saline for in vivo experiments.

Bacteria

Listeria monocytogenes, strain EGD, were kept virulent by continuous mouse passage. Bacteria were grown in trypticase-soy broth for 18 hrs, centrifuged, washed, and heat-killed. Heat-killed Listeriae (HKL) were used as antigen.

T Cell/Antigen Interactions

Specific interactions between T cells and antigen were measured according to Farr et al. (3). In short, syngeneic (B6 x DBA2)F1 (B6D2) mice from our own breeding facilities were injected i. v. with 4 x 10^3 living Listeriae. Seven days later, peritoneal exudates were induced by i.p. injection of 2 ml of a 10% protease peptone solution. Exudate cells were washed out and the T cells enriched by passaging them over nylon wool. These cells are called PETLEs (peritoneal exudate T lymphocytes enriched).

5 x 10^3 peritoneal macrophages from normal syngeneic (B6D2) mice were preincubated with 2 x 10^7 HKL for 5 hrs. Subsequently, the macrophages were cultured in 96 well flat bottom tissue culture dishes (Nunc) together with 2.5 x 10^5 PETLEs from Listeria-immune mice. Final volume was 0.2 ml per well. Tissue medium used was RPMI 1640 supplemented with 5% FCS and 2 mM L-glutamine. The substance to be tested was added at concentrations indicated. Incubation was done in 5% CO_2 at 37°C. After 2 days of incubation, 1 mc Ci ^{3}HTdR (specific activity: 2 Ci/mM, Radiochemical Center, Amersham, U. K.) was added to the wells and incubation continued for another 18 hrs. Cells were collected on glass fiber filters (Skatron Multiple Cell Culture Harvester, Flow Laboratories) and ^{3}HTdR incorporation measured using a liquid scintillation counter. ^{3}HTdR is a measure of T cell proliferation and, therefore, in this system, of a secondary immune response of Listeria-specific T cells in vitro.

Delayed Hypersensitivity to Sheep Red Blood Cells

Sensitization. Sheep red blood cells (SRBC) were purchased commercially and kept in Alsever's Solution until use. Immediately before use, cells were washed and diluted to appropriate concentrations. SRBC were injected i.v. into the tail vein in a volume of 0.2 ml.

Challenge. DTH was elicited and measured as described in (7). In short, mice received a challenge inoculum of 10^8 SRBC s. c. into one hind foot pad. The degree of swelling was measured 24 hrs. later using a dial gauge caliper (Schnelltaster, H. C. Kroplin, Schluchtern, FRG).

The difference between sham-injected and antigen-injected footpads served as a measure of DTH (units of 0.1 mm). Routinely, challenge controls were done by injecting non-immune mice; in these the degree of swelling never exceeded two units.

Antibiotic Treatment of Test Animals. The following substances were tested with respect to their influence on DTH in the dosages given below:

Doxycyclin	0.1 mg/mouse
	1.0 mg/mouse
	2.5 mg/mouse
	5.0 mg/mouse
Ciprofloxacin	0.025 mg/mouse
	0.25 mg/mouse
	2.5 mg/mouse

RESULTS

In Vitro Experiments

Dose-Response Relationship of the Influence of Ofloxacin, Ciprofloxacin, Doxycyclin, and HR 221 on Antigen-Specific T Cell Proliferation In Vitro. When Ofloxacin, Ciprofloxacin, Doxycyclin, or HR 221, respectively, were present at various concentrations in the reaction mixture during the whole incubation period, there was no inhibition by HR 221 at any concentrations tested. Ciprofloxacin and Ofloxacin exerted slightly inhibitory effects at concentrations of 25 µg/ml. At 50 µg/ml inhibition by both quinolones was marked.

Doxycyclin, on the other hand, in keeping with published evidence (8), started to show marked inhibitory effects at 12.5 µg/ml, and at 25 µg/ml, suppression of T cell proliferation was almost complete (Table 1).

Table 1. Dose-Response-Relationship of the Effects of Ciprofloxacin, Ofloxacin, Doxycyclin, and Penicillin G on Listeria-Specific T Cell Proliferation In Vitro

Incubation Mixture Containing	Concentration (µg/ml) of Test Substance[1]							
	0	1.56	3.12	6.25	12.5	25	50	100
PETLEs[2]								
MØ[3]								
HKL[4] + Penicillin G	100	85	89	84	84	107	130	110
" + HR 221	100	103	90	106	101	89	85	93
" + Ciprofloxacin	100	109	103	113	97	79	35	0.4
" + Ofloxacin	100	97	104	95	78	81	54	29
" + Doxycyclin	100	150	95	108	15	0.4	0.3	0.1
HKL + Ø	100							
PETLES								
MØ + Ø	10							
PETLEs								
HKL + Ø	49							

[1]Data are expressed as percentages of positive control (= 100%)
[2]PETLEs = 2.5 x 10^5 [3]Macrophages = 5 x 10^3 [4]HKL = 2 x 10^7

Table 2. Proliferation of Listeria-Specific T Cells after Test Substance Had Been Present During Antigen Uptake Phase (4 hrs.) Only

	± (cpm)	± in % of Controls
Penicillin G	103.492 ± 11.774	108
HR 221	103.043 ± 9.005	108
Ciprofloxacin	99.125 ± 4.622	103
Ofloxacin	103.348 ± 9.587	108
Doxycyclin	91.044 ± 7.944	95
<u>Controls</u>:		
PETLEs Macrophages HKL	95.836 ± 3.796	100
PETLEs Macrophages	66.155 ± 5.170	69
PETLEs HKL	76.645 ± 9.951	80

Concentration of each test substance was 50 μg/ml.

<u>Influence of Test Substances When Present During Antigen Uptake Only.</u> In specific T cell/antigen interactions, the phase of antigen uptake and processing can be separated from the phase of antigen recognition and T cell proliferation. In the following experiment, the question was investigated whether the test substances, when present during the antigen pulsing phase only, exert any influence on subsequent T cell proliferation. Antigen was added to normal macrophages. Test substances were added and kept in the mixture for 4 hrs. After 4 hrs antigen as well as test substances were washed out and replaced by T cells in fresh medium. T cell concentration was 2.5×10^5/well, incubation time 66 hrs. ^{3}HTdR was added 18 hrs before the end of incubation and proliferation measured at the end of the incubation period.

The results of this experiment are summarized in Table 2. They show that none of the test substances influences the capacity of macrophages to subsequently stimulate T cell proliferation.

<u>In Vivo Experiments</u>

<u>In In Vivo Experiments Measuring DTH, Only Ciprofloxacin and Doxycyclin Were Used.</u> The effects of both substances are summarized in Tables 3 and 4. Ciprofloxacin did not negatively influence DTH reactions, either when given in the sensitization phase or when given at a time close to challenge. Doxycyclin, on the other hand, suppressed DTH reactions significantly, but only when given at extremely high doses corresponding to 100 times the therapeutic dosage.

DISCUSSION

A variety of assay systems measuring the immune reactivity have recently been employed to measure the influence of antibiotics on parameters of the immune response. We have chosen two parameters of specific interactions between T cells and antigens, one in vitro and one in vivo system.

The in vitro assay used was originally described by Farr et al. (3). It allows to measure the in vitro interaction between antigen-specific T cells and antigens. In this system, <u>Listeria</u> <u>monocytogenes</u> antigen is

Table 3. Influence of Ciprofloxacin given on Various Days with Respect to Sensitization (10^6 SRBC i.v.) on DTH to SRBC in Mice

Dosage (mg)	appli- cation	day	Ciprofloxacin[1]	control[1]	significance
0.025	i. v.	d-1	0.97 ± 0.12	1.06 ± 0.14	n. s.
0.025	i. v.	d+1	1.13 ± 0.15	1.29 ± 0.16	n. s.
0.025	i. v.	d+3	1.06 ± 0.32	1.10 ± 0.19	n. s.
0.25	i. v.	d-1	1.09 ± 0.24	1.06 ± 0.14	n. s.
2.5	i. p.	d-1	1.0 ± 0.14	1.06 ± 0.14	n. s.
0.25	i. v.	d+1	1.26 ± 0.21	1.29 ± 0.16	n. s.
2.5	i. p.	d+1	1.25 ± 0.14	1.29 ± 0.16	n. s.
0.25	i. v.	d+3	1.0 ± 0.16	1.06 ± 0.32	n. s.
2.5	i. p.	d+3	0.96 ± 0.19	1.06 ± 0.32	n. s.

[1]5 mice per group

presented by macrophages to T cells, and the latter react by proliferation. It is commonly thought that this system reflects the in vivo antigen specific interaction between T cells of helper type and antigen presenting macrophages.

Ciprofloxacin and Ofloxacin, two newly developed quinolones, showed some suppression of T cell proliferation at concentrations exceeding therapeutic dosages. The β-lactams, HR 221, and Penicillin G, did not interfere with T cell proliferation whereas Doxycyclin showed marked inhibitory effects at 12.5 μg/ml. There were no effects seen when the agents were present during the antigen uptake only and were washed out subsequently.

Table 4. Influence of Doxycyclin, Given on Various Days with Respect to Sensitization (10^6 SRBC i.v.) on DTH to SRBC in Mice

Dosage (mg)	appli- cation	day	Doxycyclin[1]	control[1]	significance
0.1	i. v.	d-1	1.3 ± 0.15	1.24 ± 0.12	n. s.
0.1	i. v.	d+1	1.1 ± 0.13	1.19 ± 0.22	n. s.
0.1	i. v.	d+3	1.1 ± 0.31	1.1 ± 0.28	n. s.
1.0	i. v.	d-1	1.16 ± 0.22	1.24 ± 0.12	n. s.
2.5	i. p.	d-1	1.03 ± 0.18	1.14 ± 0.13	n. s.
5.0	i. v.	d-1	0.9 ± 0.06	1.02 ± 0.2	n. s.
1.0	i. v.	d+1	1.13 ± 0.15	1.19 ± 0.22	n. s.
2.5	i. p.	d+1	1.2 ± 0.24	1.23 ± 0.19	n. s.
5.0	i. v.	d+1	1.17 ± 0.21	1.29 ± 0.16	n. s.
1.0	i. v.	d+3	0.98 ± 0.15	1.06 ± 0.32	n. s.
2.5	i. p.	d+3	1.1 ± 0.3	1.06 ± 0.32	n. s.
5.0	i. p.	d+3	0.59 ± 0.15	1.1 ± 0.28	n. s.

[1]5 mice per group

The in vitro data were confirmed, albeit to a less marked degree, when the influence of the agents on DTH reactions was tested. Here, too, Doxycyclin showed a suppressive effect on DTH whereas the quinolones and β-lactam substances did not exert such effects.

Taken together, our results show that β-lactams and quinolones at therapeutic concentrations do not negatively influence the T-cell mediated functions, T cell proliferation and DTH. Doxycyclin showed suppressive effects, both in vitro (at concentrations slightly higher than therapeutic ones) and, at supratherapeutic doses in vivo as well.

REFERENCES

1. G. Banck and A. Forsgren, Antibiotics and suppression of lymphocyte function in vitro, Antimicrob. Agents and Chemother. 16:554 (1979).
2. U. -U. Eickenberg, H. Hahn and W. Opferkuch, eds., "The Influence of Antibiotics on the Host Parasite Relationship," Springer (1982).
3. A. G. Farr, J. -M. Kiely and E. R. Unanue, Macrophage-T cell interactions involving Listeria momocytogenes - Role of the H-2 gene complex, J. Immunol. 122:2395 (1975).
4. A. Forsgren, G. Banck, H. Beckmann and A. Bellahsene, Antibiotic-Host defense interaction in vitro and in vivo, Scand. J. Infect. Dis. 24:195 (1980).
5. A. Forsgren, D. Schmeling and G. Banck, Effect of antibiotics on chemotaxis of human polymorphonuclear leukocytes in vitro, Infection 6(Suppl. 1):102 (1978).
6. A. Forsgren, D. Schmeling and P. G. Quie, Effect of tetracycline on the phagocytic function on human leucocytes, J. Infect. Dis. 130:412 (1974).
7. H. Hahn, S. H. E. Kaufmann, E. T. Miller and G. B. Mackaness, Peritoneal exudate T lymphocytes with specificity to sheep red blood cells. I. Production and characterization as to function and phenotype, Immunology 36:691 (1979).
8. H. Hahn and M. Mielke, Influence of antibiotics on interactions between Listeria-specific T cells and antigen in vitro, Zbl. Bakt. Suppl. 13:143 (1985).
9. W. E. Hauser and J. S. Remington, Effect of antibiotics on the humoral and cell-mediated immune response, in: "In Action of Antibiotics in Patients," L. D. Sabath, ed., Hans Huber, Stuttgart, Bern, Wien. (1982).

INFLUENCE OF ANTIBIOTICS ON MITOGEN-STIMULATED AND NON-STIMULATED MURINE SPLENIC LYMPHOCYTES

J.-W. Wittke, B. H. Andresen and U. Ullmann

Department of Medical Microbiology
University of Kiel
Kiel, F.R.G.

INTRODUCTION

The question whether antibiotics have immunomodulating side effects has been investigated for several years. This is especially so since clinical situations constantly arise in which there is some kind of deliberate or unintended immunosuppression due to more frequent and prolonged periods of antibiotic treatment (2,3). Of the various immunologic parameters that have been established in order to deal with this question, the lymphocyte transformation test (6) has proven to be an expressive tool to investigate the extent to which mitogen-stimulated lymphocytes are influenced by antibiotics in their blast formation. In order to detect immuno-enhancing effects, however, non-stimulated cells must be used (5). Thus, the aim of this study was to investigate the impact of antibiotics on the blast formation of maximally and moderately stimulated as well as of non-stimulated murine lymphocytes.

MATERIALS AND METHODS

The following antibiotics were investigated: Tetracycline (Hoechst, Frankfurt, F.R.G.), cefmenoxime (Grünenthal, Stolberg, F.R.G.), ceftazidime (Glaxo, Bad Oldesloe, F.R.G.), and clavulanic acid (Beecham-Wulfing, Neuss, F.R.G.).

Spleen cell cultures were prepared following the methods described by Oppenheim and associates (6) and Bähr and Ullmann (1). Spleens were taken from syngeneic male C3H mice; lymphocytes were separated by density gradient centrifugation (Ficoll-Paque, Pharmacia, Uppsala, Sweden), washed thrice in Hank's solution and resuspended in RPMI 1640 (both solutions obtained from Biochrom, West Berlin), supplemented 10% (v/v) with heat-inactivated fetal bovine serum and 2 mMol/l L-glutamine. When mitogen was used, phytohaemagglutinin (PHA) (Wellcome, Beckenham, England) was added to give final concentrations of 1.0 mg/l (maximal stimulation) or 0.15 mg/l (submaximal stimulation).

Geometrical serial dilutions of the employed antibiotics were added to the lymphocyte suspension. Samples of 0.2 ml - 2×10^6 cells/ml, 12 aliquots for each dilution step were incubated in flat bottomed microtiter plates (Flow, Irvine, Scotland) for 72 or 96 hours at 37°C and 5% CO_2.

After the addition of 0.4 mcCi/well ^{3}H-thymidine (Amersham Buchler, Braunschweig, F.R.G.) and further incubation for 12 hours, the cells were collected by a cell harvester (Titertek, Skatron, Norway). The beta emission was measured by a liquid scintillation counter (Beckman, Irvine, CA, USA). Evaluation of significance was performed by the student's t-test.

RESULTS

Tetracycline showed the well-known (4,7) inhibition of lymphocyte transformation under maximal PHA stimulation (1.0 mg/l), starting at a concentration of around 32 mg/l (Figure 1, I). Moderately stimulated lymphocytes (0.15 mg/l PHA) revealed a stimulation by tetracycline concentrations between 8 and 32 mg/l, almost quadrupling the control value (without tetracycline) at 16 mg/l (Figure 1, II). Non-mitogen-stimulated lymphocytes reacted with a more than six-fold increase of the thymidine uptake under incubation with 8 mg/l tetracycline, compared to control without antibiotic (Figure 1, III).

Concentrations of 80 or more mg/l cefmenoxime were necessary to inhibit fully PHA-stimulated lymphocytes (Figure 2a, I), while 40 or more mg/l

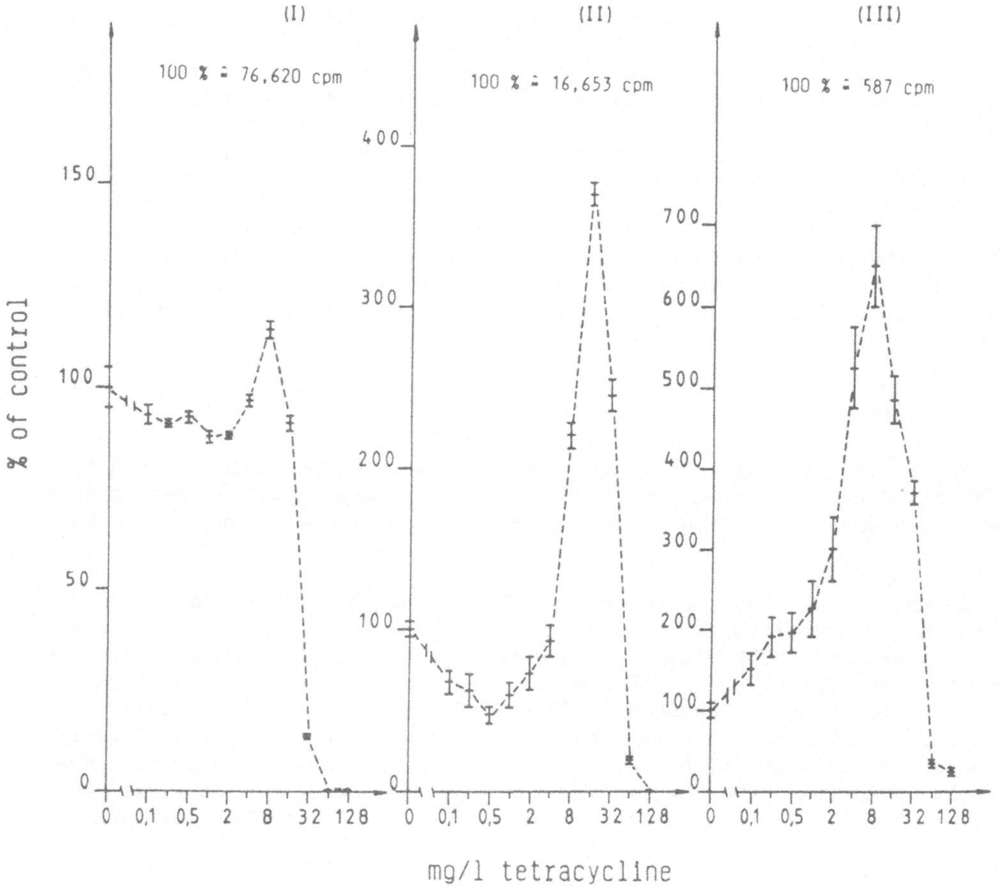

Figure 1. Influence of tetracycline on the ^{3}H-thymidine incorporation
Incubation time = 72 h; n = 12; I ≙ $\bar{X} \pm$ SEM
I) 1.0 mg/l PHA II) 0.15 mg/l PHA III) 0 PHA

cefmenoxime inhibited moderately stimulated lymphocytes (Figure 2a, II). With the latter, a weak enhancement of ^{3}H-thymidine incorporation at low concentrations could be detected.

Non PHA-stimulated lymphocytes reacted with a slight increase of ^{3}H-thymidine uptake at a concentration range between ca. 5 and 20 mg/l cefmenoxime (Figure 2b, I). Prolongation of incubation to 96 hours prior to radioactive labelling led to an even slightly higher thymidine incorporation (Figure 2b, II).

Ceftazidime hampered the blast transformation of maximally PHA-stimulated lymphocytes at concentrations of 32 mg/l or more (Figure 3, I), while submaximally stimulated lymphocytes were already inhibited at concentrations of 4 mg/l or more (Figure 3, II). No impact on the blast formation of unstimulated lymphocytes could be detected (Figure 3, III).

Clavulanic acid inhibited maximally stimulated cells at concentrations of more than 10 mg/l (Figure 4, I). Moderately stimulated lymphocytes

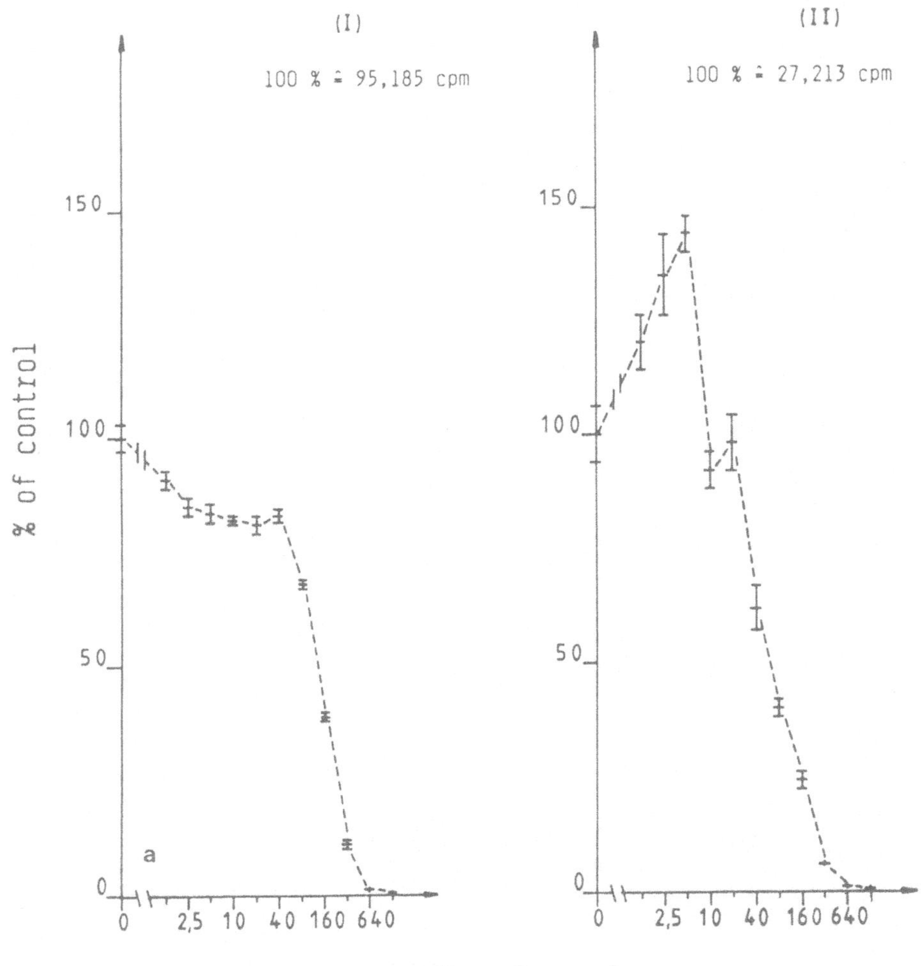

Figure 2a. Influence of cefmenoxime on the ^{3}H-thymidine incorporation
Incubation time = 72 h; n = 12; I ≙ $\bar{X} \pm$ SEM
I) 1.0 mg/l PHA II) 0.15 mg/l PHA

reacted with an increase of up to 250% at lower concentrations, again followed by a decrease at 10 or more mg/l clavulanic acid (Figure 4, II). Unstimulated lymphocytes also showed a decrease of activity in this concentration range.

DISCUSSION

With some of the antibiotics investigated (tetracycline, cefmenoxime, clavulanic acid), different degrees of augmented thymidine incorporation could be detected. It is well known that some weak mitogens need a long incubation time in order to show an effect (6). Thus, the incubation time of cefmenoxime was prolonged in order to show the stimulative effect more clearly. This could be of importance for future investigations of other antibiotics.

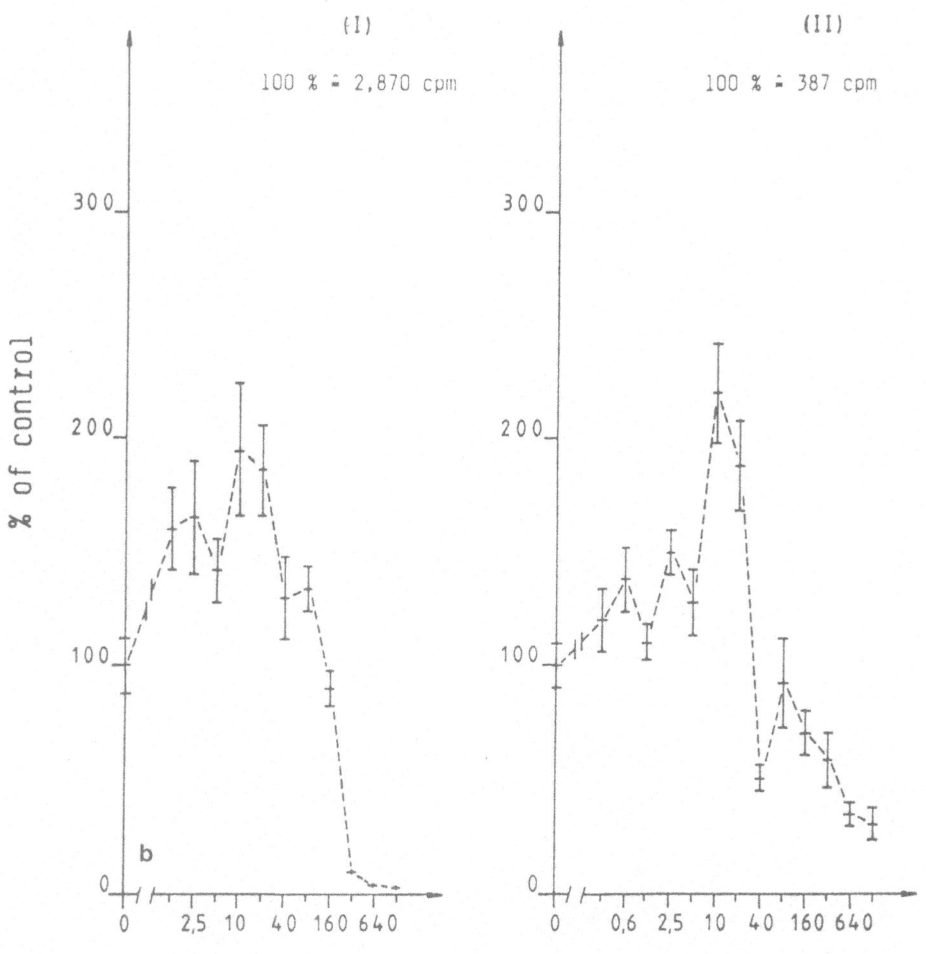

Figure 2b. Influence of cefmenoxime on the ^{3}H-thymidine incorporation 0 PHA; n = 12; Ī ≙ X̄ ± SEM. I) Incubation time 72 h II) Incubation time 96 h.

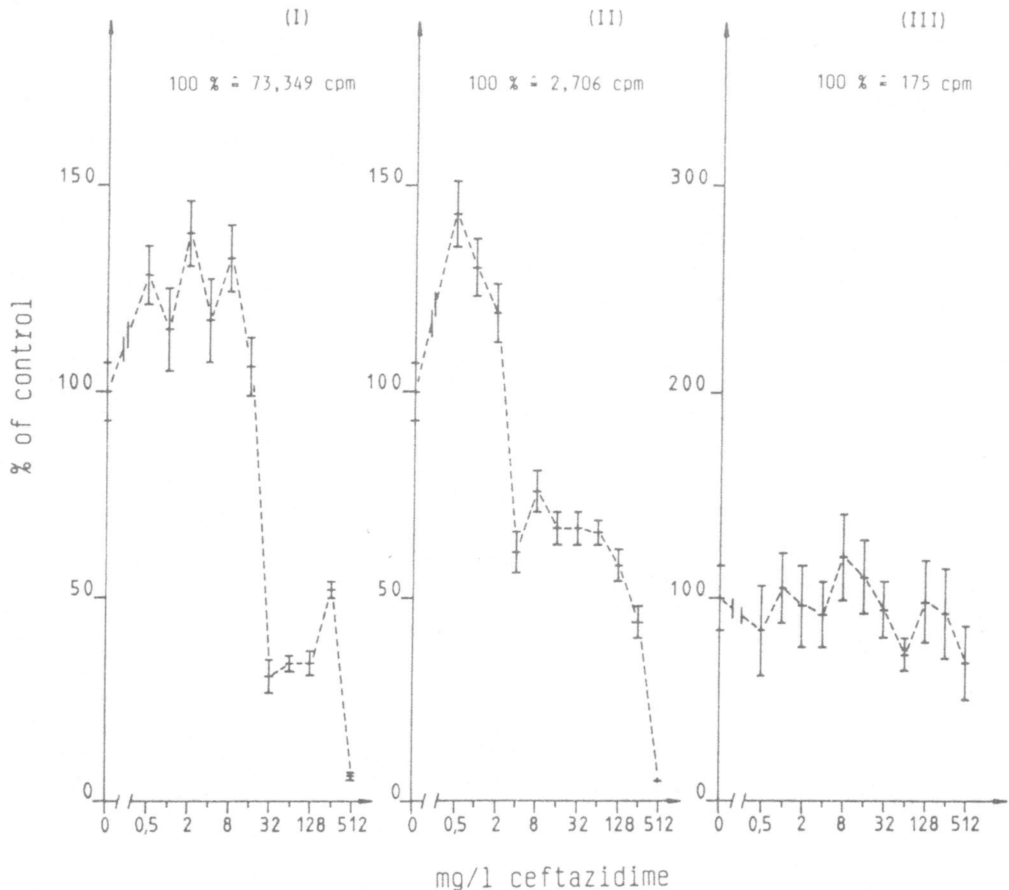

Figure 3. Influence of ceftazidime on the ^{3}H-thymidine incorporation
Incubation time 72 h; n = 12; I ≙ $\bar{x} \pm$ SEM
I) 1.0 mg/l PHA II) 0.15 mg/l PHA III) 0 PHA

The ^{3}H-thymidine uptake of murine lymphocytes parallels the one of human lymphocytes under comparable conditions (8). Therefore, it might be expected that the stimulative effects of tetracycline, cefmenoxime and clavulanic acid, which could be achieved by therapeutical concentrations, actually play a role at least during long term treatment with these substances.

Except for ceftazidime, the dosage required for a depression of lymphocyte transformation is beyond the therapeutic level (tetracycline, cefmenoxime) or only reachable for a short period of time following bolus injection (clavulanic acid) and should thus be of lesser importance for antibiotic treatment.

REFERENCES

1. V. Bähr and U. Ullmann, The influence of metronidazole and its two main metabolites on murine in vitro lymphocyte transformation, Eur. J. Clin. Microbiol. 2:568 (1983).
2. E. A. Chaperon, Suppression of lymphocytes by cephalosporins, in: "The Influence of Antibiotics on the Host-Parasite Relationship," H.-U.

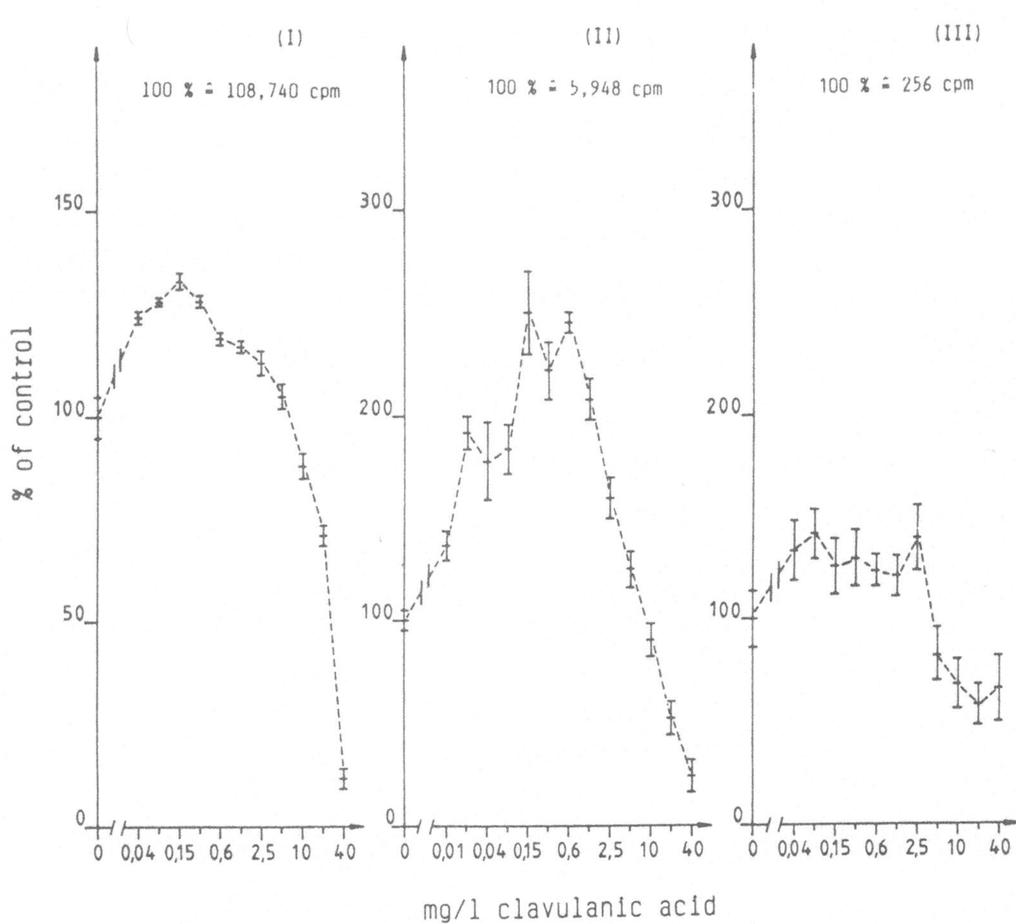

Figure 4. Influence of clavulanic acid on the ^{3}H-thymidine incorporation Incubation time 72 h; n = 12; Ī ≙ $\bar{X}$ ± SEM
I) 1.0 mg/l PHA II) 0.15 mg/l PHA III) 0 PHA

Eickenberg, H. Hahn and W. Opferkuch, eds., Springer-Verlag, Berlin, Heidelberg, New York (1982).
3. R. Finch, Immunomodulating effects of antimicrobial agents, J. Antimicrob. Chemother. 6:691 (1980).
4. A. Forsgren and G. Banck, Influence of antibiotics on lymphocyte function in vitro, Infection 6(Suppl. 1):91 (1978).
5. G. Leyhausen, G. Seibert, A. Maidhof and W. E. G. Muller, Differential stimulation of lymphocyte cell growth in vitro by cephalosporins, Antimicrob. Agents Chemother. 26:752 (1984).
6. J. J. Oppenheim, S. Dougherty, S. P. Chan and J. Baker, Use of lymphocyte transformation to asses clinical disorders, in: "Laboratory Diagnosis of Immunological Disorders," G. N. Vyas, ed., Grune & Stratton, New York (1975).
7. R. C. Potts, H. A. A. Hassan, R. A. Brown, A. MacConnachie, J. H. Gibbs, A. J. Robertson and J. Swanson Beck, In vitro effects of doxycycline and tetracycline on mitogen stimulated lymphocyte growth, Clin. Exp. Immunol. 53:458 (1983).
8. C. Schutt, Lymphozytentransformationstest (LTT), in: "Immunologische Arbeitsmethoden," H. Friemel, ed., G. Fischer Verlag, Stuttgart (1980).

STIMULATION OF SUPPRESSOR CELL ACTIVITY BY CEFADROXIL

Jacques P. Clot and Catherine Pelous

Laboratoire d'Immunologie, Hôpital Saint-Eloi
Montpellier, France

INTRODUCTION

The interaction between antimicrobial agents and the human immune system is still poorly understood. However, many in vitro effects of antibiotics have been reported in experimental systems (7,15). Some antibiotics have been shown to decrease some immunological parameters such as neutrophil functions (8), lymphocyte responsiveness to polyclonal mitogens (2,3,14), or natural killer cell activity (9).

While adverse effects of penicillin are well documented, the literature yet reveals that there are comparatively few systemic immune reactions associated with the use of cephalosporins (6). We hypothesized that such an observation could be related to the effects of cephalosporins on some lymphocyte subpopulations. In animals, as well as in humans, Type I hypersensitivity reactions involve cell-to-cell interactions between T lymphocyte subsets, B lymphocytes and antigen-presenting cells (11). Thus, the production of immunoglobulin E is closely dependent on T suppressor lymphocytes (16).

In the present work we examined the activity of three cephalosporins, a tetracycline and a macrolide on T cell subsets and functions. The results showed that one of the cephalosporins, cefadroxil, was a potent stimulator of suppressor cell activity.

EXPERIMENTAL PROCEDURES

Antibiotics

Three cephalosporins were used: cefadroxil (Laboratories Bristol, France), cefalexine (Laboratoires Glaxo, France), and cefaclor (Laboratoire Eli-Lilly, France). The tetracycline used was doxycycline (Laboratoire Sarget, France), and the macrolide, josamycine (Laboritoires Pharmuka, France). Appropriate concentrations were made up in RPMI 1640 culture medium.

Preparation of Peripheral Blood Mononuclear Cells

Blood samples were obtained from healthy volunteers. Peripheral blood mononuclear cells (PBMC) were prepared from heparinized blood centrifuged (400g, 30 min, 20°C) on Ficoll-Hypaque gradient. The lymphocyte yield was always greater than 75%. The cell suspension contained 80-90% of small lymphocytes and 10-20% of monocytes, as judged by peroxidase staining. The cell suspension was adjusted to a concentration of 10^6 cells/ml.

Cell Viability Test

A 1% solution of ethidium bromide-acridine orange (Sigma Chemical Co) was mixed with an equal volume of PBMC suspension. Under UV microscope, live cells had a green fluorescence, and dead cells fluoresced orange.

Lymphocyte Membrane Markers

PBMC which were not stained by peroxidase unlike monocytes, were detected according to classical techniques (5). Total T cells were enumerated by E-rosette forming cells. T4 cell subset was detected by Leu3a monoclonal antibody (MCAb, IgG1) from Becton-Dickinson. T8 cell subset was detected by BL15 MCAb (IgG2b, kindly provided to us by J. Brochier, INSERM U80, Lyon). The binding of MCAb to corresponding lymphocytes was revealed by fluoresceinated anti-mouse class specific Ig goat antibodies. Surface membrane Ig-bearing B cells were enumerated by membrane immunofluorescence using fluoresceinated anti-human IgM+IgG+IgA goat F(ab')2 fragments. HLA-DR-bearing B cells were detected by BL2 MCAb (IgG2a, J. Brochier, Lyon).

Lymphocyte Stimulation by Mitogens

PBMC washed three times were resuspended at a concentration of 10^6 cells/ml in RPMI 1640 culture medium buffered with Hepes and supplemented with penicillin (100 units/ml), streptomycin (100 μg/ml), and 15% inactivated fetal calf serum. Microcultures were set up as four replicates with 2 x 10^5 cells into each well of microculture plates (Microtest II, Falcon). In addition to unstimulated controls, lymphocyte cultures were stimulated with the following mitogen: phytohemagglutinin (PHA-P, Difco) at 10 μg/ml, and concanavalin A (Con A, Pharmacia) at 10 μg/ml. These optimal final concentrations of mitogens were previously determined by studies using dose-response curves of lymphocyte cultures from normal donors.

The cultures were incubated at 37°C in an humidified atmosphere of 5% CO_2. After incubation for three days, 1 μCi of ^{3}H-thymidine (1Ci/mmol specific activity, CEA, Saclay, France) was added to each well 16 hrs before harvesting the cells with a Skatron apparatus (Flow Laboratories). The blastogenesis was estimated by ^{3}H-thymidine incorporation as measured by liquid scintillation counting. The results were expressed as mean disintegration per minute (dpm) $\pm$ S.E. and as a stimulation index, i.e., the ratio between ^{3}H-thymidine incorporated in the presence of mitogens and that incorporated in the absence of mitogen.

The possible immunomodulating effect of an antibiotic was expressed as a percentage of variation = 1 - (dpm of cultures pre-incubated with a molecule) / (dpm of normal cultures) x 100.

In some experiments, cultures were performed in the presence of 1 μg/ml of indomethacin (Sigma Chemical Co) which blocks prostaglandin (PG) synthesis by inhibition of cyclooxygenase.

Depletion of Adherent Cells

Adherent cells (monocytes-macrophages) were removed from PBMC by incubating the cells in RPMI 1640 containing 20% fetal calf serum in Falcon culture dishes for 1 hr at 37°C in an humidified atmosphere of 5% CO_2. The non-adherent cells were removed by gentle aspiration and two washes. Less than 5% of peroxidase positive cells were recovered in the so-called non-adherent cell suspension (1).

RESULTS

After cell viability tests the various antibiotics were used at pharmacotherapeutic concentrations giving more than 95% of viable PBMC during the incubation period (from 1 hr to 72 hrs). The concentrations used were: a) cefadroxil: 0-100 μg/ml; b) cefalexine: 0-100 μg/ml; c) cefaclor: 0-100 μg/ml; d) doxycycline: 0-20 μg/ml; e) josamycine: 0-10 μg/ml. Such experimental concentrations are consistent with serum levels observed in vivo 1 hr after the administration of cephalosporins (10-30 μg/ml), doxycycline (2-4 μg/ml), and josamycin (1-2 μg/ml).

No significant modification of the expression of lymphocyte membrane markers was noted when the various molecules of antibiotics were pre-incubated with PBMC for 30 and 60 min before each test (data not shown).

PBMC were pre-incubated with various concentrations of the antibiotics for 30 min at 37°C before adding mitogens. The results are reported in Figure 1. The three cephalosporins had a dose-dependent inhibitory effect on lymphoproliferative responses to PHA and, to a lesser extent, to Con A. However, the inhibitory capacity of cefadroxil was more impressive than that of cefalexine and cefaclor. Josamycine did not affect mitogenic stimulation, but doxycycline was able to strongly inhibit responsiveness to both PHA and Con A.

To further investigate the inhibition of lymphocyte stimulation induced by cefadroxil, various experiments were undertaken. The results (Table 1) showed that cefadroxil decreased the PHA responsiveness of PBMC, but did not affect the response of purified lymphocytes previously depleted of adherent cells.

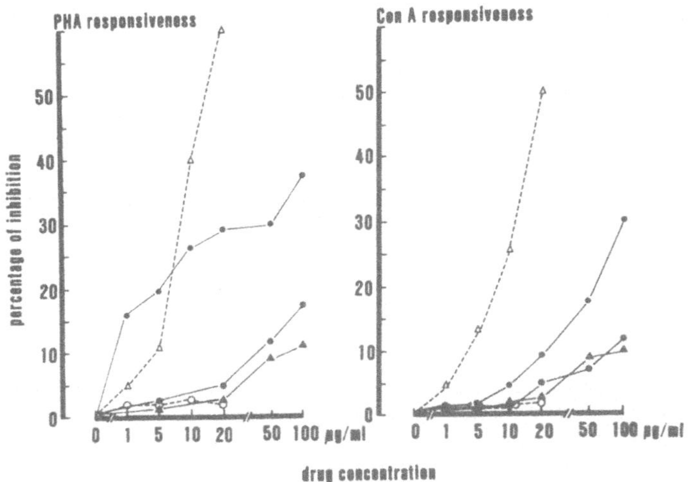

Figure 1. Percentage of inhibition of peripheral blood mononuclear cell cultures stimulated either by 10 μg/ml of phytohemagglutinin (PHA responsiveness), or by 10 μg/ml of concanavalin A (Con A responsiveness). The cells were previously incubated with various concentrations of the following drugs: cefadroxil (●—●); cefalexine (▲—▲); cefaclor (✱—✱); doxycycline (△—△); josamycine (O—O).

Table 1. Modulating Effect of Cefadroxil on Peripheral Blood Mononuclear Cells (PBMC) and on Adherent Cell-Depleted Lymphocytes Incubated With or Without Indomethacin

	Thymidine incorporation of cells stimulated with 10 μg/ml PHA	Percentage of variation*
PBMC alone	98640 ± 6857	
Adherent cell-depleted lymphocytes alone	97108 ± 6640	
PBMC with indomethacin	117107 ± 6191	+ 18.7
PBMC + 50 μg/ml of cefadroxil	68945 ± 4112	- 30.1
Adherent cell-depleted lymphocytes + 50 μg/ml of cefadroxil	99043 ± 5198	
PBMC with indomethacin + 50 μg/ml of cefadroxil	113324 ± 9449	+14.9

The results are expressed as mean ±S.E. of disintegrations per minute of 5 experiments.

*The percentage of variation = 1 - (dpm of PBMC pre-incubated with a molecule) / (dpm of PBMC alone) x 100. + = an increased response; - = a decreased response.

Such data suggested that the target cell for cefadroxil could be of the monocyte-macrophage lineage. PBMC were then stimulated by PHA in the presence of indomethacin. This inhibitor of cyclooxygenase classically enhances ^{3}H-thymidine incorporation in PHA cultures (10) by blocking PG synthesis by adherent cells (12). When cefadroxil was added to PBMC in the presence of indomethacin, no inhibition of PHA responsiveness occurred, suggesting that the target cell of this mitogen was a PG-producing suppressor cell.

In a last set of experiments, PBMC were incubated with each antibiotic, in the presence of indomethacin, and stimulated by PHA (10 μg/ml). The results (Table 2) showed that cephalosporin-induced inhibitors of the PHA response was always reversed by indomethacin. No change was noted when PBMC were incubated with josamycine. In contrast, the strong doxycycline-induced inhibition of PHA responsiveness was not abolished by indomethacin, suggesting that doxycycline directly interfered with the lymphocyte stimulation process.

DISCUSSION

The data herein reported further emphasizes the possible role of certain antimicrobial agents in the human immune response. Most earlier reports underline disturbances of normal immune functions by antibiotics. We were able to confirm, for example, the potent suppression induced by doxycycline (tetracycline) on mitogen responsiveness of human lymphocytes (14). However, in our hands, a macrolide such as josamycine had no effect on lymphocyte cultures.

Cephalosporins were previously shown to be inhibitors of lymphocyte stimulation by mitogens (3,4). We report that cefadroxil particularly was

Table 2. Modulating Effect of Various Molecules of Antibiotics on Peripheral Blood Mononuclear Cells Incubated With and Without 1 μg/ml of Indomethacin

	Thymidine incorporation of cells stimulated with 10 μg/ml PHA	Percentage of variation*
PBMC alone	107789 ± 9070	
PBMC + 50 μg/ml of cefadroxil	73835 ± 3730	- 31.5
PBMC with indomethacin + 50 μg/ml of cefadroxil	117107 ± 6191	+ 8.6
PBMC + 50 μg/ml of cefalexine	98087 ± 10130	- 9.0
PBMC with indomethacin + 50 μg/ml of cefalexine	126303 ± 3738	+ 17.2
PBMC + 50 μg/ml of cefaclor	102399 ± 8166	- 5.0
PBMC with indomethacin + 50 μg/ml of cefaclor	129696 ± 7744	+ 20.3
PBMC + 10 μg/ml of doxycycline	63037 ± 9246	- 41.5
PBMC with indomethacin + 10 μg/ml of doxycycline	66685 ± 8048	- 38.1
PBMC + 10 μg/ml of josamycine	106834 ± 6940	- 0.9
PBMC with indomethacin + 10 μg/ml of josamycine	112679 ± 3563	+ 4.5

The results are expressed as mean ± S.E. of disintegrations per minute of 5 experiments.
*The percentage of variation = 1 - (dpm of PBMC pre-incubated with a molecule) / (dpm of PBMC alone) x 100. + = an increased response; - = a decreased response.

able to decrease ^{3}H-thymidine incorporation of PBMC stimulated by PHA. The inhibition of Con A responsiveness was less impressive.

The human lymphocyte in vitro responses to polyclonal mitogens involve cell-to-cell interactions and soluble mediators. Two signals are required to stimulate T helper lymphocytes. One is the mitogen itself which binds to carbohydrates on the lymphocyte membrane. The other one is a monokine, provided by adherent cells, namely Interleukine-1. These two signals induce the production of Interleukine-2 by T helper cells and the initiation of the cell cycle (13). In addition, adherent cells (monocytes-macrophages) produce prostaglandins, among them PGE2 which stimulates the activity of T suppressor cells (10).

We herein show that cephalosporins, and cefadroxil in particular, were able to stimulate PG-producing suppressor cells. The decrease of mitogen responsiveness was thus due to a stimulation of suppressor cell functions.

Such data could account for the relative paucity of adverse immune reactions associated with the use of cefadroxil. This cephalosporin could limit or decrease IgE production, by stimulating suppressor cells.

ACKNOWLEDGMENTS

We gratefully acknowledge Mrs. Christine Perez for her secretarial assistance.

REFERENCES

1. P. Aubas, B. Cosso, P. Godard, F. B. Michel, and J. Clot, Decreased suppressor cell activity of alveolar macrophages in bronchial asthma, Am. Rev. Respir. Dis., 130:875 (1984).
2. G. Banck and A. Forsgren, Antibiotics and suppression of lymphocyte function in vitro. Antimicrobiol. Agents chemother., 16:554 (1979).
3. E. A. Chaperon and W. E. Sanders, Suppression of lymphocyte response by cephalosporins, Inf. Immun., 19:451 (1978).
4. E. A. Chaperon, Suppression of lymphocytes by cephalosporins, in: "The Influence of Antibiotics on the Host-Parasite Relationship," J. Eickenberg, H. Hahn and W. Opferkuch, eds., Springer-Verlag, Berlin (1982).
5. J. Clot, E. Charmasson, and J. Brochier, Age-dependent changes of human blood lymphocytes subpopulations, Clin. Exp. Immunol., 32:346 (1978).
6. A. L. De Weck, Penicillins and cephalosporins, in: "Allergic Reactions to Drugs," A. L. De Weck and H. Bundgaard, eds., Springer-Verlag, Berlin (1983).
7. R. Finch, Immunomodulating effects of antimicrobial agents, J. Antimicrobial. Chemother., 6:691 (1980).
8. A. Forsgren, D. Schmeling, and P. G. Quie, Effect of tetracycline on the phagocytic function of human leucocytes, J. Infect. Dis., 130:412 (1974).
9. D. H. B. Goh and A. Ferrante, In vitro inhibition of natural killer cell activity by doxycycline, Int. J. Immunopharmac., 6:51 (1984).
10. J. S. Goodwin and J. Ceuppens, Regulation of the immune response by prostaglandin, J. Clin. Immunol., 3:295 (1983).
11. K. Ishizaka, Regulation of IgE synthesis, Ann. Rev. Immunol., 2:159 (1984).
12. J. I. Kurland and R. Bockman, Prostaglandin E production by human blood monocytes and mouse peritoneal macrophages, J. Exp. Med., 147:952 (1978).
13. E. L. Larsson, Mechanism of T cell activation. II. Antigen and lectin-dependent acquisition of responsiveness to TCGF is a nonmitogenic, active response of resting T cells, J. Immunol., 126:1323 (1981).
14. Y. H. Thong and A. Ferrante, Inhibition of mitogen-induced human lymphocyte proliferative responses by tetracycline analogues, Clin. Exp. Immunol., 35:443 (1979).
15. Y. H. Thong and A. Ferrante, Effect of tetracycline treatment on immunological responses in mice, Clin. Exp. Immun., 39:728 (1980).
16. T. Watanabe, M. Kimoto, S. Maruyama, T. Kishimoto, and Y. Yamamura, Regulation of antibody response in different immunoglobulin classes, V. Establishment of T cell hybrid cell line secreting IgE class-specific suppressor factor, J. Immunol., 121:2113 (1978).

ANTIBIOTICS AND SUPPRESSION OF LYMPHOCYTE RESPONSE IN VITRO: PROTECTION BY THIOL COMPOUNDS

Jean-Jacques Pocidalo, Yvon Roche, Maryse Levacher, and
Marie-Anne Gougerot-Pocidalo

Unitè de Recherches 13 INSERM
Hôpital Claude Bernard
Paris, France

INTRODUCTION

Treatment with antibiotics may have a direct effect on both bacterial virulence as well as host defense systems. Indeed several antimicrobial agents are known to affect immunological responses significantly (10). Certain antibiotics can suppress lymphocyte function in vitro (1,6). The present investigation was undertaken to evaluate the effects of two antibiotic families, macrolides and new quinoline carboxylic acid derivatives on mitogen-stimulated human peripheral blood mononuclear leucocyte (MNL) responses. We demonstrated that erythromycin, spiramycin, ciprofloxacin, pefloxacin and ofloxacin suppressed significantly lymphocyte transformation. In a second part, we evaluated the effects of thiol compounds as antioxidant agents, essentially 2-Mercaptoethanol (2-ME) on protection of the depressed immune response induced by high antibiotic concentrations. Our results clearly showed that 2-ME can partially protect the lymphocyte proliferation depressed by these antibiotics.

MATERIALS AND METHODS

Reagents

Antibiotics. Only preservative-free antibiotics were used, kindly provided by Specia (spiramycin), Abbott (erythromycin), Roussel Uclaf (ofloxacin), Bayer (ciprofloxacin) and Roger Bellon (pefloxacin). Fresh serial dilutions of drugs were prepared on the day of each experiment in RPMI 1640 culture medium.

Mitogen. Phytohaemagglutinin (PHA P Difco) was used in cultures at a final concentration of 5, 10, 20 μg/ml. Pokeweed mitogen (PWM Difco) was used at dilutions of 1/1000, 1/500 and 1/100.

Reagents. 2-Mercaptoethanol, reduced glutathione, L-cysteine and selenomethionine (SeMet) were purchased from Sigma Chemical Company (USA). For each thiol compound tested the optimal concentration was chosen with respect to increasing mitogenic response (data not shown).

Cell Preparations

Human mononuclear leukocytes (MNL) were isolated from heparinized blood of healthy adult donors by the method of Boyum on a Ficoll-Isopaque gradient. MNL obtained by this method usually comprised 75 to 85% lymphocytes and 10 to 20% monocytes.

Cell Cultures

MNL were cultivated in RPMI 1640 (Gibco) supplemented with 25 mM Hepes, 2 mM Glutamine, 100 mM pyruvate, 1% non essential amino-acids and 10% heat inactivated autologous serum. Cultures were set up in microtest plates (Falcon, Microtest II). 10^6 cells/ml in 0.2 ml culture medium were incubated in triplicate with or without mitogen at different concentrations as indicated in the results. Antibiotics were added at concentrations ranging from 0 to 100 µg/ml at the onset of culture. The plates were incubated at 37°C in 95% air, 5% CO_2 for 72 hrs. (PHA stimulation) or 96 hrs. (PWM stimulation). In order to examine the effects of the addition of spiramycin (Sp) or erythromycin (Er) to cell cultures after the addition of PHA (5 µg/ml) MNL were placed in microtiter wells with or without mitogen and 100 µg/ml of Sp or Er were added at the same time or at 4, 6, 8, 10, 12, 24 or 48 hrs after the addition of mitogen. Cells to which no antibiotic had been added served as control cultures. All cell cultures were incubated for 72 hrs. The effects of pre-incubation of MNL in the presence of Sp were also examined, MNL were preincubated for 1, 4, 8 or 24 hrs with 10 or 100 µg/ml Sp. The cells were then washed in phosphate buffered saline and cultured in antibiotic-free medium for 72 hrs.

Incorporation of ^{3}H-Thymidine (^{3}H-TdR) and ^{3}H-Uridine (^{3}H-UdR)

Cells were pulsed with 1 µCi of ^{3}H-TdR (2 Ci/mmol, CEA France) during the last 6 hrs of culture, or with 0.25 µCi of ^{3}H-UdR (5 Ci/mmol, Amersham, England) for 24 hrs during mitogen stimulation. Harvesting onto glass fiber filters was performed using a multiple sample harvester. The filters were then dried and placed in scintillation vials containing 4 ml of toluene scintillator (Packard). ^{3}H-TdR and ^{3}H-UdR incorporation were measured by counting in a liquid scintillation spectrometer (Intertechnique). The mean count for triplicate cultures was expressed as a percentage of that obtained for antibiotic free controls.

Cell Viability

Determination of cell viability as measured by trypan blue exclusion and the lactic dehydrogenase release test, was carried out at the end of each culture.

Oxygen Exposure

Cultures were first incubated at 37°C in a humidified atmosphere containing 95% O_2-5% CO_2 in a leak-proof chamber which had been tested prior to experimentation. The cells were exposed to O_2 for periods varying from 24 to 48 hrs with or without antibiotics, after which incubation was completed at 37°C in 5% CO_2 enriched humidified air atmosphere (Heraus, France). Total cultivation time was fixed at 72 hrs. Cells cultivated in ambient air for 72 hrs served as control culture.

RESULTS

The cell viability as measured by trypan blue exclusion and the lactic dehydrogenase release test was not altered at any of the drug concentrations used with different antibiotics.

Table 1. Sp and Er Depressed ^{3}H-TdR Incorporation of MNL Induced by PHA

Doses (μg/ml)	1	5	10	50	100
Sp (%)	88 ± 2.0	72 ± 1.5	70 ± 1.2	68 ± 2.0	35 ± 0.5
Er (%)	85 ± 2.0	75 ± 2.0	68 ± 2.0	60 ± 1.5	37 ± 0.5

Percentage of stimulation expressed by the following ratio: ^{3}H-TdR incorporation (at any antibiotic concentration) to ^{3}H-TdR in control medium (without antibiotic) x 100. Both PHA (10 μg/ml) and antibiotics were added at the beginning of culture. ^{3}H-TdR was added at 72 hrs. Each result is the mean ± SD of 3 experiments performed in triplicate.

Effects of Spiramycin (Sp) and Erythromycin (Er) on MNL Response to PHA

The effects of Sp and Er added at the onset of culture on MNL response to PHA are indicated in Table 1. A decrease in ^{3}H-TdR uptake was observed in cultures containing Er and Sp. Suppression of MNL proliferation increased as the concentration of Sp or Er present in the medium was raised. Maximum inhibition was observed at a suboptimal concentration of PHA (5 μg/ml). Inhibition of DNA synthesis as demonstrated by the decrease in ^{3}H-TdR uptake appeared after the addition of 1 μg/ml of Sp or Er and was significant at a dose of 5 μg/ml. There was no difference between MNL responses to the antibiotics at 5 and 10 μg/ml. Significant dose-response correlations were obtained for both Sp and Er ($p \leq 0.01$ and ≤ 0.001 using concentrations 1 to 100 μg/ml).

Table 2. Effects of Sp and Er on MNL Response to PWM After 5 μg/ml PHA Stimulation

PWM Concentration		1/1000	1/500	1/100
Drug concentration		(μg/ml)		
Sp	0	0	0	0
	1	85%	91%	96%
	10	67%	81%	79%
	50	42%	61%	70%
	100	6%	3%	8%
Er	0	0	0	0
	1	85%	88%	92%
	10	71%	78%	86%
	50	68%	70%	65%
	100	37%	33%	34%

Each figure represents the mean of three experiments performed in triplicate and is expressed as a percentage of the stimulation observed in control cultures.

Table 3. Effect of Different Doses of Quinolone Antibiotics on ^{3}H-TdR (cpm) Incorporation into PHA Stimulated MNL

Antibiotic	Pef	Cip	Ofl
Control	135 ± 8	137 ± 10	138 ± 9
0.1 µg/ml	124 ± 11	121 ± 8	121 ± 11
1 µg/ml	131 ± 9	130 ± 9	125 ± 7
10 µg/ml	127 ± 7	132 ± 11	128 ± 8
25 µg/ml	102 ± 10	109 ± 6	122 ± 9
100 µg/ml	27 ± 3	7 ± 1	79 ± 6

Effects of Pef, Cip and Ofl at different dosages on ^{3}H-TdR uptake by PHA (5 µg/ml) stimulated MNL. Each figure represents the mean ± SD of three experiments performed in triplicate and expressed cpm x 10^3.

Effects of Sp and Er on MNL Responses to PWM

The effects of Sp and Er added at the onset of culture MNL response to PWM are presented in Table 2. Inhibition of DNA synthesis by Sp or Er occurred at all drug concentrations and was similar at all levels of PWM stimulation. Significant dose-response correlations were obtained for both Sp and Er ($p \leq 0.01$ and ≤ 0.001 respectively) using concentrations of 1, 10, 50 and 100 µg/ml.

Effects of Quinolones on MNL Responses to PHA

The effects of three different quinoline carboxylic acid derivatives were studied (Table 3): pefloxacin (Pef), ciprofloxacin (Cip) and ofloxacin (Ofl) added at the onset of culture on MNL depressed PHA (5, 10, 20 µg/ml) responses displayed only at high concentrations (25 and 100 µg/ml antibiotics).

Table 4. Incorporation of ^{3}H-TdR by MNL Induced by PHA in Presence of Sp With or Without 2-ME (Air Culture)

PHA µg/ml	5	10	20
Control	134 ± 12	172 ± 11	181 ± 12
+ 2-ME (5.10^{-6}M)	120 ± 11	153 ± 13	164 ± 10
100 µg/ml Sp	51 ± 6	93 ± 8	97 ± 7
100 µg/ml Sp + 2-ME (5.10^{-6}M)	72 ± 5*	102 ± 6*	121 ± 9*

Each figure represents the mean ± SD of three experiments performed in triplicate and expressed as cpm x 10^3. The conditions of air culture were defined previously (see Methods).
*$p \leq 0.01$ between responses at 100 µg/ml Sp with or without 2-ME (5.10^{-6}M).

Table 5. Incorporation of ^{3}H-TdR by MNL Induced by PHA (5 μg/ml) in Presence of Ofl, Per or Cip With or Without 2-ME (Air Culture)

	Ofl	Pef	Cip
Control	138 ± 9	135 ± 8	137 ± 10
+ 2-ME (5.10^{-6}M)	121 ± 8	130 ± 9	121 ± 8
100 μg/ml antibiotic	79 ± 6	27 ± 3	7 ± 1
100 μg/ml antibiotic + 2-ME (5.10^{-6}M)	104 ± 7*	42 ± 5*	15 ± 3*

For legend see Table 4.

Effect of 2-Mercaptoethanol on the PHA Response of MNL With or Without Antibiotic

The antioxidant properties of a thiol compound like 2-ME was tested first on the depressed PHA response of MNL induced by macrolides. As seen in Table 4, the PHA proliferative responses with 2-ME were not modified in control culture conditions, but were enhanced in presence of high dose of spiramycin (100 μg/ml); Table 5 represents the PHA responses of MNL in presence of Ofl, Pef or Cip at 100 μg/ml concentration. We noted a larger depressive action of Pef and Cip than that of Ofl. But the protective action of 2-ME is significant with the three quinolone antibiotics.

Effects of 2-ME on MNL Response to PHA Depressed by Antibiotics in Hyperoxic Conditions

We previously found that oxygen concentrations modulated the proliferative response to ConA of rat lymphoid cells (13,14). We confirmed these results on human MNL response to PHA, as seen in Table 6. In these conditions, 2-ME can be considered as an efficient antioxidant agent. The protection obtained at 2-ME optimal concentration was time dependent (lower after 48 hrs. than 24 hrs.), partial but highly significant ($p \leq 10^{-3}$). In presence of Sp, Pef, Cip and Ofl, the results were summarized in Table 7.

In hyperoxic conditions, the ^{3}H-TdR incorporation of MNL was depressed after PHA stimulation. Addition of different antibiotics increased these depressive responses. In spite of the presence of high antibiotic concentra-

Table 6. Effect of O_2 Exposure (FiO_2 = 0.95; $FiCO_2$ = 0.05) on ^{3}H-TdR Incorporation (cpm) by PHA Stimulated Human MNL

Culture medium	0.5	0.3	0.3
2-ME (5.10^{-6}M)	1	0.5	0.5
PHA (10 μg/ml)	135	67	9
PHA + 2-ME (5.10^{-6}M)	130*	100*	32*

For legend see Table 4.

Table 7. Effects of 2-ME on MNL Response to PHA Depressed by Sp, Pef, Cip and Ofl in Hyperoxic Cultures

	Sp	Pef	Cip	Ofl
^{3}H-TdR incorporation (cpm) after 24 hr. O_2 exposure	55 ± 3	51 ± 4	60 ± 5	64 ± 5
In presence of 100 μg/ml antibiotic	25 ± 3	8 ± 0.8	2 ± 0.3	42 ± 4
In presence of 100 μg/ml antibiotic + 2-ME (5.10^{-6}M)	51 ± 3	26 ± 3	15 ± 2	76 ± 7

For legend see Table 4.

tion, 2-ME, at optimal concentrations, showed a more or less protection of the DNA proliferation (Ofl > Sp > Pef > Cip).

DISCUSSION

The present work confirmed the fact that some antimicrobial agents from different antibiotic families were able to exhibit in vitro immunosuppressive properties on human MNL. Macrolides and quinolones derivatives studied here showed depressed phytohaemagglutinin (PHA) responses at various concentrations. In addition, a reducing thiol compound, the 2-Mercaptoethanol may partly protect the mitogens MNL responses, particularly with spiramycin or Ofloxacin. Modification of proliferative responses in the presence of macrolide or quinolone antibiotics could be due to penetration and intracellular accumulation effects. Macrolide antibiotics are known for their good penetration into eukaryote cells (5), but also in vitro into phagocytic cells (12,17) and in vivo into alveolar rat macrophages (16).

Although Sp and Er exhibited some similar pharmacokinetic properties (e.g. intracellular penetration), intracellular half-life and accumulation rate were different: Sp has a much longer half-life than Er (16). In spite of these differences, the dose response correlations of mitogen responses were not affected. Increasing linearly with the macrolide antibiotic concentration, the inhibiting effect was already significant at low concentration (close to the concentrations obtained in vivo during an antibiotic treatment). The suppressor effects induced by each of the two macrolides were observed after both PHA and PWM stimulation. PHA is known to be a T cell mitogen (11) while PWM stimulates blast formation of B cells in the presence of T helper cells (9). Consequently it could be hypothesized that T and/or B cells participate in macrolide-induced suppression of the proliferative response. Interactions between different cells and particularly those involving macrophages are a pre-requisite for lymphocyte activation by specific and non-specific mitogens (18). Penetration of phagocytic cells by Er or Sp might also modify these accessory cells. The immunosuppressive effects of the three quinolone antibiotics tested here (Pef, Cip and Ofl) were not dose related; low concentrations (close to the concentration obtained in vivo during an antibiotic treatment) have no inhibiting effect against the PHA-induced proliferation of MNL. This inhibiting effect appeared with high doses of quinolone antibiotic showing significant differences between the three drugs tested. At an antibiotic concentration of 100 μg/ml, the PHA-induced proliferation of MNL is practically abolished with Cip, highly decreased with Pef; the effect of Ofl was moderate and close to that of the macrolide antibiotics.

We previously studied the changes in intraphagocytic concentration which occurred following the administration of different Pef doses in rats and showed the good intracellular penetration of this quinolone derivative. All quinolone antibiotics must be concentrated by leucocytes, but the pharmacokinetic characteristics (such as half-life) could be different from those of macrolide antibiotics. Trypan blue exclusion and the lactic dehydrogenase release test revealed that neither macrolides nor quinolones affected the cell viability, even at high antibiotic concentration; but these results do not exclude an ultimate metabolic and/or toxic cellular effect. 2-Mercaptoethanol (2-ME) is a well-known antioxidant thiol compound, used for a long time for murine immunological technics (4). We have previously shown that 2-ME protected against the inhibition of the mitogen-induced proliferation of splenic cells in mice or rat exposed to normobaric oxygen exposure (7,8). In order to explore if the immunodepressive effects of antibiotics, described above, were related to an oxidant injury, we tested the effect of 2-ME on the antibiotic-immune cell interactions in presence of mitogen. We demonstrated a significant protective effect of 2-ME with all the tested antibiotics added at high doses to the MNL culture stimulated by PHA in air (with 5% CO_2) and in hyperoxia (O_2 = 95%; CO_2 = 5%) conditions. But the degree of the effect varied with the different antibiotics tested. 2-ME was more efficient on Sp and Ofl immune responses than Pef and especially Cip. Therefore the protective effects of a reducing thiol compound is in accord with the hypothesis of an oxidant injury induced by the antibiotics inhibiting mitogen immune response of human MNL. We know neither the cause of the difference in effects of 2-ME with different tested drugs, nor the mechanism of the antibiotic oxidant effect.

Intracellular accumulation of these antibiotics could be in favor of the hypothesis of cellular toxicity, (especially accessory cells) induced by a high dose of the drug. Presently we should test in vitro other reducing thiol compounds to confirm this hypothesis. The therapeutic interest of the above results should be further evaluated in animal models, such as those obtained with rifampin or fusidic acid in mice (2). The antioxidant drugs able to protect the immune system from an eventual antibiotic injury could then be evaluated in vivo. This hypothetic oxidant injury could be related either to a direct effect of an N-oxide antibiotic metabolite and/or to a modification of a metabolic pathway, as a perturbation of the glutathione cycle.

SUMMARY

Macrolides and quinolones demonstrated, as other antibiotic families, immunosuppressive properties, particularly on the mitogen proliferative response of human mononuclear leucocytes (MNL). We studied erythromycin (Er) and spiramycin (Sp) effects: both exhibited the same dose-related inhibition of DNA synthesis. This inhibition was already significant at low antibiotic concentration (1-10 μg/ml) and was more pronounced at high antibiotic concentration. Similar results were observed whatever mitogen was used, PHA or PWM. Different quinolone carboxylic acid derivatives, pefloxacin (Pef), Ofloxacin (Ofl) and Ciprofloxacin (Cip) were tested. The inhibition of the proliferative response was obtained only with high antibiotic concentration (over 25 μg/ml) but not with therapeutic antibiotic doses (0.1 to 10 μg/ml). The addition of the thiol compound, 2-Mercaptoethanol (2-ME) in the culture medium with high doses of all the above antibiotics significantly protected the immune response (Sp = Ofl > Pef > Cip). The antioxidant properties of 2-ME are well demonstrated. We can hypothesize that this type of antibiotic immune injury could be partly mediated by an oxidant injury. The mechanism of this injury could be related to an oxidant metabolite which is derived from the antibiotic demethyl metabolites. The drugs able to protect the immune cells from an oxidant stress could then represent a new family of immunomodulator agents.

ACKNOWLEDGMENTS

We are grateful to Mrs. Michèle Despalin for preparing and typing this manuscript.

REFERENCES

1. G. Bänk and A. Forsgren, Antibiotics and suppression of lymphocyte function in vitro, Antimicrob Agents Chemother. 16:554 (1979).
2. A. Bellahsene and A. Forsgren, Effect of fusidic acid on the immune response in mice, Infect Immun. 29:873 (1980).
3. A. Boyum, Isolation of mononuclear cells and granulocytes from human blood, Scand. J. Clin. Lab. Invest. 21:77 (1968).
4. J. D. Broome and M. W. Jeng, Promotion of replication in lymphoid cells by specific thiols and disulfides in vitro. Effects of mouse lymphoma cells in comparison with splenic lymphocytes, J. Exp. Med. 138:574 (1973).
5. K. N. Brown and A. Percival, Penetration of antimicrobials into tissue culture cells and leukocytes, Scand. J. Infect. Dis. 14:251 (1978).
6. E. A. Chaperon and W. E. Sanders, Suppression of lymphocyte responses by cephalosporins, Infect. Immun. 19:378 (1978).
7. M. A. Gougerot-Pocidalo, M. Fay and J. J. Pocidalo, In vivo normobaric oxygen exposure depresses spleen cell in vitro ConA response. Effects of 2-mercaptoethanol and peritoneal cells, Clin. Exp. Immunol. 58:428 (1984).
8. M. A. Gougerot-Pocidalo, M. Levacher, L. Kraus, E. Azoulay-Dupuis, H. Mansour and J. J. Pocidalo, Agression oxydante et immunitè spècifique, in: "Infections, Causes et Dèficits Immunitaires," J. J. Pocidalo and J. P. Coulaud, eds., Arnette, Paris (1984).
9. M. F. Greaves, G. Janossy and M. Doehnoff, Selective triggering of human T and B lymphocytes in vitro by polyclonal mitogens, J. Exp. Med. 140:1 (1974).
10. W. E. Hauser and J. S. Remington, Effects of antibiotics on the immune response, Am. J. Med. 72:711 (1982).
11. G. Janossy and M. F. Greaves, Lymphocyte activation. I. response of T and B lymphocytes to phytomitogens, Clin. Exp. Immunol. 9:483 (1971).
12. J. O. Johnson, W. L. Hand, J. B. Francis, N. Ying-Thompson and R. W. Corwin, Antibiotic uptake by alveolar macrophages, J. Lab. Clin. Med. 95:424 (1980).
13. L. Kraus, Ph. Lacombe, M. Fay and J. J. Pocidalo, High concentrations of oxygen modulate in vitro ConA responses of rat lymphoid cells. Effects of 2-mercaptoethanol, Immunol. Letters in press (1985).
14. L. Kraus, M. A. Gougerot-Pocidalo and J. J. Pocidalo, Depression of ConA proliferative response of immune cells by in vitro hyperoxic exposure. Protective effects of thiol compounds, Int. J. Immunopharmacol. in press (1985).
15. H. Ohmori and I. Yamamoto, Mechanism of augmentation of the antibody response in vitro by 2-ME in murine lymphocytes. I. 2-ME induced stimulation of the uptake of cysteine, an essential amino acid, J. Exp. Med. 155:1277 (1982).
16. J. J. Pocidalo, F. Albert, J. F. Desnottes and S. Kernbaum, Intraphagocytic penetration of macrolides. In vivo comparison of erythromycin and spiramycin, J. Antimicrob. Chemother. in press (1985).
17. R. C. Prokesch and W. L. Hand, Antibiotic entry into human polymorphonuclear leukocytes, Antimicrob. Agents Chemother. 21:373 (1982).
18. E. R. Unanue, The regulatory role of the macrophage in antigenic stimulation. II. Symbiotic relationship between lymphocytes and macrophages, Adv. Immunol. 31:17 (1981).

SECTION VI
RELATIONSHIP BETWEEN IMMUNE STIMULATORS AND ANTIBIOTICS

AMPHOTERICIN B - A MODEL MURINE IMMUNOSTIMULANT

J. R. Little, S. H. Stein and K. D. Little

The Jewish Hospital at Washington University Medical Center
and the Department of Microbiology & Immunology
Washington University School of Medicine
St. Louis, Missouri

INTRODUCTION

Amphotericin B (AmB) was first isolated from the fermentation products of Streptomyces nodosus in 1956 (35). Its broad spectrum of antifungal activity and therapeutic efficacy made it possible to treat successfully a number of fungal infections that previously had been almost invariably fatal (6,17,33). Nearly 30 years after its discovery, AmB remains the most important agent in the treatment of systemic fungal infections. In addition to its direct antifungal properties, studies have indicated that AmB can stimulate murine host resistance to certain nonfungal infections (22,32) and to several kinds of tumors (18,34). The exact mechanism of these host protective effects has not been established but it seems probable that the stimulation of lymphoid cells by AmB plays a significant role.

Several studies from our laboratories have shown that in many mouse strains, AmB or its derivative, amphotericin B methyl ester (AME), can stimulate cell mediated (27,28) as well as humoral immunity (1,16,30) with a potency comparable to complete Freund's adjuvant. Among the in vitro immunostimulant effects, murine polyclonal B cell activation (PBA) was first reported by Hammarstrom and Smith (11,12) and these results have been confirmed and extended (15). Lin et al. have reported stimulation of murine macrophages in vivo as well as in vitro (14) and our laboratory has shown that AmB stimulates interleukin-1 (IL-1) production by normal murine macrophage cultures (29).

In the studies reported here, we provide new evidence that optimal stimulation of lymphocytes by AME in vitro requires the participation of accessory cells. In addition, we show that the stimulation of lymphoid cells by AmB or AME can be related to the formation of reactive oxygen metabolites, especially H_2O_2.

MATERIALS AND METHODS

Mice

AKR/J and C3H/HeJ 6-8 week old female mice were obtained from the Jackson Laboratories, Bar Harbor, ME. A/J and C57BL/6J (B/6) females were obtained from the Animal Resources Facility, The Jewish Hospital at Washington University Medical Center.

Reagents

AME (SQ 14,518; batch NN013ND) as the aspartate salt was supplied by W. E. Brown (E. R. Squibb and Sons, Princeton, NJ). AmB was purchased as Fungizone (Squibb) and reconstituted in 5% dextrose just before use. *A. niger* catalase and animotriazole (AT) were the products of Sigma Chemical Co. (St. Louis, MO), lipopolysaccharide (LPS) from *E. coli* 0127-B8 was obtained from Difco Laboratories, Detroit, MI. Purified protein derivative (PPD), batch RT32, lot 16, was obtained from Statens Seruminstitut, Copenhagen, Denmark.

Polyclonal B Cell Activation

Spleen cell suspensions were prepared from 4-6 normal female mice. Cells were pooled, washed by centrifugation and incubated for 48 hrs in RPMI 1640 containing 10% fetal calf serum (FCS) (Reheis-Armour Pharmaceutical, Kankakee, IL) and various stimuli (AME, LPS or PPD). After incubation, each culture was washed and scored for direct plaque forming cells (PFC) (36) with trinitrophenylated (TNP) sheep erythrocytes used as indicator cells (26). Control cultures containing no mitogen were included in each experiment. The catalase effect was observed with spleen cell suspensions that had been preincubated in catalase (1000 U/ml) for 1 hr at 37°C then washed twice and resuspended in RPMI 1640 with 10% FCS and incubated 48 hrs in the presence or absence of a B cell mitogen before scoring for anti-TNP PFC.

IL-1 Assay

This assay was performed as described by Mizel (19). Macrophage culture supernatants were diluted 1:4, 1:8 and 1:16 with RPMI 1640 with 5% FCS, 2×10^{-5} M 2-mercaptoethanol, 1% glutamine, penicillin, streptomycin, and 12 mM Hepes buffer, pH 7.2. The assay system consisted of 1.5×10^{6} C3H/HeJ thymocytes per culture in RPMI 1640 with 5% FCS and 1 µg/ml PHA in flat bottom microtiter cultures performed in sets of four. After 48 hrs, 0.5 µCi ^{3}H-thymidine (5 Ci/mMole, New England Nuclear, Boston, MA) was added to each culture for the final 24 hr incubation. Cultures were harvested automatically on Whatman 934-AH glass fiber filters and the radioactivity (cpm) incorporated into DNA was estimated from the filter bound cpm, determined with a Packard Tricarb Scintillation Spectrometer.

Macrophage Cultures

Murine bone marrow macrophage cultures were derived and propagated as described previously (13) and P388.D1 cells were obtained from the American Type Culture Collection (Rockville, MD). The untransformed macrophage cell lines were serially cultured in Dulbecco's Modified Eagle's Medium with high glucose/high bicarbonate, 10% FCS (HyClone Laboratories, Logan, UT), 5% horse serum, and 10% L cell conditioned medium.

^{35}S-Methionine Labeling of Macrophage Secretions

A/J and B/6 macrophage cell lines were incubated in flat bottom microtiter plates (5×10^{4} cells/well) in Dulbecco's Modified Eagle's Medium with high glucose/high bicarbonate and 10% L cell conditioned medium. After 24 hrs at 37°C in 5% CO_2, the medium was aspirated and replaced with methionine-free medium without FCS or horse serum, but containing dialyzed 1% L cell conditioned medium. To this was added AmB (5 µg/ml) or additional media (control cultures). After 48 hrs, approximately 4.4 µCi of ^{35}S-meth-

Table 1. Effect of X-Irradiated Filler Cells on AME-Induced B Cell Activation[a]

Viable spleen cell Density	X-Iradiated spleen cell Density	Mitogen	Average PFC (SE) per 10^7 viable SC
1×10^7/ml	-	0	28.4 (2.7)
1×10^7/ml	-	AME, 75 μg/ml	482.5 (8.5)
1×10^6/ml	-	AME, 75 μg/ml	50.2 (4.3)
1×10^6/ml	9×10^6/ml	0	77.5 (5.1)
1×10^6/ml	9×10^6/ml	AME, 75 μg/ml	350.0 (10.8)

[a]AKR spleen cells were cultured 48 hrs in 1.0 ml medium as described in Materials and Methods. Spleen cells from the same pool as viable cells were x-irradiated with 3000 R just prior to initiation of the cultures. Control cultures containig 1×10^7 irradiated spleen cells alone yielded <15 PFC/culture in the presence or absence of AME.

ionine (>800 Ci/mMole, Amersham Corp., Arlington Heights, IL) were added to each culture. Culture supernatants were harvested 24 hrs. later and aliquots of each supernatant were analyzed on 13% polyacrylamide slab gels (PAGE) containing 1% sodium dodecyl sulfate (SDS). The gels were fixed in 50% methanol-10% acetic acid, dried and autoradiograms were prepared with Kodak SB-5 (Rochester, NY) x-ray film. The developed autoradiograms were scanned in an E-C Densitometer, the height of each band on triplicate scans was measured, averaged and the percent change from the control in each band was calculated. The molecular weight of each radioactive band was estimated from 14C standards (m.w. = 14,000 - 200,000, Amersham) on the same gel.

RESULTS

Splenic Adherent Cells Augment AME-induced Polyclonal B Cell Activation (PBA)

Previously published results showed a striking dependency of AME-induced murine PBA on the density of cells in culture (15). The optimum spleen cell density was found to be 1×10^7 cells/ml. AME added to splenocyte cultures at a density of 1×10^6 cells/ml induced no detectable B cell proliferation. This result suggested that cell-to-cell proximity or direct cellular contacts were required for B cell activation and proliferation. To determine if accessory cells were required for AME-induced PBA, x-irradiated normal spleen cells were added to cultures of syngeneic viable spleen cells containing AME. The data in Table 1 indicate that a culture containing 90% x-irradiated cells markedly augmented the PBA response of 1×10^6 viable spleen cells.

The experiment in Table 2 was performed to determine if isolated splenic adherent cells (mainly macrophages) would reconstitute adherent-cell depleted spleen cell cultures stimulated by AME. Following the depletion of adherent cells, the PBA response of 1×10^7 lymphocytes per ml was much reduced and was increased greater than two-fold by the addition of 10% splenic adherent cells.

Table 2. Adherent Cells Reconstitute AME-Induced PBA[a]

Adherent cell depleted lymphocytes[b] (cells/ml)	Adherent cells (cells/ml)[c]	AME concentration (μg/ml)	Average IgM PFC per culture	P value[d]
1×10^7	-	0	4.8 (1.0)	
1×10^7	-	75	83.3 (14.2)	
1×10^7	-	25	91.2 (11.9)	
-	1×10^6	75	<1.0	
1×10^7	1×10^6	0	10.0 (6.0)	
1×10^7	1×10^6	75	216.0 (8.9)	<0.05
1×10^7	1×10^6	25	134.3 (6.7)	<0.05

[a]AKR females were used as donors of splenic lymphocytes and 2 hr adherent cells.
[b]Splenic lymphocytes were harvested as nonadherent cells after 2 hr incubation at 37°C of whole spleen cell suspensions (5×10^6 cells/ml) in polystyrene petri dishes.
[c]Adherent cells were harvested by a jet spray technique (13) from polystyrene petri dishes following removal of the nonadherent cell fraction.
[d]P values were derived from student's t-test. Each P value represents a comparison between indicated culture and corresponding adherent cell depleted control (i.e., 10^7 lymphocytes/ml + 75 μg/ml or 25 μg/ml AME).

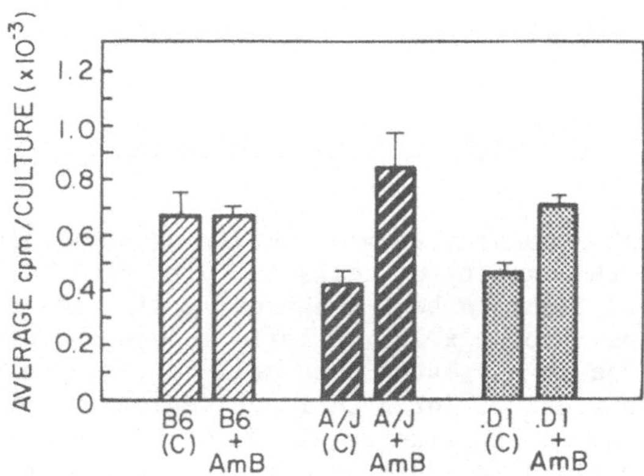

Figure 1. AmB stimulated IL-1 secretion. Bone marrow derived macrophages from A/J and B/6 mice or P388.D1 (.D1) cells were cultured in 1 ml growth medium (22) in 24 well plates. 1×10^6 cells/ml were inoculated into each well and after 24 hr cell adherence, the medium was apirated and replaced by 1 ml RPMI 1640 without serum $\pm$ 0.5 μg/ml AmB. After 1 hr incubation with or without AmB, the medium was aspirated and replaced with fresh RPMI 1640 + 5% FCS for 24 hr incubation at 37°C in 5% CO_2. These 24 hr culture supernatants were then harvested for IL-1 bioassay on C3H/HeJ thymocytes as described by Mizel (21).

AmB Simulates Macrophage Secretion In Vitro

AmB-induced adjuvant effects in vivo and the PBA responses to AME and AmB in vitro were induced in most but not all inbred mouse strains (15). There was complete concordance between those inbred strains showing strong adjuvant responses and the strains whose normal spleen cells showed vigorous PBA during stimulation by AME in culture. The low or non-responding strains in both assays were also concordant. In view of the adherent cell dependency of the PBA response (Table 2), we tested the capacity of AmB to stimulate isolated macrophages from various strains in culture. Figure 1 shows the results of bioassays (murine thymocyte comitogenesis) of IL-1 activity in 24 hr macrophage culture supernatants collected after a 1 hr incubation in AmB. Macrophage cultures exhibited a statistically significant increase in IL-1 activity following incubations in 0.5 - 10 µg/ml AmB. B/6 and other strains related to C57BL were consistent exceptions. B/6 macrophage supernatants showed no change in IL-1 activity after 1 hr incubation in 0.5 µ g/ml AmB. Higher AmB concentrations (e.g. 5 µg/ml) regularly produced a reduction in IL-1 activity secreted by B/6 macrophages under the same conditions that produced an increase (up to six-fold) in the IL-1 activity secreted by A/J, AKR, DBA/2 or CBA macrophages. Also shown (Figure 1) is the increase in IL-1 secretion by the transformed macrophage line P388.D1 (19,20).

Figure 2 shows that AmB stimulated the secretion of several other polypeptides by cultured macrophages from A/J mice, a typical AmB-high responder

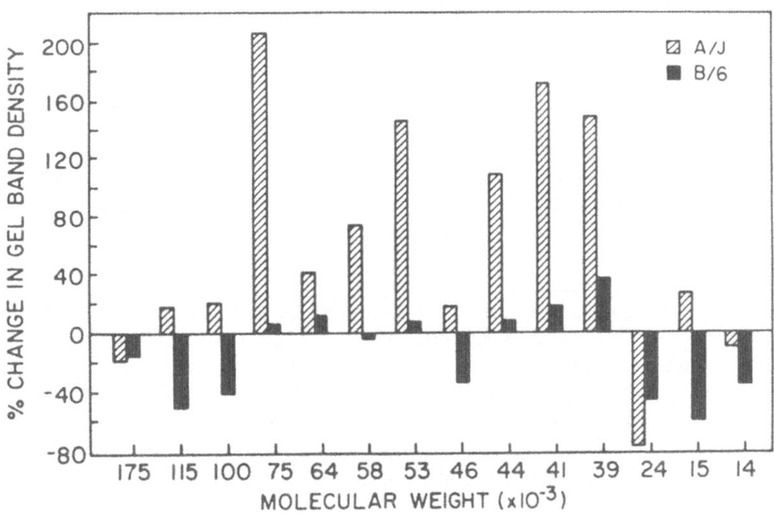

Figure 2. SDS-PAGE autoradiogram densitometry of culture supernatants from AmB-treated macrophages. Bone marrow derived A/J and B/6 macrophages were cultured in microtiter plates (5×10^4 cells/well) at 37°C in 5% CO_2. After adherence at 24 hr, the medium was aspirated, each well was filled with methionine-free medium and AmB (5 µg/ml) or medium (control). At 48 hrs, approximately 4.4 µCi of 35S-methionine were added to each well. Culture supernatants were harvested at 72 hr and analyzed on 13% SDS-PAGE slab gels followed by autoradiography and densitometry scanning of the x-ray film. The height of each band on triplicate scans was measured and averaged. The percent change in each band density produced by AmB (ordinate) is shown for A/J (cross-hatched bars) and B/6 (solid bars) cells. The molecular weight of each band (abscissa) was estimated from ^{14}C molecular weight standards on the same gel.

Table 3. Effect of Catalase Preincubation on Polyclonal B Cell Mitogenicity

Pretreatment of spleen cells[a]	Mitogen	Average IgM PFC/culture (SE)	% of mitogen response	P value[b]
None	-	48.5 (3.5)	-	-
None	AME-75	471.7 (12.8)	100	
CAT-1000	AME-75	221.0 (4.2)	47	<0.01
None	LPS-100	554.5 (37.5)	100	
CAT-1000	LPS-100	161.0 (20.8)	29	<0.01
None	PPD-100	216.7 (50.2)	100	
CAT-1000	PPD-100	92.0 (5.6)	42	<0.05

[a]Spleen cells from female AKR mice were preincubated 1 hr in 1000 U/ml catalase (CAT-1000) from A. niger at 37°C in RMPI-1640, 10%FCS or in medium alone (no pretreatment). The cells were then washed twice and resuspended in fresh medium containing either no mitogen, 75 μg/ml AME, 100 μg/ml LPS, or 100 μg/ml PPD. After 48 hr incubation at 37°C in 5% CO_2, the cells from each culture were washed by centrifugation and scored for direct PFC using TNP-SRBC as indicator cells.
[b]P values were calculated for comparison of PFC responses in the presence or absence of catalase by Students' t-test.

strain. Newly synthesized and secreted radiolabeled peptides produced in A/J or B/6 macrophages were displayed in adjacent lanes of an SDS-PAGE slab gel. Densitometric scanning of an x-ray film autoradiogram permitted a comparison of the AmB-induced increase or decrease in the secretion of individual polypeptides from A/J or B/6 macrophages.

AmB stimulated the secretion of most of the major peptide products formed by A/J macrophages under the same conditions that resulted in unchanged or depressed secretion by B/6 macrophages. Companion results from this experiment (data not shown) indicated that A/J macrophages were more resistant to the toxicity of higher concentrations of AmB (10-20 μg/ml) than were B/6 macrophages.

H_2O_2 Participates in the B Cell Stimulation Induced by AME In Vitro

Studies by Brajtburg et al. of AmB-induced erythrocyte lysis (2) indicated that reactive oxygen metabolites were involved in the lytic process. These results suggested the possibility that oxygen metabolites might also participate in the immunostimulant properties of AmB. The results shown in Table 3 support this hypothesis. Catalase added to PBA cultures of AKR spleen cells had a marked inhibitory effect on AME stimulation. Catalase also inhibited the PPD- or LPS-induced PBA of AKR spleen cells (Table 3).

Because catalase consistently inhibited PBA responses to AME in spleen cell cultures from all the AmB-high responder strains tested and because these same strains have also been reported to exhibit high liver cell catalase activity (25), we next examined the effect of 3-amino-1,2,4-triazole (AT), a selective catalase inhibitor, on AME-induced spleen cell PBA. The results of two experiments are presented in Table 4. AT treatment of AKR spleen cells in vitro or the i.p. injection of AKR mice with AT resulted in a reduction of AME induced PBA. In experiment 2 (Table 4), a selective

Table 4. Aminotriazole Inhibits AME-induced PBA

Treatment	Mitogen	Average PFC/culture (SE)	% of mitogen response	P value[b]
Experiment 1 - Aminotriazole in vitro (spleen cells)[a]				
None	0	18 (5)		
25mM AT, 1h, 37°C	0	12 (2)		
None	AME	226 (10)	100	
25mM AT, 1h, 37°C	AME	143 (9)	63	< 0.01
Experiment 2 - Aminotriazole in vivo[c] (mice)				
None	0	6 (1)		
6 x 25 mg AT/mouse	0	3 (1)		
None	AME	130 (12)	100	
6 x 25 mg AT/mouse	AME	72 (4)	55	< 0.02
None	LPS	329 (25)	100	
6 x 25 mg AT/mouse	LPS	308 (34)	94	N.S.

[a]In Experiment 1, spleen cells from normal AKR female mice were preincubated at 37°C for 1 hr in 25 mM aminotriazole (AT) in 0.15 M NaCl or in NaCl alone. After washing, the cells were resuspended in medium ± 75 μg/ml AME and incubated for 48 hrs before PFC scoring.

[b]p values were determined by Student's t-test. Comparison is between experimental (AT) samples and the corresponding mitogen response without AT treatment.

[c]Normal female AKR mice were injected i.p. twice daily for 3 days with AT (25 mg/mouse) in 0.15 M NaCl solution. Control mice received 0.15 M NaCl i.p. by the same schedule. All mice were sacrificed for PFC assay 15 hrs after the last injection. Mitogen concentrations used in the cultures were 75 μg/ml AME or 100 μg/ml LPS.

effect on B cell stimulation by AME was observed since LPS-induced PBA was undiminished in aliquots of spleen cells from the same AT recipient mice that showed a 45% reduction of the AME response.

DISCUSSION

Our results indicating modulation of AME-induced PBA by adherent accessory cells are at variance with the results from Hammarstrom and Smith (11). The difference can probably be explained by the failure of macrophage depletion techniques to ablate the PBA response and the much weaker PBA induced by AmB (used by Hammarstrom and Smith) compared with AME (Tables 1 and 2). Although we did not succeed in reducing the PBA response to background following adherent cell depletion, it was sufficiently low that reconstitution of B cell stimulation by adding back splenic adherent cells was successful (Table 2).

The experimental results in Tables 1 and 2 suggest that macrophages serve as the modulating accessory cell in murine B cell stimulation by AME in vitro. Macrophages are the most prevalent adherent cells in the spleen; accessory cell activity is x-irradiation resistant (Table 1) and macrophages are known to be required for optimal responses to several other murine B and T lymphocyte mitogens (3,9,10). We cannot exclude the possibility that dendritic cells are important in AME-induced mitogenicity since they would have been retained in the adherent cell fraction (31) used in Table 2. We have shown previously that T cells were not required for AME-induced PBA, since good responses were obtained with spleen cells from severely T cell deficient nude mice (data not shown) as well as anti-thy-1 treated AKR spleen cells (15). This conclusion is in accordance with that of Hammarstrom and Smith (11).

The finding that AmB stimulated IL-1 secretion from murine macrophages in vitro (Figure 1), provides support for a unitarian hypothesis for the immunostimulant effects of AmB in vivo as well as in vitro. Immune stimulation by enhanced IL-1 secretion would be in accordance with the physiological role of IL-1 to enhance T cell growth factor stimulation of helper T cells (24) and to augment B cell activation and proliferation in vitro (7).

Enhancement of IL-1 production has been shown for LPS (5) and muramyl dipeptide (MDP) (23) and it has been suggested that stimulation of IL-1 secretion is a common property of immunoadjuvants (4). The failure of AmB to stimulate IL-1 secretion from B/6 macrophages may also explain the failure of this strain and related C57BL inbred strains to exhibit the adjuvant effects of AmB while preserving responses to other adjuvants (16).

The results in Figure 2 indicated that AmB also stimulated secretion of peptides other than IL-1 that were formed by macrophages from AmB-high responder mouse strains. The presence of increased ^{35}S-protein in the supernatants of macrophages incubated in AmB cannot be attributed to cell leakage. Cellular toxicity would be expected to result in less, not more, protein synthesis and secretion. Also, if cell permeabilization by AmB were the cause of increased labeled protein in the macrophage supernatants, it would be expected to result in preferential leakage of low molecular weight species, yet the amount of the 14 Kd product in the supernatant of AmB treated macrophages was less than in untreated control macrophages. The major results of this experiment were that AmB stimulated the secretion of a variety of macrophage protein products and that the macrophages from an AmB-high responder strain (A/J) were more stimulated than macrophages from the low responder strain (B/6). The strain specific effects of AmB could be explained in a relatively simple fashion if the cells from B/6 and other low responder strains were more sensitive to AmB-induced toxicity than the corresponding cells from high responders. Other experiments from our laboratory (data not shown) support this interpretation.

A striking inhibition of mitogenic activity was observed when catalase was continuously present throughout the 48 hr incubation in AME (data not shown). However, this result could have been explained by an interaction between catalase and AME blunting the AME stimulation. The results in Table 3 were obtained with spleen cells preincubated 1 hr in catalase, washed and then stimulated in culture by three different B cell mitogens. These conditions reduce the probability of a direct mitogen-catalase interaction. Significant inhibition of PBA responses by catalase pretreatment was observed for all three of these chemically diverse mitogens (Table 3). These results strongly suggest that H_2O_2 is required in the final pathway to B cell proliferation stimulated by mitogens in vitro.

The hypothesis that H_2O_2 may produce stimulatory effects on certain kinds of lymphocytes also provided a clue to a possible mechanism for the low or absent immunostimulant effects of AmB in the C57BL strains. The same strains that are low responders to AmB are also reported to have low tissue catalase activity (25). Since catalase functions as an important scavenger of H_2O_2, cells with reduced catalase would be expected to be more susceptible to membrane damage via peroxidation. The concentrations of H_2O_2 required for AME induced PBA (Table 3) may be toxic for lymphoid cells from low catalase mouse strains.

The excellent correlation between mouse strains that show high responses to AmB and high tissue catalase activity (15,25) suggests that a high intracellular catalase concentration is required for lymphoid cell stimulation by AmB. On the other hand, catalase added to the medium probably had two effects. It protected against membrane peroxidation (2) but it also degraded the extracellular H_2O_2 to concentrations too low to promote mitogen induced lymphocyte proliferation. The data in Table 4 also support this line of reasoning. AT has been used extensively to inactivate cellular catalase. One hour incubation in 25 mM AT has been reported to reduce murine macrophage catalase >90% (21). Table 4 indicates that following in vitro (exp. 1) or in vivo (exp. 2) exposure to AT, the AME-induced PBA was significantly depressed. Although these results are in accord with the speculation that reduced cellular catalase is associated with reduced PBA responses, the results also suggest that catalase is not the only determinant of AmB reactivity. Liver (25) and macrophage (data not shown) catalase levels in the C57BL strains were about one-half those found in high catalase strains and the AME-induced PBA response of these strains was regularly <10% of high responders. In the results shown in Table 4, treatment with AT was sufficient to reduce cellular catalase to very low levels, yet, the AME responses were less than 50% reduced and the LPS response (exp. 2) was unaffected.

SUMMARY

AmB-induced murine immunostimulation provides a promising model system for studies of the mechanisms of adjuvant effects. Like many other immune stimuli, accessory cells seem to play an important role in AME responses. Inbred mouse strains bearing the C57BL background genes (regardless of MHC genotype) do not exhibit the immunostimulant effects of AmB. Hybrid offspring of an AmB high responder strain (e.g. AKR) and a low responder (C57BL/6) show low responses (15). Catalase inhibits AME-induced PBA, suggesting a critical role for H_2O_2 in the stimulation of lymphoid cells. The mouse strain distribution of tissue catalase activity reported by others (25) correlates directly with AmB responsiveness (15). Genetic dominance of the low AmB responder phenotype is also in accordance with the pattern of liver catalase expression in hybrids of high and low catalase parents in which the low catalase phenotype is dominant (8). We interpret these results to indicate that the magnitude of AmB responsiveness is related to differences in peroxidative damage among different inbred mouse strains and that the concentrations of H_2O_2 that are required for lymphoid cell stimulation by AmB are toxic for C57BL strains because of their low cellular catalase activity. We also conclude that the immunostimulant effects of AmB may play a significant role in the therapeutic efficacy of AmB in the treatment of systemic fungal infections.

ABBREVIATIONS USED

AmB, Amphotericin B; AME, Amphotericin B methyl ester; PBA, polyclonal B cell activation; IL-1, interleukin-1; AT, 3-amino-1,2,4-triazole; LPS, lipopolysaccharide from E. coli 0127-B8; PPD, purified protein derivative derived from M. tuberculosis; FCS, fetal calf serum; TNP, the 2,4-6-trinitrophenyl group; cpm, counts per minute; PAGE, polyacrylamide gel electrophoresis; SDS, sodium dodecyl sulfate; and MDP, muramyl dipeptide.

ACKNOWLEDGMENTS

This work was supported by U. S. Public Health Service Grants CA-15665 and AI-15353 and 5T32-CA-09118 from the National Institute of Health and by a grant from the American Cancer Society (IM-371).

REFERENCES

1. T. J. Blanke, J. R. Little, S. F. Shirley and R. G. Lynch, Augmentation of murine immune responses by amphotericin B, Cell. Immunol. 33:180 (1977).
2. J. Brajtburg, G. Medoff and G. S. Kobayashi, Action of amphotericin B on inbred mouse strains. I. Toxic effects are mouse strain dependent (submitted for publication) (1985).
3. C. Cortel and F. Melchers, Requirement for macrophages or for macrophage- or T cell-derived factors in the mitogenic stimulation of murine B lymphocytes by lipopolysaccharides, Eur. J. Immunol. 13:528 (1983).
4. C. A. Dinarello, Interleukin-1, Rev. Infect. Dis. 6:51 (1984).
5. G. W. Duff and E. Atkins, The detection of endotoxin by in vitro production of endogenous pyrogen: Comparison with limulus amebocyte lysate gelation, J. Immunol. 52:323 (1982).
6. G. Edwards and C. J. P. LaTouche, The treatment of bronchopulmonary mycoses with a new antibiotic - primaricin, Lancet 1:1349 (1964).
7. R. J. M. Falkoff, A. Muraguchi, J-X Hong, J. L. Butler, C. A. Dinarello and A. S. Fauci, The effect of interleukin-1 on human B cell activation and proliferation, J. Immunol. 131:801 (1983).
8. R. E. Ganschow and R. T. Schimke, Murine catalase phenotypes, Biochem. Genetics 4:157 (1970).
9. D. K. Greineder and A. L. Rosenthal, The requirement for macrophage-lymphocyte interaction in T lymphocyte proliferation induced by generation of aldehydes on cell membranes, J. Immunol. 115:932 (1975).
10. S. Habu and M. C. Raff, Accessory cell dependence of lectin-induced proliferation of mouse T lymphocytes, Eur. J. Immunol. 7:451 (1977).
11. L. Hammarstrom and E. Smith, Mitogenic properties of polyene antibiotics for murine B cells, Scand. J. Immunol. 5:37 (1976).
12. L. Hammarstrom and E. Smith, In vitro activating properties of polyene antibiotics for murine lymphocytes, Acta Pathol. Microbiol. Scand. (C) 85:277 (1977).
13. C. R. Johnson, D. Kitz and J. R. Little, A method for the derivation and continuous propagation of cloned murine bone marrow macrophages, J. Immunol. Methods 65:319 (1983).
14. H-S. Lin, G. Medoff and G. S. Kobayashi, Effects of amphotericin B on macrophages and their precursor cells, Amtimicrob. Agents Chemother. 11:154 (1977).
15. J. R. Little, A. Abegg and E. Plut, The relationship between adjuvant and mitogenic effects of amphotericin methyl ester, Cell. Immunol. 78:224 (1983).
16. J. R. Little, E. J. Plut, J. Kotler-Brajtburg, G. Medoff and G. S. Kobayashi, Relationship between the antibiotic and immunoadjuvant effects of amphotericin B methyl ester, Immunochemistry 15:219 (1978).
17. W. R. Lockwood, J. F. Busey, E. B. Blair and F. Allison, Preferred treatment of blastomycosis with 2-hydroxy-stilbamidine, Clin. Res. 10:60 (1962).
18. G. Medoff, F. Valeriote, R. G. Lynch, D. Schlessinger and G. S. Kobayashi, Synergistic effect of amphotericin B and 1,3-Bis(2-chloroethyl)-1-nitrosourea against a transplantable AKR leukemia, Cancer Res. 34:974 (1974).

19. S. B. Mizel, Production and quantitation of lymphocyte-activating factor (Interleukin 1), in: "Manual of Macrophage Methodology," H. Herscowitz, H. Holden, J. Bellanti and A. Ghaffar, eds., Marcel Dekker, Inc., New York, NY (1981).
20. S. B. Mizel and D. Mizel, Purification to apparent homogeneity of murine interleukin 1, J. Immunol. 126:834 (1981).
21. H. W. Murray, C. F. Nathan and Z. A. Cohn, Macrophage oxygen-dependent antimicrobial activity. IV. Role of endogenous scavengers of oxygen intermediates, J. Exp. Med. 152:1610 (1980).
22. G. R. Olds, S. J. Stewart and J. J. Ellner, Amphotericin B-induced resistance to Schistosoma mansoni, J. Immunol. 126:1667 (1981).
23. J. J. Oppenheim, A. Togawa, L. Chedid and S. Mizel, Components of mycobacteria and muramyl dipeptide with adjuvant activity induced lymphocyte activating factor, Cell. Immunol. 50:71 (1980).
24. A. Rao, S. B. Mizel and H. Cantor, Disparate functional properties of two interleukin-1 responsive Ly-1+2- T cell clones: Distinction of T cell growth factor and T cell replacing factor activities, J. Immunol. 130:1743 (1983).
25. M. Rechcigl and W. E. Heston, Tissue catalase activity in several C57BL substrains and in other strains of inbred mice, J. Nat. Cancer Inst. 30:855 (1963).
26. M. B. Rittenberg and K. L. Pratt, Antitrinitrophenyl (TNP) plaque assay. Primary response of BALB/c mice to soluble and particulate immunogen, Proc. Soc. Exp. Biol. Med. 132:575 (1969).
27. S. F. Shirley and J. R. Little, Immunopotentiating effects of amphotericin B. I. Enhanced contact sensitivity in mice, J. Immunol. 123:2878 (1979).
28. S. F. Shirley and J. R. Little, Immunopotentiating effects of amphotericin B. II. Enhanced in vitro proliferative responses of murine lymphocytes, J. Immunol. 123:2883 (1979).
29. S. Stein and J. R. Little, Importance of interleukin-1 (IL-1) in the immunostimulation produced by amphotericin B (Abstr.) Fed. Proc. 43:1747 (1984).
30. S. H. Stein, E. Plut, T. J. Shine and J. R. Little, The importance of different murine cell types in the immunopotentiation produced by amphotericin methyl ester, Cell. Immunol. 40:211 (1978).
31. R. M. Steinman and M. C. Nussenzweig, Dendritic cells: features and function, Immunol. Rev. 53:127 (1980).
32. M. Z. Thomas, G. Medoff and G. S. Kobayashi, Changes in murine resistance to Listeria monocytogenes infection induced by amphotericin B, J. Infect. Dis. 127:374 (1973).
33. J. P. Utz, J. E. Bennett, M. W. Brandriss, W. T. Butler and G. J. Hill, Amphotericin B toxicity. Combined clinical staff conference at the National Institutes of Health, Ann. Intern. Med. 61:334 (1964).
34. F. Valeriote, G. Medoff, S. Tolen and J. Diekman, Amphotericin B potentiation of the cytotoxicity of anticancer agents on normal hematopoietic leukemia cells in mice, Cancer Res. 73:475 (1984).
35. J. Vandeputte, J. L. Wachtel and E. T. Stiller, Amphotericins A and B, antifungal antibiotics produced by a streptomyces. II. The isolation and properties of the crystalline amphotericins, in: "Antibiotics Annual 1955-1956," Medical Encyclopedia, Inc., New York, NY (1956).
36. H. Yamada and A. Yamada, Antibody formation against 2,4-dinitrophenyl-hapten at the cellular level. Hemolytic plaque-in-gel assay for lymphoid cells producing anti-2,4-dinitrophenyl-hapten antibody, J. Immunol. 103:357 (1969).

ATTEMPTS TO EXPLAIN IMMUNOLOGICAL SIDE EFFECTS OF ANTIBIOTICS ON THE PRODUCTION OF CELLULAR MEDIATORS

Günther Gillissen

Department of Medical Microbiology
Medical Faculty
Aachen, F.R.G.

INTRODUCTION

A prerequisite for an optimal therapeutic effect of antimicrobial chemotherapy is not only an adequate antibiotic but also a functionally intact immune system (2,3,72). The latter requirement applies to bacteriostatic drugs as well as to bactericidal ones. A state of primary or secondary immunodeficiency may, therefore, impair the therapeutic effect of antibiotics (22,43,56). In this context, the question arose if antibiotics influence immune defense mechanisms by themselves, i.e., besides their proper antimicrobial activity, immune defense mechanisms (19). Since methods for evaluating the immune status are increasingly available, this problem has become an area of growing interest. Many antibiotics have been assayed in vitro and in vivo with regard to their influence on different immunological parameters (15,16,23-25,27,28,39). The aim of these experiments was to obtain predictive results whether an antibiotic will induce by itself, independent of its antimicrobial effect, an enhancement or depression of immune response.

An overview shows that antibiotics may display both enhancing or depressing effects on immunological parameters (15,24,28,39). The results, however, were by no means homogeneous even when similar test systems were used and were not conclusive in respect to clinical experiences (7,12,14,17,44,51). In many cases the immunomodulating effect of different antibiotics did not correlate sufficiently with the findings in experimental infections using primary resistant microorganisms (22). Some examples are listed in Table 1.

With regard to a possible clinical significance of immunological side effects of antibiotics, the use of such in vivo models has been postulated (23). The results show that the influence of antibiotics on particular immunological parameters may outline, but do not necessarily reflect a comparable effect in experimental infections. Cefoxitin, as an example, inhibited antibody production, stimulated the footpad swelling reaction as a model of cellular immune response (22), had no effect on phagocytosis in vivo (23) but enhanced mortality rate in experimental infections with Cand. albicans significantly (26). This result has been explained by an immunosuppressive effect of the antibiotic because it could be abrogated by a concomitant treatment with an immunostimulator (26). Furthermore, it could be shown that the immunosuppressive effect of cefoxitin was equally abrogated if animals were concomitantly treated with indomethacin, an inhibitor of the cyclooxygenase pathway of arachidonic acid metabolism, indicating

Table 1. Comparison of Immunological Side Effects of Antibiotics and Influence on Experimental Infection with Primary Resistant Microorganisms (7,12,17,22,23,38,40,44,51)

Drugs	DPFC	FPST	Clearance test[a]	Experimental infection
Cefoperazone	↑	↑/0[b]	↓	⇡
Cefotetan	↓	↑/0[b]	±0	⇡
Cefmenoxime	↓	↑/0[b]	↑	⇡
Cefoxitin	↓	↑/0[b]	±0	↓
Cefotaxime	↑	↑	↑	↑
Cefsulodin	⇡ n.s.	↑[c]	↓	⇡
Cefaclor	↑	↑[c]	—	⇡
Tetracycline	⇡ n.s.	↓[c]	—	⇣

[a]Phagocytosis in vivo
[b]Dependent on the day of application relative to the day of immunization.
[c]No influence on or a suppression of secondary response of T cells to macrophage-bound antigen.
DPFC = direct plaque forming, IgM producing spleen cells.
FPST = footpad swelling test.

an influence of the antibiotic on mediator formation by immunocompetent cells (30). In the affirmative case, not only the influence of antibiotics on the production of different cellular mediators has to be considered, but also their interactions and feedback mechanisms.

The hypothesis to explain immunological side effects of antibiotics by their influence on the release of pharmacological mediators is based on the effect of indomethacin (see above) together with the well known observation of the inhibitory effect of prostaglandins of the E series (PGE_2) and of cyclic 3',5'-adenosine monophosphate (cAMP) (5,18,37,42,53,54), (but not of $PGF_{1\alpha}$ or $PGF_{2\alpha}$) on most of the immune response parameters as blastogenic response of lymphocytes (20,31,32,34,52), Ig-production (13,50), or the cytolytic activity of macrophages (MØ) (49). In this context, the influence of antibiotics on receptor formation must also be considered. The presence of PGE_2 receptors on lymphocytes could be demonstrated using cAMP response as a sensitive parameter (10,11,35). A particular high density of these receptors was apparently found on T_G (T suppressor) cells (33) and it was suggested that in this case PGE_2 activates these cells resulting in an inhibition of other lymphocyte populations (31,33,35,71).

Bacteria and bacterial products may act on mediator release (66-68) as well as on receptor formation (e.g., β-adrenergic receptors) (59,60,65,68). It might therefore be suggested that antibiotics may act also by the ways outlined in Figure 1.

A decrease of immune response might be induced by activation of adenylate cyclase or an inhibition of cAMP-phosphodiesterase. On the other hand, an increase could be expected by an activation of ATPase or of guanylate cyclase or by an inhibition of cGMP (cyclic 3',5'-guanosine monophosphate)-phosphodiesterase because cGMP enhances immune response phenomena (37).

Besides PGE_2 production and sensitivity, there are other cellular mediators to be considered such as the monokine interleukin-1 (IL-1). This factor stimulates T-helper cells by itself (57,58) and enhances the mitogenic effect of PHA-P (4,41,46,47,73). IL-1 initiates the IL-2 production by other lymphocytes inducing the generation of cytotoxic T-cells and other effector cells (61,62,64,69,70).

Hypothetically, it may be that the mechanisms of immunological side effects of antibiotics are concerned with their influence on the arachidonic acid metabolism, particularly the PGE-production as the substance of the cyclooxygenase pathway, the expression of PGE-receptors on lymphocytes demonstrable by their PGE-sensitivity and/or with an influence on IL-1 production. MØ are capable of synthesis and secretion of arachidonic acid oxygenation products derived from both cyclooxygenase and lipoxygenase pathways (8,9). They are the main producers of PGE_2 and produce equally IL-1 particularly when activated by phagocytosis. Three antibiotics have been examined in this respect and compared with their effect on experimental infection with Cand. albicans: cefoxitin, cefotaxime and cefaclor, the first one depressing and the two others rather enhancing immune defense in experimental infections (22).

MATERIALS AND METHODS

For all assays, male BALB/cABOM mice (Bomholtgard, Ry, Denmark) of 20 ± 1 g were used. Therefore, the influence of antibiotics on PGE_2 and IL-1 production by resident MØ was investigated. Thymocytes were used to examine the PGE_2-sensitivity.

Resident MØ were obtained and incubated with opsonized zymosan in the presence of antibiotics for 1 hour as described previously in detail (30). The PGE_2 content in the supernatant was evaluated using the ^{135}J-RIA-kit

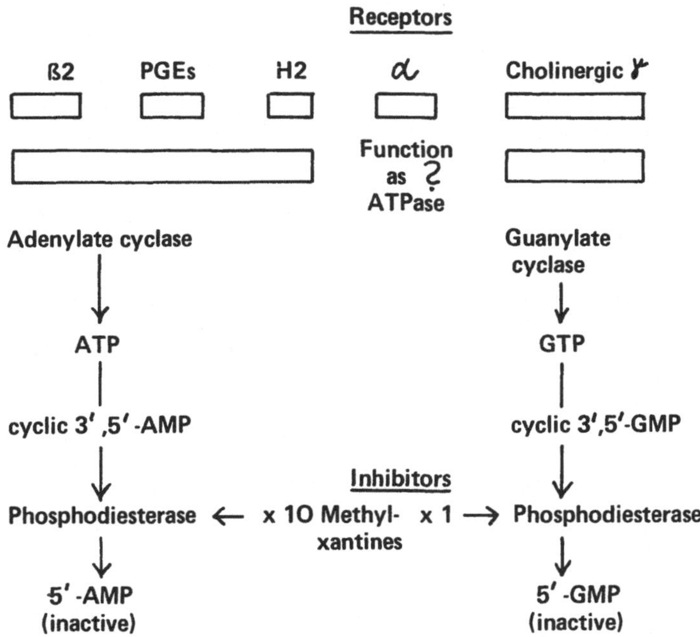

Figure 1. Possible ways of influence on cAMP and cGMP production as regulatory mediators of immune response (50-52).

Table 2. Zymosan-induced PGE_2 Production in the Presence of Antibiotics (In Vitro). Factor = Antibiotic + Opsonized Zymosan:Antibiotics Alone

µg/ml	Cefoxitin	Cefotaxime
control without antibiotics	7.17	8.61
15	6.39	12.68
30	8.00	10.07
60	5.37	8.76
control without antibiotics	8.77	8.77
120	4.95	7.75
150	-	-
200	5.63	8.28
300	5.16	7.33
400	4.65	10.00

system (NEN/USA) and calculated for 10^6 MØ. In vivo experiments were performed by treating animals with antibiotics and testing in vitro the zymosan induced PGE_2 production of MØ.

PGE_2 sensitivity of thymocytes is defined by the concentration of PGE_2 needed for a 50 per cent reduction of lymphocyte transformation induced by an optimal concentration of 10 µg PHA-P per ml (31,36). As described previously (29,30), thymocytes were isolated and incubated with PGE_2 (Sigma Chemicals/USA) in concentrations of 10^{-5} to 10^{-9} M together with different concentrations of antibiotics. The PGE_2 dependent decline of transformation rate evaluated by the ^{3}H-thymidine uptake of thymocytes permitted the extrapolation of the PGE_2 concentration necessary for a 50 per cent reduction of transformation. In vivo experiments were performed correspondingly by treating animals with antibiotics and testing thymocytes in the absence of these drugs for PGE_2 sensitivity.

IL-1 produced by phagocytizing MØ (1,6,45,61) can functionally be characterized by stimulating T cells and particularly by enhancing the mitogenic effect of PHA-P in low concentrations (co-stimulating activity) (47,48). As described previously in detail (29), resident MØ were isolated and incubated with opsonized zymosan and indomethacin (Sigma Chemicals/USA) in concentrations of 3×10^{-6} mol/l in the absence or presence of different concentrations of antibiotics. After an incubation time of 24 hours, the supernatants were filtered, extensively dialyzed and assayed in a 1:2 dilution for transformation activity in the presence of 1 µg PHA-P per ml using 2×10^6 thymocytes per well. In vivo experiments were performed by pretreating animals with antibiotics instead of treating MØ in vitro.

RESULTS

Opsonized zymosan enhanced as expected PGE_2 production of MØ considerably as demonstrated by a high stimulation factor (Table 2). The presence of cefoxitin reduced zymosan induced PGE_2 production particularly in concen-

Table 3. Influence of Antibiotics In Vitro on PGE_2 Sensitivity of Thymocytes

	Control	Cefoxitin µg/ml 150	300	400	Cefotaxime µg/ml 150	300	400
transformation factor[a]	5.6	1.9	1.01	-	2.4	1.6	-
PGE_2 sensitivity	1.2nM	120nM	∿400nM	-	2000nM	1000nM	-
transformation factor[a]	1.8	1.8	1.9	2.2	1.8	2.0	1.3
PGE_2 sensitivity	4500nM	50nM	∿400nM	1000nM	1400nM	700nM	>10000nM

[a] ^{3}H-thymidine uptake by 2 x 10^6 thymocytes in the presence of 10 µg/ml PHA-P per ml relative to controls.
[b] PGE_2 concentration reducing PHA-P induced lymphocyte transformation by 50%.

trations beyond 60 µg per ml. In contrast, cefotaxime enhanced PGE_2 production in concentrations of 15 and 30 µg per ml; higher concentrations were less effective (Table 2).

If the MØ donors were pretreated with antibiotics the zymosan induced PGE_2 production was only enhanced in case of cefotaxime whereas cefoxitin and cefaclor treatment had neither an enhancing nor an inhibiting effect (Figure 2).

In contrast to these results, the influence of antibiotics on PGE_2 sensitivity of thymocytes showed a quite different pattern. In vitro, cefotaxime induced a considerable increase in PGE_2 resistance demonstrable by higher PGE_2 concentrations needed for a 50 per cent reduction of PHA-P induced transformation (Table 3). On the other hand, cefoxitin increased PGE_2 sensitivity of thymocytes (lower PGE_2 concentrations needed for a 50 per cent reduction of PHA-P induced transformation) or - in case of a decrease - the absolute values of PGE_2 sensitivity in nM were clearly below

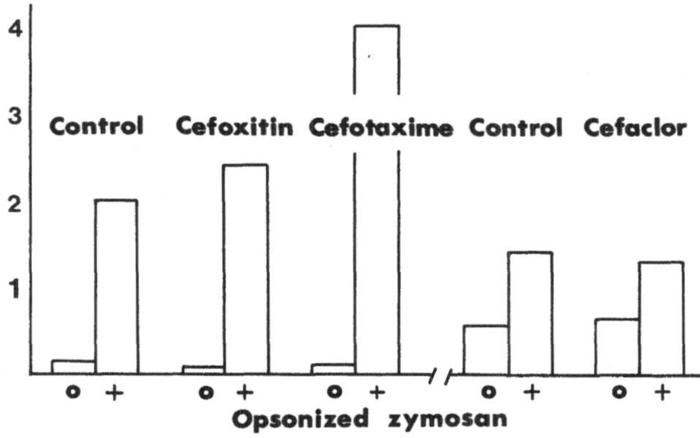

Figure 2. PGE_2 production by zymosan-activated resident macrophages (PGE_2 x 10^3 per 10^6 MØ) of mice pretreated with antibiotics. Treatment: cefoxitin and cefotaxime were given intravenously in doses of 50 mg/kg and cefaclor in doses of 30 mg/kg twice the day before and 1 hr before cells were taken.

Table 4. PGE_2 Sensitivity of Thymocytes Taken from Animals Pretreated with Antibiotics

	Control	Cefoxitin[c]	Cefotaxime[c]	Control	Cefaclor[c]
Transformation factor[a]	2.8	3.9	3.03	2.8	1.35
PGE_2 sensitivity[b]	22 nM	52.5 nM	220 nM	20 nM	55 nM

[a] and [b] see Table 3. [c]Doses of 30 mg per kg were injected intravenously twice the day before and once 1 hour before cells were taken.

those obtained with cefotaxime in parallel experiments (Table 3). The extent of PGE_2 sensitivity is apparently related to target cell responsiveness shown by different PHA-P induced transformation factors in controls.

If cell donors were pretreated with antibiotics and thymocytes assayed for PGE_2 sensitivity, the following results were obtained: a ten-fold increase in PGE_2 resistance was observed after treatment with cefotaxime whereas cefoxitin or cefaclor treatment resulted only in a two-fold increase (Table 4).

IL-1 production of MØ activated by opsonized zymosan was evaluated by its transformation promoting activity on thymocytes. In vitro, cefotaxime increased IL-1 production by a factor of 10 in concentrations of 150 µg per ml; higher concentrations had decreasing effects (Table 5). In contrast, cefoxitin in concentrations of 150 µg per ml rather inhibited IL-1 production and was stimulatory by a factor of 2-3 in higher concentrations (Table 5).

With regard to clinical conditions, the influence of an antibiotic treatment on IL-1 production of resident MØ in vitro activated by opsonized zymosan was examined. It could be shown (Table 6) that cefoxitin had no

Table 5. Influence of Antibiotics In Vitro on IL-1 Production by Resident Macrophages Not Stimulated (1) and Stimulated (2) by Opsonized Zymosan; Evaluation by Thymocyte Transformation in Presence of 1 µg PHA-P/ml

	Stimulation Factor			
	Cefoxitin		Cefotaxime	
µg/ml	(1)	(2)	(1)	(2)
150	2.32[a]	0.85	2.60[b]	9,97[b]
300	1.08[a]	3.07[b]	3.67[b]	8.25[b]
400	2.24[b]	2.03[b]	1.02	0.76

Stimulation factor is calculated relative to values obtained in analogous assays without antibiotics.
[a]$P < 0.02$
[b]$P < 0.01$

Table 6. IL-1 Production by Resident Macrophages (Activated) by Opsonized Zymosan) of Pretreated Animals*

Antibiotic	c.p.m.[a]	Groups compared	Factor
1) Control	692 ± 222	2:1	1.08
2) Cefoxitin	750 ± 412		
3) Cefotaxime	2317 ± 355	3:1	3.35[b]
4) Control	715 ± 55	4:5	2.57[b]
5) Cefaclor	1834 ± 349		

*30 mg/kg antibiotic in 0.5 ml saline injected intravenously twice the day before and 1 hr before cells were taken. Evaluation of IL-1 activity by its effect on thymocyte (2×10^6) transformation in presence of 1 μg PHA-P/ml.
[a]Counts per minute; 5 assays per group.
[b]$P < 0.01$

effect at all whereas cefaclor and particularly cefotaxime increased IL-1 production significantly.

DISCUSSION

Cefotaxime and cefaclor rather reduced mortality rate in experimental infections with primary resistant microorganisms as with Candida whereas cefoxitin enhanced it (22,26,29). This phenomenon was explained by immunological side effects of antibiotics independent of their proper antimicrobial activity. Because the immunodepressive effect of cefoxitin was abrogated by a concomitant treatment with indomethacin (30) it was supposed that the mechanism of such immunological side effects might be based on or connected with an influence on production and secretion of immunopharmacological mediators as monokines or products of the arachidonic acid metabolism.

The experiments showed that cefotaxime enhanced PGE_2 production by phagocytizing MØ in vitro more than cefoxitin. This observation is contrary to the hypothesis that the immunodepressive effect of cefoxitin in experimental infections is due to a heightened PGE_2 production, an inhibitor of immune response parameters (13,20,31,32,34,50,52). Comparable results were obtained if cell donors were treated with these antibiotics. Also in this in vivo model, the zymosan-induced PGE_2 production by MØ was increased after pretreatment with cefotaxime. In contrast, cefoxitin or cefaclor treatment had no significant effect when compared with controls.

In this context, not only PGE_2 production but also PGE_2 sensitivity of immunocompetent cells has to be considered because a higher sensitivity is indicative of a more pronounced inhibition of immune response (32,33,52). The experiments showed that in vitro cefotaxime increased PGE_2 resistance considerably when compared with cefoxitin. The extent of this effect is, however, dependent on the condition of target cells (20) as shown by different PHA-P induced transformation rates of controls. In case of a low transformation rate, the PGE_2 resistance is high and vice versa. In any experiment, however, cefotaxime induced a higher PGE_2 resistance than cefoxitin.

If thymocytes of cell donors pretreated with antibiotics were examined comparable results were obtained. Also in this case, cefotaxime induced the highest PGE_2 resistance. This might be the reason why an increase of PGE_2 production is without effect in experimental infection. On the other hand, cefoxitin and cefaclor both induced a small increase of PGE_2 resistance and to a quite similar degree although the first one increased and the latter reduced mortality rate in experimental infections. It could be suggested that receptor expression for PGE_2 on immunocompetent cells varies not only with the application of antibiotics but additionally with infection, which remains to be examined.

IL-1 production by MØ is enhanced by cefoxitin as well as by cefotaxime in vitro, in the latter case, however, comparably more. In vivo experiments showed that only cefotaxime and, to a lesser degree, cefaclor (21) increased IL-1 production whereas cefoxitin had no effect. If IL-1 production is taken as an indicator for some aspects of immune defense the corresponding effect of cefotaxime and cefaclor correlates with that in the model of experimental infection. Cefoxitin, however, did not reduce IL-1 production relative to controls as should be expected if this parameter correlates directly with its effect in experimental infection. It might be, as in case of PGE_2 sensitivity, that the condition of target cells plays an additional role that has not yet been examined in detail.

SUMMARY

Cefotaxime, cefoxitin and cefaclor have been examined in vitro as well as in vivo with respect to their influence on PGE_2 and IL-1 production by macrophages and on PGE_2 sensitivity of thymocytes. In vitro, cefotaxime enhanced PGE_2 production by zymosan activated macrophages whereas cefoxitin did not. Pretreatment of cell donors with cefotaxime equally enhances PGE_2 production in contrast to cefoxitin and cefaclor. PGE_2 resistance of thymocytes has considerably been increased by cefotaxime compared with cefoxitin both in vitro as well in vivo. In vivo, cefaclor induced a similar change of PGE_2 resistance of thymocytes as did cefoxitin. IL-1 production of macrophages has particularly been increased by cefotaxime in vitro and, to a smaller degree, by cefoxitin. In vivo experiments showed that cefotaxime and cefaclor enhanced IL-1 production considerably whereas cefoxitin had no effect. These results have been compared with the effect of antibiotics in experimental infections using primary resistant microorganisms. With regard to the formation and secretion of products of the arachidonic acid metabolism or cytokines, it was suggested that direct influences of antibiotics may additionally be modulated or superposed by infectious processes.

REFERENCES

1. L. A. Aarden, Revised nomenclature for antigen-nonspecific T cell proliferation and helper factors, J. Immunol. 123:2928 (1979).
2. D. Adam, P. Philipp and B. H. Belohradsky, Studies on the influence of host defence mechanisms on the antimicrobial effect of chemotherapeutic agents. Effect of antibiotics on phagocytosis of mouse-peritoneal-macrophages in vitro, Arztl. Forsch. 25:181 (1971).
3. D. Adam, F. Staber, B. H. Belohradsky and W. Marget, Effect of dihydrostreptomycin on phagocytosis of mouse-peritoneal macrophages in vitro, Infect. Immun. 5:537 (1972).
4. A. C. Allison, Mechanisms by which activated macrophages inhibit lymphocyte responses, Immunol. Rev. 40:3 (1978).
5. W. B. Anderson and I. Pastan, Altered adenylate cyclase activity: its role in growth regulation and malignant transformation of fibroblasts, Adv. Cyclic Nucleotide Res. 5:681 (1975).

6. F. Arenzana-Seisdedos and J. L. Virelizier, Interferons as macrophage-activating factors. II. Enhanced secretion of interleukin 1 by lipopolysaccharide-stimulated human monocytes, Eur. J. Immunol. 13:437 (1983).
7. G. Banck and A. Forsgren, Antibiotics and suppression of lymphocyte function in vitro, Antimicrob. Agents Chemother. 16:554 (1979).
8. R. J. Bonney and J. L. Humes, Physiological and pharmacological regulation of prostaglandin and leukotriene production by macrophages, J. Leukocyte Biol. 35:1 (1984).
9. H. R. Bourne, L. B. Epstein and K. L. Melmon, Lymphocyte cyclic adenosine monophosphate (AMP) synthesis and inhibition of phytohemagglutinin-induced transformation, J. Clin. Invest. 50:10a (1971).
10. H. R. Bourne, L. M. Lichtenstein, K. L. Melmon, C. S. Henney, Y. Weinstein and G. M. Shearer, Modulation of inflammation and immunity by cyclic AMP, Science 184:19 (1974).
11. S. J. Bromberg, S. Goodwin and G. T. Peake, Receptors for prostaglandin E on human peripheral blood mononuclear cells, Clin. Res. 27:321A (1979).
12. E. A. Chaperon, Suppression of lymphocytes by cephalosporins, in: "The Influence of Antibiotics on the Host-Parasite Relationship," U. Eickenberg, H. Hahn and W. Opferkuch, eds., Springer-Verlag, Berlin, Heidelberg, New York (1982).
13. J. Ceuppens and J. S. Goodwin, Endogenous prostaglandin E enhances polyclonal immunoglobulin production by tonically inhibiting T suppressor cell activity, Cell. Immunol. 70:41 (1982).
14. G. J. Damert and P. G. Sohnle, Effect of chloramphenicol on in vitro function of lymphocytes, J. Infect. Dis. 139:220 (1979).
15. H. U. Eickenberg, H. Hahn and W. Opferkuch, eds., "The Influence of Antibiotics on the Host-Parasite Relationship," Springer-Verlag, Berlin, Heidelberg, New York (1982).
16. R. Finch, Immunomodulating effects of antimicrobial agents, J. Antimicrob. Chemother. 6:691 (1980).
17. A. Forsgren and G. Banck, Influence of antibiotics on lymphocyte function in vitro, Infection 6(Suppl. 1):91 (1978).
18. H. Friedman, T. W. Klein and A. Szentivanyi, ed., "Immunomodulation by Bacteria and Their Products," Plenum Press, New York, London (1981).
19. C. Frugoni and G. Giunchi, Antibiotika und Immunitat bei bakteriellen Infektionen, Scientia medica 3:205 (1954).
20. D. Gemsa, E. Barlin, H. G. Leser, W. Deimann and M. Seitz, Prostaglandins and leukotrienes: physiological and pathophysiological mediators of immunity, Behring Inst. Mitt. 68:51 (1981).
21. G. Gillissen and B. Melzer, L'influence des antibiotiques sur la production de l'interleukine-1 par des macrophages, Path. Biol. (in press).
22. G. Gillissen and Z. Pusztai-Markos, Influence of antibiotics on immunological parameters: significance in experimental infections, Drugs Exptl. Clin. Res. X(11):813 (1984).
23. G. Gillissen and Z. Pusztai-Markos, Evaluation des effets modulateurs des antibiotiques in vivo sur la phagocytose chez la souris utilisant des mèthodes diffèrentes, Pathol. Biol. 32:355 (1984).
24. G. Gillissen, Antibiotika und Immunantwort - Begleiteffekte der Chemotherapie, Immun. Infekt. 8:79 (1980).
25. G. Gillissen, Nouveaux antibiotiques beta-lactam et response immunitaire, Med. et Hyg. 39:122 (1981).
26. G. Gillissen, The influence of sodium-8-chlorotheophyllinate (S8CT) on immune processes, Experientia 37:420 (1981).
27. G. Gillissen, Influence of cephalosporins on humoral immune response, in: "The Influence of Antibiotics on the Host-Parasite relationship," U. Eickenberg, H. Hahn and W. Opferkuch, eds., Springer-Verlag, Berlin, Heidelberg, New York (1982).

28. G. Gillissen, Interaktion zwischen Antibiotika und Immunabwehr, in: "Infektiologisches Kolloquium 1. Neues von 'alten' Erregern und neue Erreger," C. Kraseman, ed., Walter DeGruyter Verlag, Berlin (1983).
29. G. Gillissen, Influence of cefaclor on immune response parameters, Arzneim.-Forsch./Drug Res. 34:1535 (1984).
30. G. Gillissen, Possible mechanisms of immunological side-effects of antibiotics, Zbl. Bakt. 13(Suppl.):91 (1985).
31. J. S. Goodwin, A. D. Bankhurst and R. P. Messner, Suppression of human T cell mitogenesis by prostaglandins, J. Exp. Med. 146:1719 (1977).
32. J. S. Goodwin and J. Cueppens, Regulation of the immune response by prostaglandins, J. Clin. Immunol. 3:295 (1983).
33. J. S. Goodwin, P. A. Kaszubowski and R. C. Williams, Jr., Cyclic adenosine monophosphate response to prostaglandin E_2 on subpopulations of human lymphocytes, J. Exp. Med. 150:1260 (1979).
34. J. S. Goodwin, R. P. Messner and G. T. Peake, Prostaglandin suppression of mitogen-stimulated lymphocytes in vitro. Changes with mitogen dose and preincubation, J. Clin. Invest. 62:753 (1978).
35. J. S. Goodwin, A. Wiik, M. Lewis, A. D. Bankhurst and R. C. Williams, High affinity binding sites for prostaglandin E on human lymphocytes, Cell. Immunol. 43:150 (1979).
36. J. S. Goodwin, Changes in lymphocyte sensitivity to prostaglandin E, histamine, hydrocortisone, and X irradiation with age: studies in a healthy elderly population, Clin. Immunol. Immunopathol. 25:243 (1982).
37. J. W. Hadden, Cyclic nucleotides in lymphocyte proliferation and diferentiation, in: "Immunopharmacology," J. W. Hadden, R. G. Coffey and F. Spreafico, eds., Plenum Press, New York (1977).
38. H. Hahn and S. H. E. Kaufmann, T lymphocyte macrophage interactions in cellular antibacterial immunity, Immunobiol. 161:361 (1982).
39. W. E. Hauser, Jr. and J. S. Remington, Effect of antibiotics on the immune response, Am. J. Med. 72:711 (1982).
40. S. H. E. Kaufmann, M. M. Simon and H. Hahn, Regulatory interactions between macrophages and T cell subsets in Listeria monocytogene-specific T cell activation, Infect. Immun. 38:907 (1982).
41. G. A. Koretzky, J. A. Elias, S. L. Kay, M. D. Rossman, P. C. Nowell and R. P. Daniele, Spontaneous production of interleukin-1 by human alveolar macrophages, Clin. Immunol. Immunopathol. 29:443 (1983).
42. G. B. Mackaness and R. V. Blanden, Cellular Immunity, Progr. Allergy 11:89 (1967).
43. L. A. Mandell, Effects of antibiotic, antifungal and antiviral drugs on neutrophil function, in: "Current Chemotherapy and Immunotherapy," P. Periti and G. G. Grassi, eds., The American Soc. for Microbiol., Washington D.C. (1982).
44. M. Mielke and H. Hahn, Influence of cefsulodin and tetracycline on listeria-specific T cell macrophage interactions in vitro, in: "Proceedings of the 13th Internat. Congr. Chemother. Vienna," K. H. Spitzy and K. Karrer, eds., H. Egersmann, Vienna (1983).
45. S. B. Mizel and D. Mizel, Purification to apparent homogenicity of murine interleukin 1, J. Immunol. 126:834 (1981).
46. S. B. Mizel, J. J. Oppenheim and D. L. Rosenstreich, Characterization of lymphocyte-activating factor (LAF) produced by the macrophage cell line, $P388D_1$. I. Enhancement of LAF production by activated T lymphocytes, J. Immunol. 120:1497 (1978).
47. S. B. Mizel, D. L. Rosenstreich and J. J. Oppenheim, Phorbol myristic acetate stimulates LAF production by the macrophage cell line, $P388D_1$, Cell. Immunol. 40:230 (1978).
48. S. B. Mizel, Studies on the purification and structure-function relationships of murine lymphocyte activating factor (interleukin 1), Mol. Immunol. 17:571 (1980).

49. M. Mochizuki, J. S. Zigler, P. Russell and I. Gery, Cytostatic and cytolytic activities of macrophages. Regulation by prostaglandins, Cell. Immunol. 83:34 (1984).
50. T. Morito, A. D. Bankfurst and R. C. Williams, Jr., Studies on the modulation of immunoglobulin production by prostaglandins, Prostaglandins 20:383 (1980).
51. A. M. Munster, C. B. Loadholdt, A. G. Leary and M. A. Barnes, The effect of antibiotics on cell-mediated immunity, Surgery 81:692 (1977).
52. R. C. Page, J. A. Clagett, L. D. Engel, G. Wilde and T. Sims, Effects of prostaglandin on the antigen- and mitogen-driven responses of peripheral blood lymphocytes from patients with adult and juvenile periodonitis, Clin. Immunol. Immunopathol. 11:77 (1978).
53. C. W. Parker, T. J. Sullivan and H. J. Wedner, Cyclic AMP and the immune response, Adv. Cyclic Nucleotide Res. 4:1 (1974).
54. I. H. Pastan, G. S. Johnson and W. B. Anderson, Role of cyclic nucleotides in growth control, Ann. Rev. Biochem. 44:491 (1975).
55. M. Plaut and L. M. Lichtenstein, Cellular and chemical basis of the allergic inflammatory response, in: "Allergy, Principles and Practice, Vol. I," E. Middleton, Jr., C. E. Reed and E. F. Ellis, eds., The C. V. Mosby Co., St. Louis, Toronto (1983).
56. J. A. Raeburn, Antibiotics and immunodeficiency, Lancet 4:954 (1972).
57. M. Rollinghoff, Interleukine: ihre Rolle und Wirkung bei der immunologischen Abwehrreaktion, Allergologie 6:397 (1983).
58. M. Rollinghoff, Interleukine: Signalstoffe des Immunsystems, Die gelben Hefte XXIII. Jahrgang, 4 (1983).
59. A. J. Schreurs and F. P. Nijkamp, Contribution of bacterial cell wall compounds to airway hyperreactivity, Int. J. Immunopharmacol. 4:294 (1982).
60. A. J. M. Schreurs, "Haemophilus Influenzae and the β-Adrenergic System," University of Utrecht Press, Utrecht, The Netherlands (1982).
61. K. A. Smith, T cell growth factor, Immunol. Rev. 51:337 (1980).
62. W. Solbach, M. Rollinghoff and H. Wagner, Die Rolle von Interleukine-2 bei der Aktivierung von zytotoxischen T-Lymphozyten, Klin. Wschr. 61:67 (1983).
63. D. P. Stites, J. D. Stobo, H. H. Fudenberg and J. V. Wells, eds., "Basic and Clinical Immunology," Lange Medical Publications, Los Altos (1982).
64. J. D. Stobo, Cellular interactions in the expression and regulation of immunity, in: "Basic and Clinical Immunology," D. P. Stites, J. D. Stobo, H. H. Fudenberg and J. V. Wells, eds., Lange Medical Publications, Los Altos (1982).
65. A. Szentivanyi, E. Middleton, Jr., J. F. Williams and H. Friedman, Effect of microbial agents on the immune network and associated pharmacologic reactivities, in: "Allergy, Principles and Practice, Vol. 1," E. Middleton, Jr., C. E. Reed and E. F. Ellis, eds., The C. V. Mosby Co., St. Louis, Toronto (1983).
66. A. Szentivanyi and C. W. Fishel, Effect of bacterial products on responses to the allergic mediators, in: "Immunological Diseases," M. Samter and H. L. Alexander, eds., Little Brown & Co., Boston (1965).
67. A. Szentivanyi und C. W. Fishel, Die Amin-Mediatorstoffe der Allergischen Reaktion und die Reaktionsfahigkeit ihrer Exfolgszellen, in: "Pathogenese und Therapie Allergischer Reaktionen: Grundlagenforschung und Klinik," G. Filipp, ed., Ferdinand Enke Verlag, Stuttgart (1966).
68. A. Szentivanyi and D. F. Fitzpatrick, The altered reactivity of the effector cells to antigenic and pharmacological influences and its relation to cyclic nucleotides. II. Effector reactivities in the efferent loop of the immune response, in: "Pathomechanismus und

Pathogenese Allergischer Reaktionen," G. Filipp, ed., Werk-Verlag, Dr. Edmund Banachewski, Grafelfing/Munich (1980).

69. H. Wagner, C. Hardt, K. Heeg, K. Pfizenmaier, W. Solbach, R. Bartlett, H. Stockinger and M. Rollinghoff, T-T cell interactions during cytotoxic T lymphocyte (CTL) responses: T cell derived helper factor (Interleukin 2) as a probe to analyse CTL responsiveness and thymic maturation of CTL progenitors, Immunolog. Rev. 51:215 (1980).

70. H. Wagner and M. Rollinghoff, T-T cell interactions during in vitro cytotoxic allograft responses: I. Soluble products from activated Ly 1^+ T cells trigger autonomously antigen primed Ly 23^+ T cells to cell proliferation and cytolytic activity, J. Exp. Med. 148:1523 (1978).

71. D. R. Webb and I. Nowowiejski, Mitogen-induced changes in lymphocyte prostaglandin levels: a signal for the induction of suppressor cell activity, Cell. Immunol. 41:72 (1978).

72. L. Weinstein and A. C. Dalton, Host determinants of response to antimicrobial agents, N. Engl. J. Med. 279:467, 524, 580 (1968).

COMBINED ACTIVITIES OF AN ANTIBIOTIC AND THE IMMUNOSTIMULATING LAUROYLTETRAPEPTIDE (R.P. 40 639) ON BACTERIAL INFECTIONS

François Floc'h, Jacques Poirier, and Georges H. Werner

Centre de Recherches de Vitry
Vitry sur Seine, France

ABSTRACT

R.P. 40 639 (lauroyltetrapeptide), a synthetic immunostimulating compound, enhances the resistance of mice against lethal bacterial infections such as Listeria monocytogenes or Klebsiella pneumoniae, when administered at doses around 1 mg/kg i.p. or s.c. one day before challenge. On the other hand, mice can be cured from Listeria infection with a 100 mg/kg s.c. dose of ampicillin. As it has been reported that antibiotics can render bacteria more susceptible to the host's immune mechanisms, we investigated the effects of combined administration of R.P. 40 639 and ampicillin. The immunostimulant was administered either prophylactically (day -1) at a normally active dose (1 mg/kg i.p.) or under less active or inactive conditions of treatment, such as 0.1 to 0.2 mg/kg s.c. on days 0 and +2 or on days -1, 0 and +3. Ampicillin was injected therapeutically (day 0) at a normally inactive dose (20 mg/kg s.c.). Results have shown that, under such conditions, combined treatments gave significant protection whereas treatments with a single agent were either inactive or less active.

It is suggested that combined immuno-chemotherapy could be a treatment of choice for chronic or recurrent infections.

PROHOST MODULATION OF IMMUNITY BY ISOPRINOSINE AND NPT 15392

Claudio DeSimone[1] and John W. Hadden[2]

[1]Clinica Malattie Infettive, Policlinico Umberto I
Rome, Italy, and [2]University of South Florida
College of Medicine, Program of Immunopharmacology
Tampa, Florida

INTRODUCTION

Antimicrobial agents which act on nucleic acids (e.g., rifampin, sulfonamides, trimethoprim, metronidazole), on ribosomes (e.g., tetracyclines, chloramphenicol, aminoglycosides) or on cytoplasmic membranes (e.g., amphotericin B, griseofulvin, polymyxin, imidazoles) positively influence the outcome of infections by acting against the offending pathogens but they may also have negative effects on the host's immunocompetence (22). Although the immunosuppressive properties of most of the antimicrobials are not sufficient to warrant restricting their use, under certain circumstances a "pro-host" immunopharmacological approach seems warranted. In this regard it is important to remember that the immune system "cures" an infection, not the antimicrobial agent, and under circumstances where antimicrobial therapy is lifesaving, the host's immune defenses are almost invariably compromised. To expedite the development of immunorestorative therapy it is important first of all to characterize the immunological deficiency which precedes, accompanies or follows a disease in order to select the appropriate immunorestorative agent. Secondly, new therapeutic strategies, where the antimicrobials are associated with prohost immunomodulating drugs, need to be studied in the appropriate animal systems.

Hopefully, in the future, antibiotic choices will include consideration not only of antimicrobial susceptibilities but also of the appropriate immunomodulating drug to be used based on the patient's underlying defect. The choices of the appropriate immunomodulating drug will include those substances which are well tolerated, safe, non-carcinogenic and effective. One class of agents under development for use in such infections are the thymomimetic drugs. Thymomimetic means that a drug has the ability to mimic the action of the thymus in the maturational and functional processes which lead the T lymphocyte to acquire its full competence as an immune cell. Many infections, particularly those involving viruses, facultative intracellular bacteria, and fungi involve defects in thymus-dependent immunity. These drugs will help to correct the immunoderegulation which accompanies such infectious diseases and in preventing antimicrobial-induced immunodepression. Two classes of compounds are considered thymomimetic (75): inducers of thymic hormones or thymic hormone-like substances (e.g., levamisole) and simulators of the action of the thymic hormones (e.g., methisoprinol, NPT 15392).

Our review will focus on this second category. Methisoprinol is licensed for clinical use in 70 countries. Although relatively high doses

(2-4 gr/day) are required, Methisoprinol is not generally toxic and is consistent in its immunopharmacologic actions. NPT 15392 is an experimental drug under development. NPT 15392 is more potent on a weight basis by a factor of 10-1000 than methisoprinol and has more prolonged actions in vivo.

METHISOPRINOL

Methisoprinol (isoprinosine, inosiplex) is a synthetic drug complex composed of inosine and of the p-acetamidobenzoate salt of N, N-dimethylamino-2-propanol (DIP - PACBA) in a molar ratio of 1:3. Studies done to evaluate tolerance and toxicity have shown, as the only side effect worthy of note, a sporadic and transitory increase of uric acid levels in urine and blood, devoid, however, of any appreciable clinical consequences (28-30,71). Between 1973 and 1978, clinical observations on experimentally infected subjects with influenza or rhinovirus showed that the drug has a favorable effect in most cases examined (4,50,58,69,82).

Since methisoprinol has been approved by the Health Ministries of France and Italy, there has been an opportunity for many clinicians to prescribe the drug in many viral diseases and immunodepressive states. After a decade of use in the clinics of these countries, the drug has proven to be one of the safest antiviral-immunomodulator drugs available. The clinical observations reported by French and Italian physicians have been confirmed by the scientists of the countries where the drug has been more recently licensed (Germany, Spain, United Kingdom and Canada). We present a brief review on the use of methisoprinol in the treatment of naturally occurring viral diseases in France and Italy.

Clinical Trials

Nervous System. Rancurel et al. (65) treated 23 patients afflicted with acute necrotic encephalitis with methisoprinol. In 12 cases the etiological agent was identified as being the herpes virus. Of the 19 cured patients, 14 showed no residual neurologic consequences (64,65). Villa and colleagues (81) described, in a comatose patient suffering from Creutzfeldt-Jacob disease, a terminal stage lasting 16 months (an unusually long survival in this type of illness) and they attributed the phenomenon to the administration of methisoprinol. The case of a 14-year old boy having a polyradiculoneuritis with prevalent bulbar incidence and with anti-coxsackie antibodies in the spinal fluid was described by Delogu et al. (13). They administered methisoprinol i.v. at the dosages of 10 g/day; respiratory autonomy was re-established after 12 days of therapy and a complete neurological recovery occurred on the twentieth day. The administration of methisoprinol, in two cases of viral meningoencephalitis, was accompanied by such a favorable and rapid clinical course that Sinardi et al. (73) hypothesized that the drug could have a fundamental role in resolving the meningoencephalitic syndrome. Recently, a report has been published on 98 patients with subacute sclerosing panencephalitis and treated with methisoprinol. They were compared with a historical control group of untreated patients for life expectancy and quality of life. In the methisoprinol-treated group the mortality rate was 43% of the non-treated subjects (47).

Respiratory Tract. Methisoprinol was employed by Danto et al. (10) to treat relapses of bronchopneumopathy following infection by respiratory syncitial virus, influenza A virus, parainfluenza B virus and *Mycoplasma Pneumoniae*. An amelioration of the symptomatology, witnessed by a more rapid resolution of the radiological picture, was reported.

The possibility of restoring the altered leukocytic functions in children affected by recurrent respiratory infections, through the use of methisoprinol, was evaluated by Azzara et al. (1). In 13 children, the clinical remission of the symptomatology, as well as the results of the in vitro assays of chemotaxis and NBT test, supports the use of the drug in patients with this type of infection. Positive results in 28 children (8 bronchiolitis, 15 bronchitis, 5 bronchopneumonia) were also reported by Loiacono and coworkers (49) following methisoprinol treatment.

Liver. D'Aquino and colleagues (11) observed a reduced confinement to bed without significant modifications in biomedical parameters in 50 subjects affected by acute HBsAg+ viral hepatitis and in 50 patients with acute HBsAg- viral hepatitis treated with methisoprinol, compared to the placebo-treated groups. Similarly, Bechi and Cini (3) reported a reduced confinement to bed as compared to the group treated with the conventional therapy. On a more conservative basis, Mansueto, et al. (78) suggest that methisoprinol should be reserved for those patients who do not recover from acute viral hepatitis within normal time limits.

Pasqui et al. (60) in a study on 50 children ranging in age from four to 16 years all affected by HBsAg- viral hepatitis, noted that therapy with methisoprinol induced a rapid disappearance of jaundice with an improvement of the clinical conditions. Vellucci et al. (80) observed a significant reduction of the serum transaminases in 22 cases of acute viral hepatitis (13 of which were HBsAg+), as compared to the control group; moreover, they reported a faster sero conversion of antibody to the HBsAg to negative. Also Frappampina et al. (25) showed in 55 subjects a more rapid clearance of the HBsAg after treatment with methisoprinol as compared with the control group, while Paffetti et al. (59) reported a reduction of the bilirubinemia in HBsAg+ viral hepatitis. In the treatment of chronic aggressive hepatitis and persistent hepatitis, methisoprinol induced only slightly significant improvements.

Skin (Except Herpes). Twenty patients with variously distributed warts with condyloma acuminatum were treated by Spadafora (74). The combination of methisoprinol and diathermocoagulation treatment interrupted the periodic reappearance of the skin manifestations whereas no improvement was noted with diathermocoagulation-treatment alone. Zagni and Cannarozzo (85) showed the efficacy of methisoprinol in inducing complete recovery and preventing relapses typical of warts and condyloma acuminatum by treating 15 patients affected with this type of pathology employing a 20% methisoprinol cream, with or without associated diathermocoagulation. Of the 84 female patients affected by condyloma, 41% of the group treated with oral methisoprinol showed a disappearance of the condylomatosis. A similar reduction of skin manifestations in this disease were reported by Signorelli and colleagues (70). In those cases where methisoprinol had been topically applied alone as a 20% ointment, 58% of the patients showed a reduction of the condylomatosis and 16% completely cleared.

Herpes Simplex (Types 1 and 2). Administration of methisoprinol significantly reduces the relapses of labial and genital herpes, as demonstrated by Galli et al. (27) in 70 patients. The same conclusions were reached by Italia and colleagues (46) (27 subjects) and by Grippaudo and colleagues (36) (25 patients); these authors found, moreover, that the drug, even when topically administered, was capable of reducing oedema, pain, itching and the frequency of the episodes.

Chicken Pox. The lapse of time it took the blistering exanthema to transform into crusts and the duration of fever were taken as parameters for the evaluation of methisoprinol's efficacy in the therapy of chicken pox by Precchia et al. (63). Both these parameters were significantly reduced in the 60 patients treated by the authors. Lento et al. (48) observed in 41 patients affected by chicken pox with prevalent intercostal and trigerminal localization, a faster regression of the painful symptomatology and an accelerated evolution of the blisters into crusts after methisoprinol administration. A reduction in the symptomatology (duration of fever, skin eruptions, the intensity of the itch, the appearance of complications and the length of hospitalization) was observed in 27 patients treated with methisoprinol by Catania and colleagues (6).

Infectious Mononucleosis, Mumps, Measles, Rubella. In mixed patient populations, and thus difficult to evaluate, the studies carried out by Santangelo (68), Precchia (63), and Lento (48), all seem to favor the use of methisoprinol in the therapy of these diseases.

AIDS. Studies are in progress on the therapeutic application of methisoprinol in AIDS and related syndromes. Up to the present time, encouraging results have been published by Glasky et al. (31,79) which report improvement of the T cell subsets and of the NK cell activity. It has been suggested that methisoprinol effects on the immune system are responsible for the beneficial clinical effects observed.

IMMUNOPHARMACOLOGICAL PROFILE

One of the major drawbacks in the acceptance of methisoprinol in the domain of antiviral drugs, despite its proven efficacy for the treatment of viral diseases, has been the difficulty to detect its antiviral action in tissue culture. Nevertheless, the replication of various RNA viruses (poliovirus, A and type B influenza, rhinovirus, ECHO virus and the Oriental Equine encephalitis virus) and DNA viruses (herpes simplex, adenovirus, and vaccinia) is inhibited in the presence of high concentrations of methisoprinol (32,33,57). The hypothesized mechanism for this is that the substance links itself to the ribosomes of the infected cells provoking a steric modification such as to render the cellular mRNA an advantage over the viral mRNA in the competition for linkage with ribosomal combining sites. Consequently there would be a nonreading or an incorrect reading with incorrect transcription of the viral genetic code, without alteration from a qualitative point of view of the cellular protein synthesis (8,12,34).

According to Ohnishi (56), methisoprinol protects the host's cells through two different mechanisms:

1. Direct Antiviral: suppression of the viral RNA synthesis and inhibition of viral growth;

2. Indirect Antiviral: potentiation of the post-viral, infection-depressed lymphocytic RNA synthesis.

The indirect antiviral mechanism, or the potentiation of the host's immune responses had been previously predicted by Hadden and coworkers (41,43). Further studies, here briefly summarized, confirmed that the principal mechanism of action of methisoprinol is of the immunopotentiating type with characteristics similar to those of the thymic hormones and of levamisole.

IMMUNOPHARMACOLOGY

Macrophage Function

Monocytes isolated from human peripheral blood when incubated in vitro with methisoprinol showed increased phagocytic properties (83). The drug is more active on monocytes than on neutrophils with regard to phagocytosis and chemotaxis. This effect is more evident in patients with herpetic infections in whom compromised monocyte function is present (52).

Lymphocyte Differentiation

Touraine and coworkers (76) demonstrated an action of methisoprinol very similar to that of the thymic hormones. Methisoprinol induces the appearance of a membrane determinant expressing maturity in precursor cells of the T lineage isolated from the bone marrow. Using athymic nu/nu homozygote mice given a single intraperitoneal injection of methisoprinol, Renoux (67) confirmed, in vivo, the above cited effect, observing the appearance of Thy-1 phenotype on about 20% of the splenocytes.

Lymphocyte Activation and Proliferation

Addition of methisoprinol at the beginning of the culture of lymphocytes stimulated with nonspecific mitogens or with specific soluble antigens, resulted in an increased incorporation of tritiated thymidine into DNA (41,55,67,83). In vivo testing of the lymphocytes from methisoprinol-treated subjects for various diseases, confirmed the above finding (16,55). That the drug acts mainly on the proliferative responses of the OKT4+ and OKM1+ cells was shown by studies conducted on lymphocyte populations depleted with various monoclonal antibodies plus complement (21). Apparently, the cyclic GMP phosphodiesterase is inhibited by high concentrations of the drug with an effect, in terms of potency, equivalent to that of inosine (37). It has been hypothesized that methisoprinol stimulates RNA synthesis through the effects of inosine on the incorporation of orotic acid into RNA (9). A 20 minute incubation of lymphocytes in the presence of the drug is sufficient to reduce nuclear refringence, an index of the early nuclear events of lymphocyte activation in vitro (62).

Activation of T Suppressor Cells

By preincubating murine splenocytes with methisoprinol, Renoux and coworkers (66) demonstrated a significant suppression of the proliferative response to an allogeneic stimulus. The activation of suppressor cell activity in the presence of Concanavalin A (Con A) and methisoprinol was confirmed by Touraine (77) using human lymphocytes. Recently, it has been hypothesized that methisoprinol acts on the Con A-inducible suppressor activity of the theophylline-resistant T cells (18). It was demonstrated, using the 5/9 monoclonal antibody that identified the T cells responsible for the proliferative response in the mixed lymphocyte cultures and with helper activity in the mitogen-induced stimulation of the B-cells, that the percentage of 5/9+ cells increases significantly after incubation with methisoprinol. Besides increasing the percentage of the 5/9+ cells, the in vitro treatment with the drug also augments the functional activity of the 5/9+ cells, as has been demonstrated by T and B lymphocyte co-culture experiments (14).

Interleukins 1, 2, γ-Interferon and Other Lymphokines

Hersey and colleagues (44) demonstrated that methisoprinol potentiates the production of interleukin 1 (IL 1) and interleukin 2 (IL 2). Time course experiments of γ-interferon (γ-IFN) production and thymidine incorporation showed that the drug accelerates the production and release of γ-IFN in vitro by lymphocytes stimulated with mitogens. Moreover, the incubation of lymphocytes from healthy donors with γ-IFN containing supernatants resulted in an increase in the natural killer cell activity (20). Hadden and Giner-Sorolla (39) demonstrated that methisoprinol is capable of increasing lymphokine production only if the T cells have been previously activated with mitogens or antigens and in an inosine-free culture medium. Lymphotoxin

(LT) production by lymphocytes from subjects with mucocutaneous infections due to herpes virus increased by about 80% after treatment with methisoprinol as shown in a study carried out by Bradshaw et al. (5).

Activation of B Lymphocytes

An increase of plaque-forming cells (PFC) belonging to the IgM and the IgG classes was demonstrated in the mouse by Renoux et al. (67). Using human lymphocytes, Morin et al. (55) obtained similar results.

Lymphocyte Surface Markers

An increase in the active E rosette-forming T cells and in autologous rosette-forming T cells was shown by Wybran (83). Following a brief period of lymphocyte incubation with methisoprinol, an increased expression of the receptors for the Fc fragment of the IgG and of the receptors for the third component of complement (C3) was demonstrated (19). Pompidou (62) has published data showing that methisoprinol increases OKT4+ cells when used at low concentrations, and increases of OKT8+ cells at higher concentrations of the drug. The cell population which increased, in both cases, was HLA-DR+. An increase in the expression of the antigens recognized by Leu 3a+ monoclonal antibody was induced by the treatment of the theophylline-resistant T cells with methisoprinol (18).

Activation of Natural Killer (NK) Cells

Goutner (35) showed a higher degree of lytic activity of human lymphocytes against the K562 cells, after incubation with methisoprinol. Preincubating the effector cells for four hours with the drug, Balestrino et al. (15) noticed an increase in NK activity two to four times greater than the control values. This phenomenon was independent of the production of interferon during the culture period. After intraperitoneal administration of methisoprinol to the mouse, similar results were obtained (23).

Interactions with Other Immunoactive Drugs

Using lymphocytes of healthy subjects and of patients with lung and gastrointestinal cancers it was possible to show that methisoprinol antagonizes the action of azathioprine in the active E rosette test (15). The simultaneous administration of methisoprinol and corticosteroids in man resulted in a potentiation of the corticosteroid-dependent immunosuppressive properties of the plasma of the treated subjects (17). Cerutti et al. (7) have shown that methisoprinol potentiates the protective effect of exogenous interferon in mice challenged with Sarcoma 180 or encephalomyocarditis virus.

NPT 15392

NPT 15392 (9-erythro-2-hydroxy-3-nonyl hypoxanthine) (hydroerythranol-Erimunol) is an hypoxanthine derivative which has been considered since its synthesis complementary to methisoprinol (38). In vitro, its effects are more subtle than those of methisoprinol and are somewhat difficult to demonstrate on mitogen-induced lymphocyte proliferation.

This compound shares, however, each of the immunopharmacological activities of methisoprinol, but at concentrations 1/10 - 1/1000 of the latter drug. NPT 15392 at 0.01 - 1 μg/ml induces prothymocyte differentiation, increases E rosette formation and modulates the proliferative, helper and suppressor functions of T lymphocytes (24,40,42,45,51). Lymphokine production and release in vitro are equally affected (40,42,51). At therapeutic dosages (0.1 - 1 mg/kg), NPT 15392 failed to show significant side effects in man and animals. Notably, the in vivo immunopharmacological effects of NPT 15392 are more easily demonstrable than those in vitro. In mice, for example, NPT 15392 augments delayed hypersensitivity and natural killer cell activity in vivo (37). In murine models, NPT 15392 (0.1 mg/kg) partially reversed tumor, virus and chemotherapy-induced immunodepression, and showed, correlating with immunorestoration, increased survival or decreased metastasis formation in sarcoma 180, T 241 fibrosarcoma, Lewis lung carcinoma, AH41c, 44, 66 and 130 tumors and P 388 leukemia. No effect was observed in L1210 leukemia or NF sarcoma (72). In immunopharmacological trials on humans with cancer NPT 15392 proved effective in augmenting lymphocyte counts, active E rosettes and natural killer cells in some but not all patients (84).

CONCLUSIONS

Many, but not all the activities of methisoprinol and NPT 15392 can be termed thymomimetic. In addition to inducing T cell differentiation and to modulating mature T cell function, these drugs induce B cell differentiation, potentiate γ-IFN, IL 1 and IL 2 production, increase natural killer cell activity and phagocytic cell function. These actions can be explained assuming that both drugs act through a receptor not restricted to T cells but common to B cells, NK cells, granulocytes, macrophages, inducing modifications of unknown enzymatic pathways.

It has been suggested that these compounds are agonists for an inosine-like P receptor or, alternatively, like methylxanthines, these compounds may turn out to be antagonists for R type receptors. Methisoprinol and NPT 15392 could be allosteric modifiers of inosine or hypoxanthine-utilizing enzymes giving rise to active analogs of xanthine and uric acid which regulate in turn the activity of adenosine deaminase (ADA), purine-nucleoside phosphorylase (PNP), 5'-nucleotidase inosine dehydrogenase or hypoxanthine-guanine phosphoribosyltransferase (HGPRT) (37).

Part of this work has been supported by a CNR grant # 84.02046.52.

REFERENCES

1. A. Azzara, A. Meozzi, G. Carulli, M. Martelli, F. Tangheroni, E. Serravalle and F. Ambrogi, Normalizzazione di funzioni neutrofiliche in bambini affetti da infezioni croniche ricorrenti dopo terapia ciclica con metisoprinolo, Chemioterapia 3:179 (1983).
2. C. Balestrino, E. Montesoro, A. Nocera, M. Ferrarini and T. Hoffman, Incremento dell' attivita NK di cellule mononucleate di sangue periferico umano dopo trattamento con metisoprinolo, Biol. Resp. Modifiers 2:577 (1983).
3. M. Bechi and A. Cini, L'impiego del metisoprinolo nel trattamento della epatite virale acuta, Clin. Europea. 20:79 (1981).
4. R. F. Betts, R. G. Douglas, S. D. George and C. J. Rinehart, Isoprinosine in experimental influenza A infection in volunteers, 78th Annual Meeting of A.S.M., Las Vegas, Nevada (1978).
5. L. J. Bradshaw, H. L. Sumner, W. H. Wickett, Jr. and E. B. Correia, Immunological and clinical studies on herpes simplex patients treated with inosiplex, 4th International Congress of Immunology, Paris, Abst. 17.7.5 (1980).
6. S. Catania, F. Zennaro, P. Vittucci and M. Monacelli, Indagine clinica sul trattamento della varicella con isoprinosina, G. Mal. Inf. 35:194 (1983).
7. I. Cerutti, C. Chany and J. F. Schlumberger, Isoprinosine increases the antitumor action of interferon, Int. J. Immunopharmacol. 1:59 (1979).

8. T. W. Chang and L. Weinstein, Antiviral activity of isoprinosine in vitro and in vivo, Am. J. Med. Sci. 265:143 (1973).
9. P. Cornaglia-Ferraris, R. Coffey and J. W. Hadden, Purine substituted analogs as immunomodulators, EOS 4:134 (1984).
10. M. Danto, R. Colella, G. Borrelli, G. LaBella and R. Mele, L'uso di metisoprinolo in corso di broncopeumopatie croniche riacutizzate, Clin. Europea. 20:130 (1981).
11. M. D'Aquino, A. Borri, E. Radin, S. Scremin and L. Caprioglio, Efficacia del metisoprinolo nella terapia delle epatiti acute virali, 11th Congr. Naz. A.M.O.I., G. Mal. Infett. 34:1746 (1982).
12. S. W. D'Arca, A. Pana and M. Grassi, Attivita del metisoprinolo nei confronti del virus rabbico: Valutazione in vitro, EOS 3:8 (1983).
13. G. Delogu, D. Meli, C. DeSimone, G. Cristina, A. Lozzi and G. DeRitis, Impiego del metisoprinolo in un caso di poliradicolonevrite virale a prevalente incidenza bulbare, XI Congresso Nazionale A.M.O.I., Napoli giugno (1981).
14. C. DeSimone, G. W. Canonica, G. Corte and D. Meli, Influence of methisoprinol on surface antigens of T lymphocytes, Curr. Chemother. Immunother. 1:1161 (1982).
15. C. DeSimone, C. Capozzi, S. Campo, D. Ricca and G. Matteucci, Effetto dell' azatioprina e dell' inosiplex sulla formazione di rosette da parte dei linfociti di soggetti sani e di pazienti con neoplasie, Ann. Sclavo. 23:116 (1981).
16. C. DeSimone, A. Cilli, S. Zanzoglu and F. Matricardi, Results of clinical trials with methisoprinol in Italy, EOS 4:108 (1984).
17. C. DeSimone, G. Delogu, L. Pugnaloni and C. Mastropietro, Methisoprinol and corticosteroids: Immunopharmacokinetic assessment, Tissue Reactions 1:101 (1984).
18. C. DeSimone, A. Koverech, L. Pugnaloni, C. Mastropietro, M. C. Salis and F. Sorice, Defective adenosine-inducible suppressor T lymphocyte generation by NPT 15392 and methisoprinol, Int. J. Immunother. 1:67 (1985).
19. C. DeSimone, D. Meli, M. Sbricoli, E. Rebuzzi and A. Koverech, In vitro effect of inosiplex on T lymphocytes: Influence on T cells with receptors for IgG (Tγ), Int. J. Immunopharmacol. 4:139 (1982).
20. C. DeSimone, L. Pugnaloni, S. DeSantis, L. Baldinelli and F. Sorice, Influence of methisoprinol on kinetics of immune interferon production and blastogenesis, Int. J. Immunopharmacol. 3:317 (1985).
21. C. DeSimone, A. Ricca, A. Lozzi and L. Lucci, Influence of methisoprinol on OKT4+, OKT8+, OKM1+, OKIa1+ cells, Int. J. Immunopharmacol. 4:291 (1982).
22. R. Finch, Immunomodulating effects of antimicrobial agents, J. Antimicrobiol. Chemother. 6:691 (1980).
23. I. Florentin, M. Bruley-Rosset, J. Schulz, M. Davigny, N. Kiger and G. Mathe, Attempt at functional classification of chemically-defined immunomodulators, in: "Advances in Immunopharmacology," J. W. Hadden, L. Chedid, P. Mullen and F. Spreafico, eds., Pergamon Press, Oxford (1981).
24. I. Florentin, E. Taylor, M. Davigny, C. Mathe and J. W. Hadden, Kinetic studies of the immunopharmacologic effects of NPT 15392 in mice, Int. J. Immunopharmacol. 4:225 (1982).
25. V. Frappamaina, L. Monno, F. Trotta and G. Pastore, Clearance sierica dell 'HB e AG nell 'epatite acuta di tipo B trattata con metisoprinolo, EOS 2:115 (1982).
26. H. Friedman, R. Calle and A. Morin, Double-blind study of isoprinosine influence on immune parameters in solid tumor-bearing patients treated by radiotherapy, Int. J. Immunopharmacol. 2:194 (1980).
27. M. Galli, A. Lazzarin, M. Moroni and C. Zanussi, Inosiplex in recurrent herpes simplex infections, Lancet 2:331 (1982).

28. T. Ginsberg, Urinary excretion of purine metabolites in macaca mulatta following administration of inosine and 1-(dimethylamino)-2-propanol, p acetamidobenzoate, 5th Congress Pharmacology, S. Francisco, CA (1972).
29. T. Ginsberg and A. J. Glasky, Inosiplex: an immunomodulation model for the treatment of viral disease, Third conference on antiviral substances, Ann. N. Y. Acad. Sci. 284:128 (1977).
30. A. J. Glasky, G. E. Friebertshauser, J. W. Halker, R. A. Settineri and T. Ginsberg, The role of cell mediated immunity in the therapeutic action of viral disease processes, Chemotherapy 6:235 (1976).
31. A. Glasky, J. Gordon, F. Hoehler, J. Wallace and J. C. Bekesi, Isoprinosine (INPX) in progressive generalized lymphodenopathy (PGC) - kinetics of action and clinical response, Int. J. Immunopharmacol. 7:318 (1985).
32. P. Gordon and E. R. Brown, The antiviral activity of isoprinosine, Can. J. Microbiol. 18:1463 (1972).
33. P. Gordon, B. Ronsen and E. R. Brown, Anti-herpes virus action of isoprinosine, Antimicrob. Agents Chemother. 5:153 (1974).
34. P. Gordon and B. Rosen, Isoprinosine: biochemical correlates of antiviral and experimental learning-enhancing activities, FASEB 29:684 (1970).
35. A. Goutner, In vitro modulation of natural killer cell activity by isoprinosine, NPT 15392, and interferon, Int. J. Immunopharmacol. 2:197 (1980).
36. G. Grippaudo, V. Diminiello and G. Fratto, Il metisoprinolo nel trattamento delle manifestazioni erpetiche intra ed extra-orali, Inform. Sanitario 4:1 (1982).
37. J. W. Hadden, P. Cornaglia-Ferraris and R. Coffey, Purine analogs as immunomodulators, in: "Progress in Immunology," Academic Press, Japan (1984).
38. J. W. Hadden and A. Giner-Sorolla, Isoprinosine and NPT 15392: Modulators of lymphocyte and macrophage development and function, in: "Augmenting Agents in Cancer Therapy: Current Status and Future Perspectives," M. Chirigos and E. Hersh, eds., Raven Press, New York (1980).
39. J. W. Hadden and A. Giner-Sorolla, Isoprinosine and NPT 15392: Modulators of lymphocyte and macrophage development and function, Prog. Cancer Res. Ther. 16:492 (1981).
40. J. W. Hadden, A. Giner-Sorolla, E. M. Hadden, S. Ikehara, R. Pahwa, R. Coffey, A. M. Castellazi, C. Jones, K. Maxwell and L. Simon, NPT 16416: A levamisole-like purine with immunomodulatory effects, Int. J. Immunopharmacol. Abst. 4:287 (1982).
41. J. W. Hadden, E. M. Hadden and R. G. Coffey, Isoprinosine augmentation of phytohemagglutinin induced lymphocyte proliferation, Infect. Immun. 13:382 (1976).
42. J. W. Hadden, E. M. Hadden, T. Spira, R. Sedlineri, L. Simon and A. Giner-Sorolla, Effects of NPT 15392 in vitro on human leukocyte functions, Int. J. Immunopharmacol. 4:225 (1982).
43. J. W. Hadden, C. Lopez, R. J. O'Reilly and E. M. Hadden, Levamisole and inosiplex: Antiviral agents with immunopotentiating action, Third Conference on Antiviral Substances, Ann. N. Y. Acad. Sci. 284:139 (1977).
44. P. Hersey, C. Bindon, M. Bradley and E. Hasic, Effect of isoprinosine on interleukin 1 and 2 production and on suppressor cell activity in pokeweed mitogen stimulated cultures of B and T cells, Int. J. Immunopharmacol. 6:315 (1984).
45. S. Ikehara, J. W. Hadden, R. A. Good and R. Pahwa, In vitro effects of two immunopotentiators, isoprinosine and NPT 15392, on murine T cells differentiation and function, Thymus 3:90 (1981).
46. G. Italia and E. Rizza, Studio clinico sull' impiego del metisoprinolo

nell' herpes genitalis, Quad. Clin. Ostetrica Ginecologia 37:129 (1982).
47. C. E. Jones, P. R. Dyken, P. R. Huttenlocher, J. T. Jabbour and K. W. Maxwell, Inosiplex therapy in subacute sclerosing panencephalitis: A multicentre non-randomised study in 98, Lancet 1:1034 (1982).
48. F. G. Lento, S. Tandurella, C. Baretti, G. Cannata and R. Salerno, Pazienti affetti da herpes zoster trattati con metisoprinolo, G. Ital. Pat. 28:9 (1983).
49. F. Loiacono, D. Agnello, R. Malizia and M. Balsamo. Il metisoprinolo nel trattamento di alcune affezioni delle vie respiratorie del bambino, Aggior. Pediat. 33:85 (1982).
50. S. Longley, R. L. Dunning and R. H. Waldman, Effect of isoprinosine against challenge with A(H3N2)/Hong Kong influence virus in volunteers, Antimicrob. Agents Chemother. 3:506 (1973).
51. V. J. Merluzzi, M. M. Walker, N. Williams, B. Susskind, J. W. Hadden and R. Faanes, Immunoenhancing activity of NPT 15392: A potential immune response modifier, Int. J. Immunopharmacol. 4:219 (1982).
52. A. Miglietta, M. T. Ventura, F. Dammacco and L. Bonomo, Effetto del metisoprinolo sulla fagocitosi dei monociti e dei granulociti neutrofili in vitro, EOS 2:13 (1981).
53. G. Migneco, C. LaCascia, S. Mansueto and S. Tripi, Analisi e valutazione delle modificazioni del quadro clinico di epatiti croniche in corso di trattamento con metisoprinolo, Riv. Parassitologia 43:331 (1981).
54. A. Morin, C. Griscelli and F. Daguillard, Effets de l' isoprinosine sur l' activation des lymphocytes humains in vitro, Ann. Immunol. 130:541 (1979).
55. A. Morin, J. L. Touraine, G. Renoux and J. W. Hadden, Isoprinosine as an immunomodulating agent, in: "International Symposium on New Trends in Human Cancer, Immunology and Cancer Immunotherapy," B. Serrou and C. Rosenfeld, eds., Doin Editeur, Paris (1980).
56. H. Ohnishi, H. Kosuzume, I. Hitoshi, O. Masatsugu, Y. Morita, H. Mochizuki and Y. Zusuki, Mechanism of host defense suppression induced by viral infection: Mode of action of inosiplex as an antiviral agent, Infec. Immun. 243:38 (1982).
57. H. Ohnishi, H. Kosuzume, H. Inaba, M. Okura, S. Shimada, H. Tajima and Y. Suzuki, The immunomodulatory action of inosiplex in relation to its effects in experimental viral infections, Int. J. Immunopharmacol. 5:181 (1983).
58. D. M. Pachuta, Y. Togo, R. B. Hornick, A. R. Schwartz and S. Tominaga, Evaluation of isoprinosine in experimental human rhinovirus infection, Antimicrob. Agents Chemother. 5:403 (1974).
59. A. Paffetti, D. Curti, V. Renda, A. Nurzia and S. Carlizzi, Il metisoprinolo nella epatite acuta virale di tipo B, Riv. Sci. Med. Farmacol. 5:361 (1983).
60. E. Pasqui, A. Alzeni, G. Verrocchi, G. Daga and A. Carta, Terapia con metisoprinolo di 50 casi di epatite virale acuta, Riv. Pat. Clin. 35:735 (1980).
61. A. Polloni, M. Carrai, A. Capria and G. Corsini, Trattamento delle epatiti croniche HB_sAg positive con metisoprinolo: Prime esperienze, Riv. Gastroent. 33:41 (1981).
62. A. Pompidou, In vitro effects of methisoprinol on human peripheral blood lymphocytes, EOS 4:112 (1984).
63. G. Precchia, M. Del Vecchio, G. Morelli, P. Tarallo, C. Ciccarello, A. Precchia and P. Amoroso, Il metisoprinolo nella terapia delle malattie viral: dati preliminari sul trattamento di un gruppo di malattie, Chemioter. Antimicrobican. 4:64 (1981).
64. G. Rancurel and A. Buge, Bull. et Mem. Soc. Med. Paris IX:49 (1981).
65. G. Rancurel, B. Lesourd, A. Pompidou, D. Denvil, C. Pontes, R. Moulias and A. Buge, Immunological status in necrotic acute encephalitis (NAW), L'infection herpetique humaine et ses traitments, Facultè de Medicine de Brest, Proceedings (1981).

66. G. Renoux, M. Renoux and D. Degenne, Suppressor cell activity after isoprinosine treatment of lymphocytes from normal mice, Int. J. Immunopharmacol. 1:239 (1979).
67. G. Renoux, M. Renoux, J. M. Guillaumin and C. Gouzien, Differentiation and regulation of lymphocyte populations - evidence for immunopotentiation induced T cell recruitment, Int. J. Immunopharmacol. 1:415 (1979).
68. G. Santangelo, S. Lombardo, S. Randazzo, N. Maccarone and M. Amato, Il Viruxan nelle infezioni virali dell' infanzia: Prospettive terapeutiche nelle infezioni virali ricorrenti dell' eta del lattante, Aggior. Pediatr. 32:1 (1981).
69. A. J. Sato, T. S. Hall and S. E. Reed, Trial of the antiviral action of isoprinosine against rhinovirus infection of volunteers, Antimicrob. Agents Chemother. 3:332 (1973).
70. I. Signorelli, G. Garbarino and S. Tampucci, Studio clinico del metisoprinolo in pazienti affette da condiloma acuminato, G. Ital. Ostet. Ginecol. 4:11 (1982).
71. L. N. Simon and A. J. Glasky, Isoprinosine: an overview, Cancer Treatment Reports 62:1963 (1978).
72. L. N. Simon, F. K. Hoehler, T. Ginsberg and J. W. Hadden, NPT 15392: A new chemically defined biological response modifier, in: "Immune Modulation Agents and Their Actions," E. Fenichel and M. A. Chirigos, eds., Marcel Dekker, Inc., New York, N.Y. (1984).
73. A. Sinardi, L. Santamaria, C. Practico, L. Siracusano and A. Martino, Su due casi di meningo-encefalite virale trattati con metisoprinolo, Clin. Europa. 22:396 (1983).
74. S. Spadafora, Il metisoprinolo in alcune virosi cutanee; nostre prime esperienze, Esp. Med. Chir. 1:83 (1981).
75. S. Specter and J. W. Hadden, Thymomimetic drugs, in: "Immunomodulation," J. W. Hadden and F. Spreafico, eds., Springer Verlag, in press (1985).
76. J-L. Touraine, J. W. Hadden and F. Touraine, Isoprinosine-induced T cell differentiation and T cell suppressor activity in humans, in: "Current Chemotherapy and Infectious Disease," J. D. Nelson and C. Grassi, eds., A.S.M., Washington, D.C. (1980).
77. J. L. Touraine, B. Serrou, J. W. Hadden, A. Morin and F. Touraine, Modulation of suppressor T cell activity by isoprinosine, in: "International Symposium on New Trends in Human Immunology and Cancer Immunotherapy," G. Serrou and C. Rosenfeld, eds., Doin, Paris (1980).
78. S. Tripi, G. Migneco and C. LaCascia, Comportamento dell' antigene di superficile del virus dell' epatite B(HB_sAg) e del suo anticorpo (HB_sAb) in pazienti con epatite acuta trattati con metisoprinolo, Riv. Parassit. 42:345 (1981).
79. K. Y. Tsang, H. H. Fudenberg, G. M. P. Golbriath, R. P. Donnelly, L. R. Bishop and W. R. Koopenen, Partial restoration of interleukin 2 production and tac (putative interleukin 2 receptor) expression in patients with acquired immune deficiency syndrome by isoprinosine treatment, J. Clin. Invest. 5:1538 (1985).
80. A. Vellucci, G. Galanti and A. Delongis, Virus epatite acuta trattata con metisoprinolo. Nostre osservazioni preliminari in 22 casi, G. Mal. Infett. 34:611 (1982).
81. G. Villa, C. Caltagirone and G. Macchi, Unusual clinical course in a case of Creutzfeldt-Jakob disease, Ital. J. Neurol. Sci. 2:155 (1982).
82. R. H. Waldman and R. Ganguly, Therapeutic efficacy of inosiplex (isoprinosine) in rhinovirus infection, Ann. N. Y. Acad. Sci. 284:153 (1977).
83. J. Wybran, A. Govaerts and J. Appleboom, Inosiplex, a stimulating agent for normal human T cells and human leukocytes, J. Immunol. 121:1181 (1978).

84. J. Wybran, B. Serrou, D. Belpomme, J. Boneterre, A. Desplaces, R. Favre, T. Ginsberg, J. M. Lang, G. Mayer, D. T. McKenzie, M. Miksche, D. C. Petit, G. Renoux, C. Rosenfeld, M. Schneider, L. N. Simon and L. Toujas, Immunomodulating of T cell and NK function by NPT 15392 in cancer patients, <u>in</u>: "Current Concepts in Human Immunology and Cancer Immunomodulation," B. Serrou, C. Rosenfeld, J. C. Daniels and J. P. Saunders, eds., Elsevier Biomedical, Netherlands (1982).
85. G. F. Zagni and C. Cannarozzo, Studio clinico sui metisoprinolo per uso topico in alcune virosi cutanee, <u>Clin</u>. <u>Europea</u>. 21:585 (1982).

MURAMYL DIPEPTIDES, HOST IMMUNITY AND ENHANCEMENT

Monique Parant and Louis Chedid

Institut Pasteur
Paris, France

INTRODUCTION

Immunopotentiating agents can be used either to enhance immunologically specific responses, and/or to activate mechanisms of nonspecific host resistance. Actually, immunopotentiating products may turn out to be of major importance in cases of problem infections, mainly in the immunocompromised host, or for the treatment of immunodeficiences concomitant to certain chronic infectious diseases and occurring under various conditions such as malnutrition and old age.

After the minimal adjuvant-active structure derived from bacterial peptidoglycan had been identified as muramyl dipeptide or MDP in 1974 (reviewed in 27), MDP was also shown to stimulate nonspecific resistance in experimental infections when given in saline before the challenge, whatever the route of administration (8,37). Since then, many reports on the induction of resistance to bacterial, fungal, or parasitic infections have been published (for review see 13 and 38), reflecting the ever-increasing efforts made by several laboratories.

The synthesis of MDP was followed by the preparation of a large number of analogues with the hope of determining structure-activity relationships (23,28), or at least of selecting immunostimulating compounds, which did not retain several side effects inherent to MDP administration (10,34). In several studies, chemically different muramyl peptides were comparatively evaluated, and their effect assessed in a variety of experimental test systems, such as acute infections in adult normal mice or rats, in T-cell depleted mice, in splenectomized mice, in neonates, in mice immunosuppressed by irradiation, corticosteroids, or cyclophosphamide, and in mice subjected to chronic protein depletion (6,13,17,21,23,30,37). However, protection by muramyl peptides depends on the size of the microbial inoculum, and on the microorganisms used. Several physico-chemical modifications of muramyl dipeptides have been used as means for enhancing anti-infectious effects such as alteration of hydrophobicity, polymerization, or conjugation to a carrier. The derivatives may display new biological activities. In addition, the efficacy of a combined treatment with muramyl peptide and a chemotherapeutic drug suggests that such a combination may be useful to enhance the effect of therapeutics, and to restore the defense mechanisms in immunocompromised patients.

ADJUVANT EFFECT AND ANTI-INFECTIOUS ACTIVITY

Although most of the muramyl peptides that induced an increased resistance to infections are also active in the adjuvant tests, both the stimulating properties can be dissociated in some experimental models. Generally, muramyl peptides are effective against infectious challenges under conditions which may lead to a depression of the immune response (37). Moreover, like most immunoadjuvants, MDP has been shown to generate a T cell-mediated immunosuppressive activity when given in repeated injections of large doses (25). Such a treatment does not impair its protective activity in mice against a Klebsiella infection (34).

In addition, there exist some examples of MDP derivatives that are ineffective, or poorly active as adjuvants, but can provide an anti-infective action, stronger than the original MDP (7,33,37). Moreover, animals that are low-responders to the adjuvant effect of MDP such as Lewis rats or C57Bl/6 mice are protected against a Klebsiella infection as effectively as high-responder animals (37).

PYROGENICITY AND ANTI-INFECTIOUS ACTIVITY

Should the elevation of body temperature be considered as a nonspecific immune reaction capable of inducing an enhanced resistance by impairing proliferation of thermosensitive organisms, and/or by the production of immunoregulatory factors (22)? Most of the immunostimulants derived from bacteria activate macrophages to produce endogenous pyrogen, and induce a fever response when administered to rabbits. Lipopolysaccharides of gram negative organisms have constituted the most representative class of bacterial pyrogens, although some peptidoglycans can also induce a marked febrile response. The molecular size of the preparation was always of crucial importance. It was therefore unexpected that some pyrogenic activity appeared to be associated with the small molecular weight MDP (24).

MDP was shown to stimulate monocytic cells to produce both endogenous pyrogen (EP) and Interleukin-1 (IL1), (see in 11), and its adjuvant effect has been ascribed to the release of IL1 it elicits from macrophages (43). Since some adjuvant-active muramyl peptides are not pyrogenic, and are obviously unable to induce the production of EP, they were used as inducers of IL1 release. Thus, when Murabutide, a butyl ester MDP derivative devoid of any pyrogenicity (6), was incubated with rabbit macrophages or with human blood monocytes, IL1 was produced although no detectable pyrogenicity could be found in the culture fluid (11). This result has provided the first indication that IL1 and EP correspond to at least two factors that can be dissociated in contrast to what had been previously postulated. Murabutide was also shown to be exempt of other MDP pharmacological effects such as induction of neutropenia, lowering of serum iron levels, and increases of SAA levels (reviewed in 10 and 34).

Comparison between MDP and Murabutide has shown that the effect on body temperature was not a prerequisite for the immunostimulant properties of muramyl peptides. Both glycopeptides displayed a comparable adjuvant effect on humoral immune responses (6), and are equally protective in animals infected with Klebsiella pneumoniae organisms as summarized in Table 1.

Another indication that fever response was not essential for the enhancement of nonspecific resistance to bacterial infection has been provided by indomethacin treatment which did not inhibit the stimulating effects of MDP (9). However, some derivatives obtained by conjugation to a carrier are more effective against bacterial infections and more pyrogenic, making likely an additive effect of fever or of pyrogenic factors.

Table 1. Protective Effect of MDP or Murabutide Against a Klebsiella pneumoniae Infection

Animal	Treatment i.v. at day -1[a]	Bacterial challenge	Survivors at day +15 No./total	Survivors at day +15 Protection[b]
Adult mice	Controls	10^4 i.v.	6/32	
"	MDP	"	23/32	53%
"	Murabutide	"	24/32	56%
7 day-old mice	Controls	10^3 s.c.	2/42	
"	MDP	"	18/42	38%
"	Murabutide	"	25/42	55%
Adult Wistar rats	Controls	10^7 i.v.	4/42	
"	MDP	"	28/42	57%
"	Murabutide	"	19/42	36%

[a] 100 μg/animal
[b] Difference between percentage of survivors in treated and control group.

POTENTIATION OF THE ANTI-INFECTIOUS EFFECT OF MDP BY CHEMICAL MODIFICATION

Several lipophilic MDP derivatives have been prepared because they mimick more closely the cell wall which has a high lipid content. Among them certain derivatives were shown to have new biological activities, such as stearoyl MDP (23), MTP-PE or muramyl tripeptide-dipalmitoyl phosphatidylethanolamine (13), 6-O-mycoloyl derivative (33), and MDP-GDP or MDP-dipalmitoyl-sn-glycerol (39). In some examples, the lipophilic compound has been shown to stimulate cell-mediated immune responses, even in the absence of an oily vehicle. Moreover, they may be administered in various dosage forms such as depot formulation or in liposomes. Thus, they have been shown to be efficient inducers of macrophage/monocyte tumoricidal activity when incorporated in liposomes (16,39). They may have another interesting biological property. For example, when solubilized in saline, MTP-PE exerts prophylactic and therapeutic anti-viral effect (12). Against bacterial challenges, lipophilic derivatives have often been shown to exhibit a protective activity stronger than the original MDP (13,23,29,32,33). Preliminary data indicate that administration in liposomes can increase the efficacy against experimental infections of only a few of these derivatives (Parant et al.; unpublished results).

By the use of cross-linked oligomers or by linking a muramyl peptide to a carrier, a higher protection than with free MDP was obtained against bacterial infection (9). The conjugation procedure to a large non-immunogenic or immunogenic carrier strongly potentiated the anti-infectious effect against various challenges such as Klebsiella, Pseudomonas or Listeria infections in mice (7,35). With the synthetic multi-poly(DL-Ala)-poly-(L-Lys) chain, it has also been shown that an inactive MDP stereoisomer MDP(D,D) could acquire a good potency against infection after coupling, although it remained inactive as immunoadjuvant (7). Other carriers such as Influenza viral subunits have also been used to prepare conjugates endowed with a similar protective activity, i.e. effective at a very low dosage level of MDP. Even more interesting is the fact that such a conjugate administered intranasally enhanced the mouse resistance against an unrelated viral infection, whereas free MDP was inactive (35). This type of investigation has a potential for developing antibacterial or antiviral agents endowed with both specific and nonspecific activities.

COMBINED USE OF MURAMYL PEPTIDES AND ANTIBIOTICS

Clinical experience has shown that for antimicrobial chemotherapy to be effective, a functional host defense system is required. The dosage determination of an antimicrobial agent cannot be based only on a value greater than, or identical to, the minimal inhibitory concentration at the site of infection. The host's capacity to contribute to eradication of the pathogen should be taken into account. Therefore, several studies were undertaken to evaluate the therapeutic usefulness of antibiotic-immunostimulant combination against infection. The potential importance of these treatments has stimulated the evaluation of muramyl peptides with regard to their possible synergistic, and/or additive effect with antibiotics. Various combinations of antibiotics and immunostimulants should be examined, and their efficacy evaluated both in normal and in immunodepressed animals.

In normal mice, the first observation of synergism has been reported with soluble glycopeptides administered subcutaneously, MDP or nor-MDP, and a cephalosporine derivative given orally. It was shown that in many types of acute infections (*K.pneumoniae*, *Pasteurella multocida*, and *Salmonella typhimurium*), the median effective dose of antibiotic was lowered by MDP or nor-MDP treatment (14). With nor-MDP, a synergistic effect was then obtained with gentamicin against an intraperitoneal infection of *Pseudomonas aeruginosa* (17). Survival data plotted for MDP in Figure 1 represent the type of response achieved with gentamicin in mice infected with *K. pneumoniae*. To maximize the protection elicited by MDP treatment, the challenge dose of bacteria was increased, and the combination of MDP and the

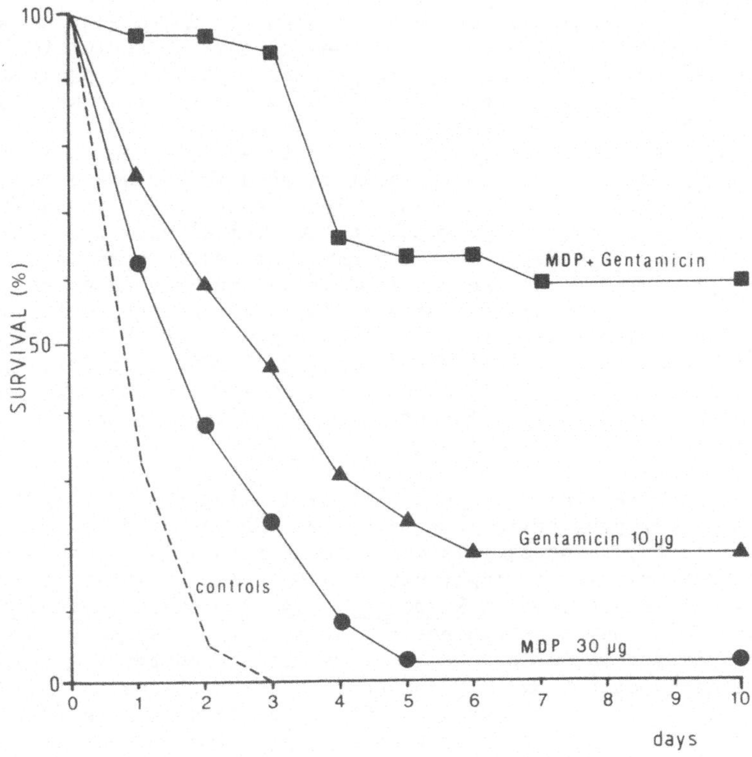

Figure 1. Survival data on animals treated intravenously with MDP or saline 24 hr before, and given one subcutaneous injection of gentamicin 2 hr after intravenous challenge with 4×10^4 *K. pneumoniae*.

Table 2. Protective Effect of Muramyl Peptides Associated with Gentamicin Against a K. pneumoniae Infection

Compound[a] (dose/mouse)	Survival at day +15[b] No gentamicin		Plus gentamicin	
Controls	0/24		4/24	
MDP 30 μg	1/24		14/24	P<0.01
MDP 100 μg	10/24	P<0.01	18/24	P<0.01
Murabutide 30 μg	2/24		12/24	P<0.01
Murabutide 100 μg	8/24		18/24	P<0.01
MDP-GDP 30 μg	4/24		14/24	P<0.01
MDP-GDP 100 μg	12/24	P<0.01	18/24	P<0.01

[a] i.v. at day -1
[b] After the challenge of 4×10^4 organisms i.v.; gentamicin 10 μg s.c. 2 hrs after challenge.

antibiotic resulted in a significant increase in the number of survivors. The efficacy of the non-pyrogenic Murabutide and of a lipophilic derivative MDP-GDP was also evaluated in the same experimental model. The data are shown in Table 2.

Treatment with the three adjuvants resulted in a similar protective activity. A local infection performed with a K. pneumoniae contaminated suture simulating surgical infection has been used by Polk et al. (40) to demonstrate an additive effect of MDP used in combination with cephaloridine or chloramphenicol. With a lipophilic derivative (6-O-stearoyl-MDP), Osada et al. (31) have also reported a marked increase in average survival time as compared with mice receiving either the stearoyl-MDP or the antibiotic alone. This effect was demonstrated with cefazolin, gentamicin, and amphotericin B, against infections with Escherichia coli, P.aeruginosa, and Candida albicans, respectively (31).

C. albicans is considered to be an important nocosomial pathogen, its establishment in patients being facilitated by corticoids, anti-tumor agents, tissue damage, and impaired cellular immunity. Experimental murine candidiasis lends itself to the assessment of nonspecific effect of immunostimulants, in that the survival time can be predetermined by adjusting the size of the inoculum. Some lipophilic MDP derivatives were superior to water soluble compounds against a candida infection, and effective even in immunosuppressed mice (31,42). Their efficacy was found to be enhanced by the simultaneous administration of anti-fungal agents (amphotericin B, fluorocytosine, papulacandin). Treatment with the MDP derivative induced a marked reduction of median effective doses of the chemotherapeutic agent (42). Against a severe challenge that killed almost all the controls within five days, the protective effect of MDP-GDP was shown by the increase in survival time as reported in Table 3. Administration of amphotericin B simultaneously with the challenge was successful in increasing protective activity (Table 3).

It is not yet possible to determine whether or not the macrophage is the principal or sole cell type which is responsible for the enhanced resistance to Candida albicans, but a linear correlation was seen between carbon clearance and anti-infective activity of several MDP analogues in normal and in immunosuppressed mice (18). Antibiotics in subinhibitory concentra-

Table 3. Protective Effect of a Lipophilic MDP Derivative Associated with Amphotericin B in Mice Infected with Candida albicans

Treatment[a]	Survivors/total at day +4	at day +15
Controls	5/24	0/24
Amphotericin B 3 μg	10/24	3/24
MDP-GDP 100 μg	22/24[b]	5/24
MDP-GDP + amphotericin B	23/24[b]	16/24[c]

[a]MDP-GDP i.v. at days -4, -3, -2, and -1 before the intravenous challenge with 4 x 10^6 C. albicans; amphotericin B s.c. at day 0.
[b]P<0.01 as compared with untreated controls.
[c]P<0.01 as compared with MDP-GDP alone.

tions may enhance the phagocytic activity of macrophages, and for example, chloramphenicol-pretreated E. coli are killed more efficiently than the controls by human leukocytes, killing that may be the result of structural changes in the outer membrane of the bacteria (41). An increased phagocytosis has also been demonstrated in vitro with Listeria monocytogenes or with E. coli in the presence of a subinhibitory amount of ampicillin or tetracyclin (1,19). In a further study, Friedman and Warren (20) have shown that administration of MDP to mice increased the ability of peritoneal macrophages to phagocytize antibiotic-treated E. coli, and that addition of MDP to normal macrophage cultures still potentiated phagocytosis of cyclacillin-treated bacteria (20). Moreover, even at low concentrations that do not significantly influence bacterial growth, certain antibiotics can affect bacterial adhesion, which represents an important factor in the pathogenesis of various infectious diseases (3,44). The choice of the antibiotic may therefore be critical and should be carefully chosen according to what is known on the pathogenicity of each bacterial strain. Since MDPs are known to stimulate macrophages, and to increase their phagocytic activity (see 26), their use in combination with antibiotics could allow decreased doses of chemotherapeutic agents, and the restoration of host defense mechanisms.

CONCLUSIONS

The great number of water soluble MDP analogues produced in several laboratories has provided a good understanding of their biological properties. Such an evaluation has allowed us to select an MDP derivative called Murabutide, which is undergoing clinical trials with conventional vaccines after its safety had been established by animal toxicological assays, and in a phase I clinical trial (10). Because of the simplicity of these molecules, and of the absence of immunogenicity, they may constitute favorable tools for a better knowledge of mechanisms involved in the stimulation of nonspecific resistance to bacterial infections, in both in vivo and in vitro studies. Minor chemical modifications have already provided compounds with different profiles, and, up to now, compounds devoid of side effects thus obtained are only water soluble MDP analogues (4,6). Moreover, though the hydrophilic MDPs are cleared rapidly from the body (36), the best timing for administration to protect against an infectious challenge is one day before, but a negative phase of higher susceptibility has never been observed.

The lipophilic derivatives of MDP seem to produce stronger side effects than most of the hydrophilic molecules, and presently have not reached the stage of clinical trials. In most cases they exhibited higher immunopotentiating activities, and even new biological properties such as antitumor or antiviral effects (14,16,39). When encapsulated within liposomes, MDP-PE was shown to enhance host's resistance to metastases after systemic injection (16). However, the antiviral effect obtained after intranasal administration of MTP-PE in saline has also opened a new way of research (13).

Conjugates containing MDP may be utilized in vaccinating preparations. Such synthetic or semi-synthetic constructs were also shown to stimulate specific and non-specific immunity (5). The pyrogenicity of MDP was increased in some of the conjugates (9), but the effective dose is far smaller than with free MDP and non-pyrogenic analogues can also be used (7). The capacity of MDP to enhance resistance to bacterial infections is strongly increased after coupling to a carrier, and was also assessed against viral infections (35). The mechanisms involved in the antiviral activity of lipophilic MDP and of conjugates are still unclear, but they may be related to a synergistic activity with endogenous interferon released after viral infection.

The synergistic combination of MDPs and antibiotics represents a positive contribution leading to a decrease in ED_{50} values of antibiotics and to an increase in the efficacy of muramyl peptides to stimulate non-specific mechanisms of resistance. Such a potentially superior application may be considered against various types of infections to lower the dose of the chemotherapeutic drugs that may possess significant inherent toxicity or immunosuppressive effect. An increasing example has been provided against Leishmania donovani since a combined therapy with an antimonial drug and a lipophilic muramyl peptide was found to be more effective than either of the two treatments applied individually (2). Moreover, the synergistic action of macrophage-activating factor (MAF) and MDPs in therapeutic studies against cancer metastases (15) may open an exciting field of research by taking advantage of the opportunity offered by modern biotechnology to produce cytokines.

REFERENCES

1. D. Adam, Enhanced in vitro phagocytosis of different pathogens by human monocytes in the presence of antibiotics, in: "The Influence of Antibiotics on the Host-parasite Relationship," H. U. Eickenberg, H. Hahn, and W. Opferkuch, eds., Springer-Verlag, Berlin (1982).
2. L. E. Adinolfi, P. F. Bonventre, M. Van der Pas, and D. A. Eppstein, Synergistic effect of glucantime and a liposome-encapsulated muramyl dipeptide analog in therapy of experimental visceral Leishmaniasis, Infect. Immun. 48:409 (1985).
3. E. H. Beachey, B. I. Eisenstein, and I. Ofek, Sublethal concentrations of antibiotics and bacterial adhesion, in: "Adhesion and Microorganisms Pathogenicity," K. Elliott, M. O'Connor, and J. Whelan, eds., Ciba Foundation Symp. 80, Pitman Medical Ltd., London (1980).
4. N. E. Byars, Two adjuvant-active muramyl dipeptide analogs induce differential production of lymphocyte-activating factor and a factor causing distress in guinea pigs, Infect. Immun. 44:344 (1984).
5. L. Chedid, and F. Audibert, New approaches for control of infections using synthetic or semi-synthetic constructs containing MDP, Springer Semin. Immunopathol. (in press).
6. L. Chedid, M. Parant, F. Audibert, G. Riveau, F. Parant, E. Lederer, J. Choay, and P. Lefrancier, Biological activity of a new synthetic

muramyl peptide adjuvant devoid of pyrogenicity, Infect. Immun. 35:417 (1982).

7. L. Chedid, M. Parant, F. Parant, F. Audibert, P. Lefrancier, J. Choay, and M. Sela, Enhancement of certain biological activities of muramyl dipeptide derivatives after conjugation to a multi-poly(DL-alanine)-poly(L-Lysine) carrier, Proc. Natl. Acad. Sci. USA 76:6557 (1979).
8. L. Chedid, M. Parant, F. Parant, P. Lefrancier, J. Choay, and E. Lederer, Enhancement of non-specific immunity to Klebsiella pneumoniae infection by a synthetic immunoadjuvant (N-acetylmuramyl-L-alanyl-D-isoglutamine) and several analogs, Proc. Natl. Acad. Sci. USA 74:2089 (1977).
9. L. Chedid, M. Parant, and G. Riveau, Immunopharmacological activities of MDP, in: "Immunopharmacology and the Regulation of Leukocyte Function," D. R. Webb, ed., Marcel Dekker, New York (1982).
10. L. Chedid, Muramyl peptides as possible endogenous immunopharmacological mediators, Microbiol. Immun. 27:723 (1983).
11. C. Damais, G. Riveau, M. Parant, J. Gerota, and L. Chedid, Production of lymphocyte-activating factor in the absence of endogenous pyrogen by rabbit or human leukocytes stimulated by a muramyl dipeptide derivative, Int. J. Immunopharmacol. 4:451 (1982).
12. F. M. Dietrich, B. Lukas, and K. H. Schmidt-Ruppin, MTP-PE (synthetic muramyl peptide): prophylactic and therapeutic effects in experimental viral infections, 13th Intern. Cong. Chemotherapy, Vienna, (1983).
13. F. M. Dietrich, W. Sackmann, G. H. Mitchell, and A. Voller, Modulation of resistance to infections by synthetic low-molecular-weight compounds endowed with immunostimulatory properties: experimental results and potential role in human medicine, in: "Chemotherapy and Immunology in the Control of Malaria, Filariasis, and Leishmaniasis," N. Anand, and A. B. Sen, eds., Tata McGraw-Hill Publ., New-Dehli (1983).
14. F. M. Dietrich, W. Sackmann, O. Zak, and P. Dukor, Synthetic muramyl dipeptide immunostimulants: protective effects and increased efficacy of antibiotics in experimental bacterial and fungal infections in mice, in: "Current Chemotherapy and Infectious Disease, vol. 2," J. D. Nelson, and G. Grassi, eds., Amer. Soc. Microbiol, (1981).
15. I. J. Fidler, and A. J. Schroit, Synergism between lymphokines and muramyl dipeptide encapsulated in liposomes: In situ activation of macrophages and therapy of spontaneous cancer metastases, J. Immunol. 133:515 (1984).
16. I. J. Fidler, S. Sone, W. E. Fogler, D. Smith, D. G. Broun, L. Tarcsay, R. H. Gisler, and A. J. Schroit, Efficacy of liposomes containing a lipophilic muramyl dipeptide derivative for activating the tumoricidal properties of alveolar macrophages in vivo, J. Biol. Resp. Modif. 1:43 (1982).
17. E. B. Fraser-Smith, and T. R. Matthews, Protective effect of muramyl dipeptide analogs against infections of Pseudomonas aeruginosa or Candida albicans, Infect. Immun. 34:676 (1981).
18. E. B. Fraser-Smith, R. V. Waters, and T. R. Matthews, Correlation between in vivo anti-Pseudomonas and anti-Candida activities and clearance of carbon by the reticuloendothelial system for various muramyl dipeptide analogs, using normal and immunosuppressed mice, Infect. Immun. 35:105 (1982).
19. H. Friedman, and G. Warren, Increased phagocytosis of Escherichia coli pretreated with subinhibitory concentration of cyclacillin or ampicillin, Proc. Soc. Exp. Biol. Med. 169:301 (1982).
20. H. Friedman, and G. Warren, Muramyl dipeptide-induced enhancement of phagocytosis of antibiotic-pretreated Escherichia coli by macrophages, Proc. Soc. Exp. Biol. Med. 176:366 (1984).

21. R. B. Galland, L. S. Trachtenberg, N. Rynerson, and H. C. Polk, Nonspecific enhancement of resistance to local bacterial infection in starved mice, Arch. Surgery 117:161 (1982).
22. M. J. Kluger, Historical aspects of fever and its role in disease, in: "Thermoregulatory Mechanisms and Their Therapeutic Implications," B. Cox, P. Lomax, A. S. Milton, and E. Schonbaum, eds., S. Karger, Basel (1980).
23. S. Kotani, H. Takeda, M. Tsujimoto, T. Ogawa, Y. Mori, T. Koga, H. Iribe, A. Tanaka, S. Nagao, J. R. McGhee, S. M. Michalek, S. Kawata, T. Shiba, and S. Kusumoto, Lipophilic muramyl peptides and synthetic lipid A analogs as immunomodulators, in: "Progress in Immunology V," Y. Yamamura, and T. Tada, eds., Academic Press, Japan (1983).
24. S. Kotani, Y. Watanabe, T. Shimono, K. Harada, T. Shiba, S. Kusumoto, K. Yokogawa, and M. Taniguchi, Correlation between the immunoadjuvant activities and pyrogenicities of synthetic N-acetylmuramyl peptides or -aminoacids, Biken J. 19:9 (1976).
25. C. Leclerc, E. Bourgeois, and L. Chedid, Demonstration of muramyl dipeptide (MDP)-induced T suppressor cells responsible for MDP immunosuppressive activity, Europ. J. Immunol. 12:249 (1982).
26. C. Leclerc, and L. Chedid, Macrophage activation by synthetic muramyl peptides, in: "Lymphokines 7," E. Pick, ed., Academic Press, New York (1982).
27. E. Lederer, Synthetic immunostimulants derived from the bacterial cell wall, J. Med. Chem. 23:819 (1980).
28. P. Lefrancier, and E. Lederer, Chemistry of synthetic immunomodulant muramyl peptides, Prog. Chem. Org. Nat. Prod. 40:1 (1981).
29. K. Matsumoto, H. Ogawa, T. Kusama, O. Nagase, N. Sawaki, M. Inage, S. Kusumoto, T. Shiba, and I. Azuma, Stimulation of nonspecific resistance to infection induced by 6-O-acylmuramyl dipeptide analogs in mice, Infect. Immun. 32:748 (1981).
30. Y. Osada, M. Mitsuyama, K. Matsumoto, T. Une, T. Otani, H. Ogawa, and K. Nomoto, Stimulation of resistance of immunocompromised mice by a muramyl dipeptide analog, Infect. Immun. 37:1285 (1982).
31. Y. Osada, M. Mitsuyama, T. Una, K. Matsumoto, T. Otani, M. Satoh, H. Ogawa, and K. Nomoto, Effect of L18-MDP(Ala), a synthetic derivative of muramyl dipeptide, on nonspecific resistance of mice to microbial infections, Infect. Immun. 37:292 (1982).
32. T. Otani, K. Katami, T. Une, Y. Osada, and H. Ogawa, Restoration by MDP-Lys (L18) of resistance to Pseudomonas pneumoniae in immunosuppressed guinea-pigs, Microbiol. Immunol. 28:1077 (1984).
33. M. Parant, F. Audibert, L. Chedid, M. Level, P. Lefrancier, J. Choay, and E. Lederer, Immunostimulant activities of a lipophilic muramyl dipeptide derivative and of a desmuramyl peptidolipid analog, Infect. Immun. 27:826 (1980).
34. M. Parant, and L. Chedid, Stimulation of nonspecific resistance to infections by synthetic immunoregulatory agents, Infection 12:230 (1984).
35. M. Parant, N. K. Masihi, W. Lange, W. Brehmer, F. Parant, M. Jolivet, and L. Chedid, Enhancement of nonspecific resistance to bacterial and viral infections by MDP conjugated to tetanus toxoid or viral subunits, submitted for publication.
36. M. Parant, F. Parant, L. Chedid, A. Yapo, J-F. Petit, and E. Lederer, Fate of the synthetic immunoadjuvant, muramyl dipeptide (^{14}C-labeled) in the mouse, Int. J. Immunopharmacol. 1:35 (1979).
37. M. Parant, Biological properties of a new synthetic adjuvant, muramyl dipeptide (MDP), Springer Semin. Immunopathol. 2:101 (1979).
38. M. Parant, Bacterial immunoregulatory agents, in: "Regulation of the Immune Response," P. L. Ogra, and D. M. Jacobs, eds., S. Karger AG, Basel (1983).

39. N. C. Phillips, M. L. Moras, L. Chedid, P. Lefrancier, and J. M. Bernard, Activation of alveolar macrophage tumoricidal activity and eradication of experimental metastases by freeze-dried liposomes containing a new lipophilic muramyl dipeptide derivative, Cancer Res. 45:128 (1985).
40. H. C. Polk, R. B. Galland, and J. R. Ausobsky, Nonspecific enhancement of resistance to bacterial infection. Evidence of an effect supplemental to antibiotics, Ann. Surgery. 196:436 (1982).
41. H. Pruul, B. L. Wetherall, and P. J. McDonald, Enhanced susceptibility of Escherichia coli to intracellular killing by human polymorphonuclear leukocytes after in vitro incubation with chloramphenicol, Antimicrob. Agents Chemother. 19:945 (1981).
42. W. Sackmann, and F. M. Dietrich, Experimental murine candidiasis: non-specific resistance induced by synthetic compounds with immunostimulatory properties, in: "Current Chemotherapy and Immunotherapy," P. Periti, and G. Grassi, eds., Amer. Soc. Microbiol. (1981).
43. M. J. Staruch, and D. D. Wood, The adjuvanticity of Interleukin-1 in vivo, J. Immunol. 130:2191 (1983).
44. K. Vosbeck, Effects of low concentrations of antibiotics on Escherichia coli adhesion, in: "The Influence of Antibiotics on the Host-Parasite Relationship," H. U. Eickenberg, H. Hahn, and W. Opferkuch, eds., Springer-Verlag, Berlin (1982).

CONTRIBUTORS

ANDREESEN, R., Department of Hematology and Oncology, University Hospital of Freiburg, 7800 Freiburg, F.R.G.

ANDRESEN, B. H., Department of Medical Microbiology, Universität Kiel, Brunswiker Str. 2-6, 2300 Kiel 1, F.R.G.

BELSHEIM, Judy, Department of Clinical Bacteriology, Gävle Central Hospital, S-801 17 Gävle, Sweden

BISTONI, Francesco, Institute of Medical Microbiology, University of Perugia, 06100 Perugia, Italy

BLOMQVIST, Charlotte, Department of Clinical Bacteriology, Gävle Central Hospital, S-801 17 Gävle, Sweden

BRANDELY, Maud, Institut Pasteur, 28 Rue du Docteur Roux, 75724 Paris, Cedex 15, France

BRUNNER, Helmut, Institute for Chemotherapy, Bayer AG, D-5600 Wuppertal 1, F.R.G.

BÜSCHER, K. H., Ruhr Universität Bochum, Medizinische Mikrobiologie und Immunologie, D-4630 Bochum, F.R.G.

CHEDID, Louis, Institut Pasteur, 28 Rue du Docteur Roux, 75724 Paris Cedex 15, France

CLOT, Jacques P., Laboratoire d'Immunologie, Hôpital Saint-Eloi, 34059 Montpellier, France

COSTERTON, J. W., Department of Biology, University of Calgary, Calgary, Alberta, Canada

DALHOFF, Axel, Institute for Chemotherapy, Bayer AG, Pharma Research Centre, P. O. Box 101709, 5600 Wuppertal-1, F.R.G.

DASCHNER, F. D., Department of Hospital Epidemiology, University of Freiburg, 7800 Freiburg, F.R.G.

DE CLERCQ, Eric, Rega Institute for Medical Research, Katholieke Universiteit Leuven, Minderbroedersstraat 10, B-3000 Leuven, Belgium

DESIMONE, Claudio, Clinica Malattie Infettive, Policlinico Umberto I, Rome, Italy

EASMON, Charles S. F., Department of Medical Microbiology, Wright-Fleming Institute, St. Mary's Hospital Medical School, London W2 1PG, England

ESCANDE, Marie Christine, Laboratoire Central de Microbiologie, Hotel Dieu Hospital, 1 Place du Parvis Notre Dame, 75181 Paris Cedex 04, France

ESCOBAR, Mario R., Medical College of Virginia, Virginia Commonwealth University, Richmond, Virginia 23298

FIETTA, Anna, Department of Chemotherapy, Institute of Respiratory Diseases, University of Pavia, 27100 Pavia, Italy

FLOC'H, François, Rhone-Poulenc Sante, Centre de Recherches de Vitry, Vitry sur Seine, France

FRIEDMAN, Herman, Department of Medical Microbiology and Immunology, University of South Florida, College of Medicine, 12901 N. 30th Street, Box 10, Tampa, Florida

GARACI, E., Institute of Microbiology, Department of Experimental Medicine, II University of Rome, Rome, Italy

GEMMELL, Curtis G., Department of Bacteriology, Medical School, University of Glasgow, Royal Infirmary, Glasgow G4 OSF, Scotland

GHIONE, Mario, Institute of Medical Microbiology, University of Milan, Via Mangiagalli, 31 - 20133 Milano, Italy

GILLISSEN, Günther, Department of Medical Microbiology, Faculty of Medicine, Rhein-Westf. Techn. Hochschule Aachen, 5100 Aachen, F.R.G.

GNARPE, Håkan, Department of Clinical Bacteriology, Gävle Central Hospital, S-801 17 Gävle, Sweden

GOUGEROT-POCIDALO, Marie-Anne, Unité de Recherches 13 INSERM, Hôpital Claude Bernard, 75944 Paris Cedex 19, France

GRASSI, Giuliana Gialdroni, Chair of Chemotherapy, Institute of Respiratory Diseases, University of Pavia, 27100 Pavia, Italy

HADDEN, John W., Program of Immunopharmacology, University of South Florida, College of Medicine, 12901 N. 30th Street, Box 19, Tampa, Florida

HAHN, Helmut, Department of Medical Microbiology, Freie Universität Berlin, D-1000 Berlin 45, F.R.G.

HURTREL, Bruno, Institut Pasteur, 28 Rue du Docteur Roux, 75724 Paris, Cedex 15, France

JUST, H.-M., Department of Hospital Epidemiology, University Hospital of Freiburg, 7800 Freiburg, F.R.G.

KUBENS, Britta, Ruhr Universität Bochum, Medizinische Mikrobiologie und Immunologie, D-4630 Bochum, F.R.G.

LAGRANGE, Philippe H., Institut Pasteur, 28 Rue du Docteur Roux, 75724 Paris, Cedex 15, France

LAMBE, Jr., Dwight W., Department of Microbiology, Quillen-Dishner College of Medicine, East Tennessee State University, Johnson City, Tennessee 37614

LEVACHER, Maryse, Unité de Recherches 13 INSERM, Hôpital Claude Bernard, 75944 Paris Cedex 19, France

LEYING, Herman, Ruhr Universität Bochum, Medizinische Mikrobiologie und Immunologie, D-4630 Bochum, F.R.G.

LITTLE, J. Russell, Departments of Medical Microbiology and Immunology and Medicine, Washington University School of Medicine and Jewish Hospital at Washington University Medical Center, 216 S. Kingshighway, St. Louis, Missouri 63110

LITTLE, K.D., Department of Medical Microbiology and Immunology, Washington University School of Medicine and Jewish Hospital at Washington University Medical Center, 216 S. Kingshighway, St. Louis, Missouri 63110

MANDELL, Lionel A., Division of Infectious Diseases, McMaster University School of Medicine, 1200 Main Street West, Hamilton, Ontario, Canada

MARCONI, P., Institute of Medical Microbiology, University of Perugia, 06100 Perugia, Italy

MARTINETTO, P., Institute of Medical Microbiology, Turin University, Turin, Italy

MAYBERRY, W. R., Department of Microbiology, Quillen-Dishner College of Medicine, East Tennessee State University, Johnson City, Tennessee 37614

MAYBERRY-CARSON, K. J., Department of Microbiology, Quillen-Dishner College of Medicine, East Tennessee State University, Johnson City, Tennessee 37614

MOTTA, Iris, Institut Pasteur, 28 rue de Docteur Roux, 75724 Paris, Cedex 15, France

NIXDORFF, Kathryn, Institut für Mikrobiologie, Technische Hochschule Schnittspahnstr. 9, D-6100 Darmstadt, Darmstadt, F.R.G.

OPFERKUCH, Wolfgang, Ruhr Universität Bochum, Medizinische Mikrobiologie und Immunologie, D-4630 Bochum, F.R.G.

PARANT, Monique, Institut Pasteur, 28 Rue du Docteur Roux, 75724 Paris Cedex 15, France

PAWELZIK, Martina, Ruhr Universität Bochum, Medizinische Mikrobiologie und Immunologie, D-4630 Bochum, F.R.G.

PELOUS, Catherine, Laboratoire d'Immunologie, Hôpital Saint-Eloi, 34059 Montpellier, France

POCIDALO, Jean-Jacques, Unité de Recherches 13 INSERM, Hôpital Claude Bernard, 75944 Paris Cedex 19, France

POIRIER, Jacques, Rhone-Poulenc Sante, Centre de Recherches de Vitry, Vitry sur Seine, France

PRESS, Andreas, Department of Medical Microbiology, Freie Universität Berlin, D-1000 Berlin 45, F.R.G.

PUCCETTI, P., Institute of Pharmacology, University of Perugia, 06100 Perugia, Italy

PUGLIESE, A., Institute of Infectious Diseases, Turin University, Turin, Italy

QUIE, Paul G., American Legion Heart Research, Dept. of Pediatrics, University of Minnesota Medical School, University of Minnesota Hospitals, Box 483, Mayo Memorial Bldg, 420 Delaware Street, S.E., Minneapolis, MN 55455

RAMOS CARNEIRO LEAO, M.T., Department of Hospital Epidemiology, University of Freiburg, 7800 Freiburg, F.R.G.

RICHET, Herve, Laboratoire Central de Microbiologie, Hotel Dieu Hospital, 1 Place du Parvis Notre Dame, 75181 Paris Cedex 04, France

ROCHE, Yvon, Unité de Recherches 13 INSERM, Hôpital Claude Bernard, 75944 Paris Cedex 19, France

ROGGE, H., Infektiologie, Center for Internal Medicine, Johann Wolfgang Goethe Universität, Theodor-Stern-Kai 7, 6000 Frankfurt 70, F.R.G.

ROWER, J., Infektiologie, Center for Internal Medicine, Johann Wolfgang Goethe Universität, Theodor-Stern-Kai 7, 6000 Frankfurt 70, F.R.G.

SALOMONE, C., Pediatric Clinic, Turin University, Turin, Italy

SCHATTSCHNEIDER, R., Infektiologie, Center for Internal Medicine, Johann Wolfgang Goethe Universität, Theodor-Stern-Kai 7, 6000 Frankfurt 70, F.R.G.

SCHELL, Sigrid, Institut für Mikrobiologie, Technische Hochschule Darmstadt, Schnittspahnstr. 9, D-6100 Darmstadt, F.R.G.

SCHROTEN, Horst, Institute for Medical Microbiology and Virology, University of Düsseldorf, F.R.G.

SHAH, Pramod M., Infektiologie, Center for Internal Medicine, Johann Wolfgang Goethe Universität, Theodor-Stern-Kai 7, 6000 Frankfurt 70, F.R.G.

SIEGMUND-SCHULTZE, Nicola, Institut für Mikrobiologie, Technische Hochschule Schnittspahnstr. 9, D-6100 Darmstadt, Darmstadt, F.R.G.

SPERLING, Uwe, Department of Medical Microbiology, Freie Universität Berlin, D-1000 Berlin 45, F.R.G.

STEIN, S. H., Department of Medical Microbiology and Immunology, Washington University School of Medicine and Jewish Hospital at Washington University Medical Center, 216 S. Kingshighway, St. Louis, Missouri 63110

STÜBNER, G., Institut für Bakteriologie und Hygiene, Krankenhaus Nordstadt, Haltenhoffstr. 41, 3000 Hannover 1, F.R.G.

SUERBAUM, Sebastian, Ruhr Universität Bochum, Medizinische Mikrobiologie und Immunologie, D-4630 Bochum, F.R.G.

SZENTIVANYI, Andor, Departments of Pharmacology and Therapeutics and Internal Medicine, University of South Florida, College of Medicine 12901 N. 30th Street, Box 9, Tampa, Florida

SZENTIVANYI, Judith, Department of Comprehensive Medicine, University of South Florida, College of Medicine, 12901 N. 30th Street, Box 41, Tampa, Florida

THOMAS, C., Infektiologie, Center for Internal Medicine, Johann Wolfgang Goethe Universität, Theodor-Stern-Kai 7, 6000 Frankfurt 70, F.R.G.

TOBER-MEYER, B. K., Division of Laboratory Animal Resources, East Tennessee State University, Johnson City, Tennessee 37614

TOVO, P. A., Pediatric Clinic, Turin University, Turin, Italy

TRUFFA-BACHI, Paolo, Institut Pasteur, 28 Rue du Docteur Roux, 75724 Paris, Cedex 15, France

ULLMANN, U., Department of Medical Microbiology, University of Kiel, Brunswiker Str. 2-6, 2300 Kiel 1, F.R.G.

UNDEUTSCH, Christian, Institute for Medical Microbiology and Virology, University of Düsseldorf, Düsseldorf, F.R.G.

VALPREDA, A., Institute of Infectious Diseases, Turin University, Turin, Italy

VECCHIARELLI, A., Institute of Medical Microbiology, University of Perugia, 06100 Perugia, Italy

VERDUCCI, G., Institute of Medical Microbiology, University of Perugia, 06100 Perugia, Italy

VERHOEF, J., Department of Medical Microbiology, Laboratory of Microbiology, University of Utrecht, Catharijnesingel 59, 3511 GG Utrecht, The Netherlands

VERINGA, Etèl, Department of Medical Microbiology, Laboratory of Microbiology, University of Utrecht, Catharijnesingel 59, 3511 GG Utrecht, The Netherlands

WARREN, George, Jefferson Medical College of Thomas Jefferson University, 1025 Walnut Street, Philadelphia, Pennsylvania 19107

WERNER, Georges, Rhone-Poulenc Sante, Centre de Recherches de Vitry, Vitry sur Seine, France

WESSLEN, Lars, Department of Clinical Bacteriology, Gävle Central Hospital, S-801 17 Gävle, Sweden

WIEMER, Christoph, Ruhr Universität Bochum, Medizinische Mikrobiologie und Immunologie, D-4630 Bochum, F.R.G.

WITTKE, J.-W., Department of Medical Microbiology, University of Kiel, Brunswiker Str. 2-6, 2300 Kiel 1, F.R.G.

WOS, Beate, Department of Medical Microbiology, Freie Universität Berlin, D-1000 Berlin 45, F.R.G.

INDEX